USMLE Step 3 Triage

USMLE Step 3 Triage

An Effective, No-nonsense Review

Kevin Schwechten, MD

Staff Physician and Family Medicine

General Leonard Wood Army Community Hospital
Ft. Leonard Wood, Missouri

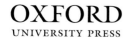

OXFORD
UNIVERSITY PRESS

2009

OXFORD
UNIVERSITY PRESS

Oxford University Press, Inc., publishes works that further
Oxford University's objective of excellence
in research, scholarship, and education.

Oxford New York
Auckland Cape Town Dar es Salaam Hong Kong Karachi
Kuala Lumpur Madrid Melbourne Mexico City Nairobi
New Delhi Shanghai Taipei Toronto

With offices in
Argentina Austria Brazil Chile Czech Republic France Greece
Guatemala Hungary Italy Japan Poland Portugal Singapore
South Korea Switzerland Thailand Turkey Ukraine Vietnam

Published by Oxford University Press, Inc.
198 Madison Avenue, New York, New York 10016

www.oup.com

Oxford is a registered trademark of Oxford University Press

Library of Congress Cataloging-in-Publication Data
Schwechten, Kevin.
USMLE Step 3 triage : an effective, no-nonsense review / by Kevin Schwechten.
p. ; cm.
ISBN 978-0-19-532847-9
1. Medicine—Examinations, questions, etc.   2. Medicine—Outlines, syllabi, etc.
I. Title.   II. Title: Step three triage. [DNLM: 1. Clinical Medicine—Outlines.
2. Licensure, Medical—Outlines. WB 18.2 S412u 2008]
R834.5.S386 2008
610.76—dc22   2007027712

The opinions and assertions contained herein are the private views of the author and are not to be construed as official
or as reflecting the views of the US Army or the US Army Service at large.

Please note: Medicine is an ever-changing science that constantly includes new discoveries and information. Although
the information in this book has been carefully reviewed for correctness of dosage, indications, and safety, neither
the author nor the publisher can accept any legal or financial responsibility for the true accuracy of any of the information contained herein. Neither the author nor the publisher, or any other associated party, makes any warranty,
expressed or implied, with respect to material contained herein. Before prescribing any medication, or rendering any
treatment, the reader must review the manufacturer's current and accurate product information pertaining to the
proper usage thereof. The information in this book in no way replaces the experience and/or judgment of a licensed,
dedicated physician.

9 8 7 6 5 4 3 2 1

Printed in China
on acid-free paper

To my wonderful wife, Dawn, whose amazing, unconditional
support made this book possible. And to my loving daughter
Ariel, who provided the best of all things, hope.

Contents

	Computer Case Simulations	3
1	Neurology	7
2	Psychiatry	39
3	Ophthalmology	63
4	Ear, Nose, and Throat	77
5	Endocrinology	91
6	Hematology	123
7	Dermatology	139
8	Musculoskeletal System	159
9	Infectious Diseases	185
10	Emergency and Trauma	223
11	Cardiovascular Diseases	247
12	Diseases of the Respiratory System	275
13	Gastroenterology	297
14	Diseases of the Kidneys and Urinary Tract	323
15	Diseases of the Male Reproductive System	339
16	Diseases of the Female Reproductive System	347
17	Pregnancy and Childbirth	371
18	Neonate	391
19	Statistics/Ethics/Health Maintenance	403
	Index	415

Preface

The most important thing to know about the USMLE Step 3 is "DO NOT UNDERESTIMATE THIS TEST." By now, those who are reading this are virtual experts in test taking and have also mastered the USMLE format. Thus, this is the last step in the long journey to become a licensed physician. Believe me when I say, "you are now the best student and test taker you will ever be." The fact you have passed the hundreds of exams to get here, you know how to study. With that said, do not study for Step 3 like you did for all those previous exams. Step 3 is set up differently with the test-makers knowing and writing the test based on what they want you to be in the future, not what you have been. That is, they want the test-taker to take the knowledge they have, apply it, and find what they are thinking. All this under a certain time constraint and under a fixed set of standardization. Approach preparation time and materials with a certain leaning toward how the background knowledge may be applied in a clinical setting. Do not forget, Step 3 is a test of performance, not knowledge. It does not reflect how good a doctor you are or will be.

This takes us to preparation. Practice with the format of the test, similar test materials, and brush up on background. First, this should focus much on practice. The USMLE publishes the best materials available for practice questions and should be considered mandatory for preparation. As well, you may be able to access additional practice questions for a fee through their website. Otherwise, there are many areas to obtain practice questions although the quality of materials varies. Judge the quality for yourself and compare with the gold standard USMLE practice questions, but do practice.

Second, background. That is the focus of this book. It has been written for the concise review of relevant medical knowledge applicable to the USMLE Step 3 by basing its content upon the published problem/disease list suggested by the USMLE. It contains the relevant knowledge you will need to pass this test. However, it is not a substitute for your prior medical training. This book will benefit most those residents who are in a residency or internship where they feel they have neither the time nor the energy to study like they did in medical school. It will also provide a broad background for residents in focused programs such as internal medicine, psychiatry, and surgery, that have not covered other areas of medicine adequately. It is at its core a review book, but also will provide some new material to everyone.

Registering for the Test

Registering to take Step 3 varies from the prior Steps 1 and 2. The main difference is the state-specific nature of the registration in that a state must be declared before taking the exam. Scores are then reported to that state's medical licensing board to qualify you for their licensure. The fee varies, but plan on a cost of approximately $700 not including hotel and transportation. The first step is to go to the website: http://www.fsmb.org and navigate to the exam services page and then to the online application where all states are listed in table format. Notice this table has various restrictions listed by state. Some states require the application of license during the registration for Step 3, some have restrictions on attempts for successful passage of Step 3, and so on. Choose the state you are interested in (which does not necessarily have to be the state you reside in) and proceed to the online application section. Make sure you meet the eligibility requirements for that particular state and that all the paperwork is prepared before application in that state. Keep in mind, it's most advantageous to pick the state you plan to practice in after residency (if your residency itself does not require you to have a license in the state you are in for the program). Planning ahead may save you the time and expense of reapplying for a new state license after training!

After registration, a scheduling permit (orange paper) will be mailed to you and will state when your 90-day eligibility period begins. Pick a date during the eligibility period and call the number (Prometric test centers) on the permit to schedule the two consecutive test days. To find the testing center nearest you, visit http://www.prometric.com, where online scheduling may also be available. Before calling to schedule (or scheduling online) have several date options you will be able to take the test, as these test centers fill up fast and scheduling two consecutive days is sometimes difficult.

Format

The USMLE Step 3 is partially arranged somewhat similarly to Steps 1 and 2 in that there are a series of blocks of multiple-choice, computer-based questions. There is only one correct answer to each question although questions may come in groups of 1, 2, or 3 based on the same vignette. However, now there are clinical settings to be considered and include: (1) Emergency Department, (2) inpatient facilities, and (3) office/health center. Questions from the ER and inpatient facilities may appear in the same block. There will be two consecutive days of testing. On day 1, there will be 7 blocks of 48 questions with each block lasting 60 min (thus, 75 s/question). The second day consists of 4 blocks of 36 questions with each block lasting 45 min (75 s/question) as well as 9 computerized case simulations for which 4 h is allotted. Each computerized case simulation has an allotted maximum time limit although it may be finished earlier. On each day, 45 min is allowed for official break time with 15 min allowed for an optional tutorial. If the tutorial is skipped, the time will be added to the break (familiarizing yourself with the format is highly encouraged as this extra break time may be useful).

You should use the practice software and cases to become very familiar with the format of the testing software. There are several useful tools including highlighting, annotations, and strikethrough, as well as navigation buttons and status bar. Make sure you are a wizard at this software before you walk into the center!

Organization

The USMLE is divided into several clinical care situations and physician tasks. Questions are then organized into these areas. The relative weight placed on each is listed below and is according to the USMLE website. You are encouraged to read more about each of these areas by going to the USMLE website, but the cited relative weight appears below.

Physician Tasks

- History and physical 8%–12%
- Diagnostic studies 8%–12%
- Diagnosis 8%–12%
- Prognosis 8%–12%
- Applying basic concepts 8%–12%
- Managing patients
  - Health maintenance 5%–9%
  - Clinical intervention 18%–22%
  - Clinical therapeutics 12%–16%
  - Legal and ethical issues 4%–8%

Clinical Care Situations

- Initial workups 20%–30%
- Continuing care 50%–60%
- Urgent intervention 15%–25%

Passing the Exam

Step 3 is reported as pass/fail although two other scores exist. These scores are a three-digit and a two-digit score. Minimum passing scores for Step 3 are 184 and 75 for respective scales. Keep in mind, neither represents a percentile. Score reporting may take up to 6 weeks, but 4–5 weeks is most typical. If you have not received your scores before then, you may contact the USMLE for score reporting.

Remember, this test is the last step in a long process of becoming an unsupervised, unrestricted physician in the United States. It has been a long road and is soon to be over. My advice is work hard, study hard, know your profession, and kill this exam. Good luck on this test and thereafter.

Kevin Schwechten, MD

USMLE Step 3 Triage

Computer Case Simulations

The computer case simulation (CCS) cases are computer-aided, user-driven interfaces between the computer and test taker, which allow both input and feedback to more closely resemble a real patient interaction. They are meant to evaluate the user's skill in the diagnosis and management of typical patient problems. In other words, they are the attempt to find out how good you are at working up a patient. Input is given in the form of reading the given history, obtaining physical exam, writing orders for labs/imaging, evaluating lab/imaging results, watching vitals, and giving treatment orders based on the situation. There are thousands of correct and incorrect input scenarios for each CCS case; thus your best strategy is to rack up as many points as possible. Be careful, however, as ordering inappropriate tests or treatments may hurt as much as it helps.

Real Time Versus Simulated Time

The CCS operates in a virtual world where time is manipulated by the user. That is, you as the test taker must advance the clock to allow time for any action or test to take place. This is a bit strange, but mastery of the time module is absolutely essential to make it work for you. Several choices in the clock control module exist so that you may choose a specific amount of time to pass, have yourself notified with the next result, or notified basically PRN. Most of the time, a notification with the return of the next result is warranted. If updates from the nurses come in while virtual time passes, it will automatically stop the clock. In real time, there is a specific time allotted for each CCS case, thus do not dilly-dally on specific sections since you cannot take forever. When or if your real time runs out, a final warning will appear with 5 min remaining instructing you to finalize your orders. The computer will then ask for a final diagnosis, enter it and you are done.

The following is an intuitive stepwise approach to the CCS cases.

Initial History

This is the area where the initial presentation is given and may be either short or long based on the case. Usually, this section has three basic steps including:

1. Chief complaint/presentation.
2. Initial vital signs.
3. More detailed history.

No questions may be asked and additional history is unavailable at this point. Take what you can from this section, but most importantly form a quick differential diagnosis. The strategy here is to jot-down (on your dry erase board supplied by the testing center) a quick list of possible diagnoses. Then move on to the next step.

Control Screen

After the initial history, you are then placed at the main control screen. Control of the simulation is done with several buttons on the navigation bar at the top. The strategy here is to order initial, quick bedside tests only if the history is suggestive of an emergent situation where these tests would be helpful. For example, a pulse ox reading on a dyspneic patient may be useful. The next step after this section is to go directly to the physical exam module and do a focused exam.

Notice what location you are working in from the top-right button on the screen. The setting gives much incite into how you should approach the patient such as time advancement and appropriate tests. For example, if the patient is in clinic, do not order a head CT and expect it to come back quickly such as in the ER.

History and Physical

This module allows you to enter, by system, the physical you would like to do. Keep in mind, time will be charged for every system you choose, thus almost never click the "complete physical" box as this will add much unnecessary time to your workup. In the results, look for problems found and abnormalities seen in the systems. Often if there is an abnormality, it will be pathopneumonic. For example, if a child comes in with the presentation of pyloric stenosis, look for a mass found in the abdomen that feels like an "olive." Otherwise, if the system is normal, the description will likely use popular phrases such as "regular rate and rhythm" or "soft, nontender, normal bowel sounds."

Initial Orders

After the initial history and physical are done, you should return to the order sheet and write initial orders. Approach this in a strategic format prioritizing your next move. Below is the order you should approach this stage:

Stabilization

Make sure any and all emergent treatments are rendered early if necessary. For example, if the patient is acutely crumping from cardiac arrest, do not waste time doing an ECG when you could be performing CPR.

The Basics

After the patient is stable, approach the basic orders by appropriateness for the setting. If in the ER, place an IV, etc. Do not assume anything! The nurses here would not automatically place oxygen or cardiac monitoring on a patient having a myocardial infarction (MI) if you do not write the order.

Diagnosis

Order your routine labs, focused labs, imaging, etc. Just like in real life, each one will take a varied amount of time to return results. An MRI will take longer than CT, etc.

After these orders are in, advance the clock.

Respond Appropriately

When the clock is advanced, the results start to come back and further decisions have to be made. Become familiar with each control button and what it can do for you by using the practice software; it makes a big difference during this management phase. There is a button at the top to check the interval history if needed or you may go to the progress notes section to review what you have seen so far. Keep in mind you may change locations if you need to admit the patient or move to a higher level of care. In addition, consultation may be in order (for the record), but do not expect any help whatsoever from the consultant. Let your training guide your decisions; and remember, the patient may worsen even despite correct treatment.

Final Orders

When the end of the case nears, you will know it either by a real-time 5-min warning "pop-up" window or the case will be obviously over. If the warning is displayed, you will have an option to write your final orders and then enter the final diagnosis. The strategy at the end is to claim as many minor points as possible. The computer is set up to enter many different health education and counseling statements, which may claim some extra points. For example, note if the patient is a smoker and counsel them to quit, counsel the family on the patient's condition, counsel the patient on advanced directives, make sure you set the patient up with follow-up, etc. These last ditch points may make the difference when the case is graded at the end.

The case will then end and you may have the option to go directly to the next one or take some break time.

Overall, the best way to approach the CCS section is with solid practice with the USMLE software and a strategy you trust. This helps with invaluable familiarization and lets you know how you will approach the unknown.

Infectious Diseases of the CNS	8
Tetanus	8
Poliomyelitis	9
Creutzfeldt–Jakob Disease	10
Rabies	10
Meningitis	12
Encephalitis	13
Brain Abscess	14
Degenerative/Hereditary Diseases of the CNS	15
Alzheimer's Disease	15
Normal Pressure Hydrocephalus	16
Parkinson's Disease	16
Multiple Sclerosis	17
Amyotrophic Lateral Sclerosis (Lou Gehrig Disease)	18
Complex Regional Pain Syndrome	18
Mental Retardation	19
Paraplegia/Quadriplegia	20
Seizure Disorder	21
Cerebral Palsy	22
Trigeminal Neuralgia (Tic douloureux)	23
Bell's Palsy	24
Myasthenia Gravis	24
Guillain–Barré Syndrome	25
Subarachnoid Hemorrhage	26
Transient Ischemic Attack	28
Ischemic Stroke	29
Malignant Intracranial Neoplasm	30
Migraine	31
Headache	32
Delirium	32
Syncope	33
Tremor	34
Insomnia	35
Coma	35
Brain Death	36

Infectious Diseases of the CNS

Tetanus

Symptoms

Classically presents with trismus (lockjaw). Actually involves several clinical presentations that are variations of muscular spasm: generalized, localized, cephalic, and neonatal. Incubation period from suspected wound infection can be extremely variable from a few days to months. Fever, malaise, and signs of local infection are common.

Diagnosis

This is a clinical diagnosis made by presentation with muscle spasm, history of wound (usually), and no history of immunization.

Labs: CBC for possible leukocytosis. Wound culture may grow *Clostridium tetani*, but infection is possible even with negative culture.

ECG to evaluate for and track possible arrhythmias.

See Table 1.1.

Treatment

- **Debridement** of wound is essential to minimize the release of further toxin. Give **penicillin** for adjunctive therapy. Metronidazole if allergic to penicillin.
- Give **tetanus immunoglobulin** to neutralize unbound toxin.
- Give **tetanus/diphtheria toxoid** for active immunization (since not conferred after disease).

TABLE 1.1 Tetanus prophylaxis by wound type

	Clean wound	Dirty wound
History of adequate vaccination with tetanus toxoid	Give toxoid if last dose of booster is given >10 years ago	Give toxoid if last dose of booster is given >5 years ago
Unknown or inadequate vaccination with toxoid	Start primary series of three toxoid doses*	Give tetanus immunoglobulin (250 units IM) **plus** start primary series of three toxoid doses*

Source: American College of Physicians Task Force on Adult Immunization and Infectious Diseases Society of America. *Guide for Adult Immunizations.* Philadelphia: American College of Physicians, 1994.

*Primary series = one dose toxoid now, repeat in 1 month, and repeat in 1 year. Adequate vaccination consists of completion of primary toxoid series.

- **Supportive care** is commonly needed and may include long-term intubation, tracheostomy, and ICU admission. Death by respiratory failure must be guarded against.

Adjunctive Treatment

- Consider sedation with **benzodiazepines** or propofol for muscle spasms. Place patient in a dark, quiet room.
- Consider muscle relaxants, classically **pancuronium**, if sedatives are inadequate.
- **Labetolol** may be used to control autonomic dysfunction, since α and β activity is so high. Avoid other β-blockers. May also consider clonidine or atropine for greater control.

Poliomyelitis

Symptoms

Uncommonly, a biphasic disease with acute illness in childhood, followed by second phase usually >35 years later. Also, 95% of cases are asymptomatic. The rest may acutely present as aseptic meningitis or encephalopathy. May progress to lasting neurological disease involving paralysis or muscle atrophy.

Types include bulbar (cranial nerves), encephalopathic, and spinal (arms/legs). The second phase, termed *postpolio syndrome* (PPS), can involve pain, weakness, fatigability, and decreased concentration. PPS always occurs in the same nerves and muscles involved in original infection. May also involve postpoliomyelitis progressive muscular atrophy (PPMA), which produces often marked atrophy of muscles innervated by affected nerves.

Diagnosis

Viral culture of pharynx or stool may demonstrate virus. CSF viral culture is the diagnostic gold standard, but is rarely performed. CSF analysis shows increased WBCs and elevated protein levels. Serum levels of antibodies are increased and classically fourfold normal.

PPS can be evaluated with EMG and muscle biopsy, but results are nonspecific and show effects of denervation.

Treatment

- In acute phase supportive care is needed. Intubation and ICU admission is warranted in a small proportion of patients. Multidisciplinary team approach is needed for any symptomatic acute infection. No specific treatment is proven effective.
- Second phase is also treated symptomatically. Nonnarcotic analgesics and physical therapy are the mainstay.

Creutzfeldt–Jakob Disease

This disease is thought to be caused by a prion infection that is often linked to ingestion or exposure to infected animal tissue (historically found in British beef). The bovine form is termed "mad cow" disease or bovine spongiform encephalopathy. Almost all cleaning techniques are ineffective in combating instruments exposed to infected tissue, including autoclave.

Symptoms

Progressive mental deterioration and myoclonus are the main features of the disease. Variants exist, which may also involve almost any other neurologic signs. Focal defect involving brainstem and cerebellar regions is more common. Dementia and mood changes are also often observed.

Diagnosis

Clinical features typical of Creutzfeldt–Jakob disease (CJD) are observed as above, but it is very difficult to make a consistent diagnosis while the patient is alive. Typical EEG with CSF assay indicative of prion disease may be found. History of rare exposure, presence in certain geologic areas, and lack of other suggested etiology point toward this disease.

Definitive diagnosis includes typical specialized histopathologic staining and genetic analysis of brain tissue derived by biopsy or autopsy specimen. These are generally only done at tertiary care laboratory centers.

Imaging: MRI with fluid-attenuated inversion recovery (FLAIR) imaging studies recognize changes in typical brain areas, and are helpful when paired with typical features of the disease.

Treatment

- Purely supportive until death, which is usually <1 year.

Rabies

Symptoms

Strong history of prior bite from wild animals or excessively angry domestic animals. Once symptoms occur, no treatment is effective. Symptoms include aphasia, **throat spasm leading to hydrophobia,** lack of coordination, fever, salivation, dysphasia, paresis, and paralysis. Progression of disease to the point of coma, disseminated intravascular coagulation (DIC), cardiac arrhythmias, and cardiac arrest is practically certain.

Diagnosis

Since the disease often manifests before antibody formation and thus detection, prophylaxis is important before laboratory diagnosis. Refer to Table 1.2 for guidelines regarding animal diagnosis and treatment. After symptoms occur, viral assay may be helpful in confirming the diagnosis of disease (see Table 1.2).

TABLE 1.2 Rabies vaccination after exposure

Animals	Evaluation consideration	Treatment
Domestic dogs and cats	Caught and observed ×10 days Escaped	If asymptomatic, no vaccination is necessary Full vaccination and rabies immunoglobulin (RIG) course
Wild animals including bats, foxes, raccoons, wolves, woodchucks	Caught and sacrificed→ brain tissue examined Escaped	If positive, full vaccination and RIG course Full vaccination and RIG course
Livestock, wild rodents, squirrels, hamsters, chipmunks, rats	Wild or domesticated	Consult local health department, but rabies is rare in these animals Remember: there is no such thing as a rabid rabbit

Treatment

- Clean and debride the wound as much as possible. **Postexposure vaccination must be both active and passive.**

- **Active:** Vaccination with one of the three available cell-cultured vaccines [human diploid cell vaccine (HDCV)]. 1.0 ml IM on days 0, 3, 7, 14, and 28. If patient has previously been vaccinated, repeat vaccination at days 0 and 3 only.

- **Passive:** Rabies immunoglobulin (RIG) 20 IU/kg injected around the site of bite (as much as anatomically possible), then the rest of the doses are given as IM.

- Rabies itself has no treatment or cure.

Q 1.1

A mother brings her 2-week-old female infant to the ER because of poor feeding and decreased interaction. She states her baby had breast fed until 1 day ago when she was noted to become sick and less responsive. On physical exam, the baby has an elevated temperature and is toxic in appearance. You suspect bacterial meningitis and perform the appropriate test. What regimen below is the appropriate empiric treatment of this patient?

A. Levofloxacin and penicillin G.
B. Ampicillin and ceftriaxone.
C. Vancomycin and imipenem.
D. Acyclovir and famciclovir.
E. Diflucan and acyclovir.

Meningitis

Symptoms

Global CNS symptoms such as headache, photophobia, confusion, irritability, decreased consciousness, lethargy, and rash may be reported.

Diagnosis

Physical exam: Nuchal rigidity, positive Kernig's and Brudzinski's signs, mental status change, and fever. Classic rash may be present, which is more common when causative organism is *Neisseria meningitidis*. Rash is classically petechial or purpuric and blanching, but presentations vary. Check retinas for possible signs of increased ICP (see Figure 1.1).

Imaging: CT to rule out mass effect from some other cause, then procede to LP.

Labs: Obtain LP evaluating for opening pressure (rarely done in practicality), glucose levels, protein levels, gram stain, antigenic testing (Wellcogens), smear, and culture (see Table 1.3).

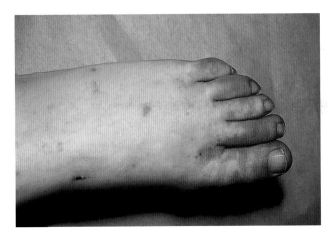

FIGURE 1.1 Characteristic purplish-red meningitis rash lesions on foot.

Problem-Orientated Clinical Microbiology and Infection. Second edition, Humphreys, H, Irving, W. Copyright 2004. Oxford University Press.

TABLE 1.3 Common CSF findings in various meningitis types

	Viral	Bacterial	Fungal
Glucose	Normal	Less than 2/3 serum glucose	Normal–low
Protein	Normal–elevated	Elevated	Elevated
Predominant cell type	Lymphocytes	polymorphonuclear neutrophils (PMNs)	Lymphocytes

Also obtain CBC, CRP, coagulation profile, blood cultures, comprehensive metabolic panel (CMP), and serum glucose levels.

Treatment

- If viral meningitis, treatment is generally supportive [unless herpes simplex virus (HSV) suspected] and full recovery is often expected. Outpatient treatment may be appropriate.

- For bacterial or fungal cause, give steroids (**dexamethasone**) to lower morbidity early on. Then give multiple antibiotic regimen IV empirically.

- Regimens differ depending on age and clinical presentation. However, treatment should be started before culture results (or other CSF analysis) are available.

- **Adults:** Include third-generation cephalosporin, **ceftriaxone (Rocephin) or cefotaxime**, plus **vancomycin** and **acyclovir** (if HSV is suspected), consider adding **ampicillin** if patient is >55 years old (to cover *Listeria*).

- **Pediatrics: Ampicillin plus cefotaxime or gentamicin.** Add acyclovir if HSV suspected.

- Tailor regimen based on CSF analysis and eventually culture.

- Provide supportive care, pain management, and antiemetics as needed. ICU admission is usually indicated.

Encephalitis

Symptoms

Viral prodrome is common, but progresses to involve global neurologic dysfunction such as lethargy, slurred speech, confusion, headaches, photophobia, seizures, and meningeal signs. May also involve focal neurologic deficit including paralysis, hearing loss, cranial nerve involvement, and gustatory/olfactory hallucinations.

Diagnosis

Labs: CSF analysis is essential and the results will be similar to viral meningitis: normal to elevated protein levels, normal glucose level, and lymphocytic predominance on microscopic analysis. **HSV PCR** is diagnostic for HSV encephalitis. Viral culture is also useful, but will take much too long to be practical before therapy. Enzyme-linked immunosorbent assay (ELISA) antibody testing in serum and CSF is useful with some cases, but may only be useful in retrospect.

Imaging: Brain CT is helpful in eliminating other causes and it looking for evidence of increased intracranial pressure (ICP). Brain **MRI** is best in detecting likely HSV by the characteristic appearance of temporal lobes.

Brain biopsy may be helpful and definitive, but may be limited by practicality and benefit.

EEG: Shows characteristic pattern termed "periodic lateralized epileptiform discharges" (PLEDs) present in HSV encephalitis.

Treatment

- Start acyclovir if viral etiology is possible. Then give corticosteroids such as dexamethasone and anticonvulsants.

- If hepatic etiology, consider lactulose (Cephulac).

- Add broad-spectrum antibiotics if bacterial cause possible.

- Remember to watch for signs of syndrome of inappropriate antidiuretic hormone (SIADH) and treat as appropriate. Otherwise, treatment is supportive and sedation may be an option to guide patient through difficult disease course.

Brain Abscess

Symptoms

Mental status changes, seizures, headache, or focal neurologic deficits are common. History is often positive for immunocompromised status (toxoplasmosis or fungus ball), postsurgery (dental) recent otitis infection, or sinusitis.

Diagnosis

Physical exam: Look for cranial nerve deficits (3rd, 6th) and papilledema, indicating increased intracerebral pressure.

Labs: Perform a CBC for elevated WBCs. ESR/CRP are elevated. Check electrolytes and basic metabolic panel (BMP) for SIADH.

Imaging: CT is classic for ring-enhancing lesions (order with contrast). MRI is more sensitive, but often takes too long (see Figure 1.2).

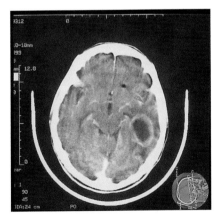

FIGURE 1.2 CT scan showing brain abscess in left temporal lobe.

Problem-Orientated Clinical Microbiology and Infection. Second edition, Humphreys, H, Irving, W. Copyright 2004. Oxford University Press.

An LP may be contraindicated because of the possibility that it might cause herniation with increased ICP.

Treatment

- Consult **neurosurgeon** as soon as possible.

- Give **dexamethasone** to reduce brain edema and ICP.

- **Antibiotics:** Prolonged course of 6–8 weeks. Different regimens exist, so culture and sensitivity should be used to guide treatment. Penicillin and chloramphenicol (Chloromycetin), or metronidazole (Flagyl) are common.

Degenerative/Hereditary Diseases of the CNS

Alzheimer's Disease

Symptoms

Progressive insidious memory loss. It commonly starts with misplacing objects, and then time disorientation and getting lost, which progresses to inability to recognize relatives. Aphasia, apraxia, and dementia follow over the course of years.

Diagnosis

Generally a clinical diagnosis is made, but may be supported by eliminating other causes of dementia and imaging. Mini-Mental Status exam useful in tracking progression. Clinically assess for depression.

Labs: Obtain CBC, CMP, vitamin B_{12}/folate, syphilis testing, TSH, HIV, and ESR/CRP. E4 allele of apolipoprotein E gene is available for prognostic and family testing, but accuracy and practicality are unestablished.

Imaging: CT may support, but MRI will accurately show, cerebral atrophy focused more on frontal lobes.

Gross exam of brain (often autopsy) shows neuritic plaques and neurofibrillary tangles.

Treatment

- Manage symptoms such as depression, psychosis, and sleep disturbance medically.

- Anticholinesterase inhibitors are the mainstay: Start with donepezil (Aricept), rivastigmine (Exelon), galantamine (Reminyl). Others in the new N-methyl-D-aspartate (NMDA) receptor antagonist class such as memantine (Namenda) have recently been found to be very effective.

- Remember to look for social aspects such as elder abuse and social support from family or friends (these are very popular on standardized tests).

Q 1.2

An 86-year-old male comes to your office clinic with his wife complaining of gradual decline in functioning. His wife states he is increasingly forgetful and seems to not know where he is driving when on routine outings. He adds to this that he has recently felt the need for a cane while walking. Upon questioning, he also admits to urinary incontinence from time to time. What is the best management for this patient's most likely diagnosis?

A. Beginning an anticholinesterase inhibitor such as donepezil (Aricept).
B. Check electrolyte levels and replace as needed.
C. MRI of head for possible structural abnormality.
D. Neurosurgery consult for possible ventriculoperitoneal (VP) shunt placement.
E. Administration of vitamin B_{12} shots for likely deficiency.

Normal Pressure Hydrocephalus

Symptoms

Classic clinical triad is **gait disturbance, urinary incontinence, and dementia,** although other diffuse signs of dementia may be present.

Diagnosis

Labs: LP is prudent to eliminate other causes of symptoms. Protein, glucose, cell count, gram stain, and culture should be normal in normal pressure hydrocephalus (NPH).
Imaging: CT and **MRI** can both be helpful showing hydrocephalus. Widened ventricles are seen.
Special testing: Miller Fisher test (also called "intermittent high-volume tap") involves the removal of 30–60 ml CSF and objectively measuring the improvement of gait symptoms. May correlate with prognosis to VP shunting.

Treatment

- **VP shunting** is the mainstay of therapy. Good response is usually achieved fairly quickly with long-term efficacy.
- No known medical therapy has shown good efficacy.

Parkinson's Disease

Symptoms

Progressive bradykinesia, masked (expressionless) facies, muscular rigidity, shuffling gait, dementia, and micrographia are classic symptoms. History in young persons may be consistent with illicit heroin use (the process of making synthetic street heroin sometimes makes 1-methyl-4-phenyl-1,2,3,6-tetrahydropyridine (MPTP), a neurotoxic by-product).

Diagnosis

Physical exam: "Cogwheel" rigidity of arms and legs, clonus, shuffling gait, and resting "pill rolling" tremor.
Imaging: None specifically.
Gross microscopic: Lewy bodies in substantia nigra.

Treatment

- Therapies are aimed at replacing or blocking the degradation of dopamine to relevant pathways. **Levodopa-carbidopa (Sinemet)** is first line. Add dopamine agonists such as bromocriptine (Parlodel), pergolide (Permax), ropinirole (Requip), and pramipexole (Mirapex) as the disease progresses. Monoamine oxidase inhibitors (MAOIs) like selegiline (Eldepryl) may be neuroprotective, and thus should be started early. Anticholinergics, amantidine (Symmetrel), catechol-O-methyltransferase (COMT) inhibitors, and selective serotonin reuptake inhibitors (SSRIs) can be started to lessen symptoms as the disease progresses.

- Multiple surgical approaches have been tried, but limited success reported. Fetal midbrain substantia nigra neuronal transplant (illegal in United States) and adrenal medullary transplant are unproven, but hopeful. Thalamotomy, stereotactic pallidotomy, and deep brain stimulation have all shown varied efficacy.

Multiple Sclerosis

Symptoms

Symptoms come and go in exacerbation/remission fashion. These symptoms are usually found in young women and often present with optic neuralgia and vision changes. Other symptoms are diplopia, gait disturbance, incontinence, vertigo, emotional lability, internuclear ophthalmoplegia, and scanning speech.

Diagnosis

Physical exam: Lhermitte's sign (electric shock down spine on neck flexion), positive Babinski sign, and vertical nystagmus.
Labs: LP reveals IgG/oligoclonal bands and myelin basic protein.
Imaging: MRI with and without contrast is diagnostic for demyelination plaques. CT and plain films are not helpful.

EMG shows characteristic slowing of conduction, but must be correlated clinically.

Treatment

- Steroids are the mainstay of medical therapy. Other medications may treat disease course, like immunosuppressive agents like azathioprine (Imuran), interferon, and cyclosporine. Other medications are aimed at symptom relief such as antispasmodics like baclofen (Kemstro). Remember to treat the accompanying disorders such as psychosis, depression, infection, and seizures.

Amyotrophic Lateral Sclerosis (Lou Gehrig Disease)

Symptoms

Progressive, insidious disease with symptoms of both upper and lower motor neuron degeneration. Classics are tongue fasciculations, dysarthria, muscle atrophy, spasticity, dysphagia, and slurred speech.
History: Family history in only 10% of patients.

Diagnosis

Physical exam: Proximal muscle weakness, hyperreflexia, spasticity, muscular atrophy, and weakness. Extraocular muscles are spared, leading to "locked in" syndrome. Eventual respiratory failure.
EMG: Widespread denervation in grouped atrophy fashion.

Treatment

- Riluzole (Rilutek) produces modest improvement in morbidity and delays mortality. Antispasmodics such as baclofen (Kemstro) may be helpful for spastic symptoms.
- Mechanical ventilator support is needed later in disease.
- Recommend advanced directive.

Complex Regional Pain Syndrome

A neurologic disease of unknown etiology most commonly manifests after an inciting event such as limb fracture/surgery, cardiac ischemia, or hemiplegia.

Type I—complex regional pain syndrome (CRPS) symptoms are without a definable nerve lesion. This type represents approximately 90% of clinical presentations.

Type II—refers to cases where a definable nerve lesion is present.

Symptoms

Pain in either the upper or lower extremities bilaterally is most common. Edema, thickening of skin, mottling, progression to limitation of movement, muscle wasting, bone demineralization, contractions of digits, cold skin, and brittle nails. Progression happens over months and generally in three stages.

Diagnosis

Autonomic testing such as resting sweat output (RSO), resting skin temperature (RST), and quantitative sudomotor axon reflex test (QSART) can all be used to measure sympathetic outflow to the limb. Simple measurement of skin temperature may also be used, but is less sensitive.

Imaging: Most helpful later in disease course. Plain radiographs may show bone demineralization, joint changes, and osteoporosis. Bone scintigraphy and MRI can also show characteristic change, but must be correlated with clinical presentation.

Treatment

- Regional sympathetic nerve block and stellate ganglion is often effective and may be diagnostic. This is usually done at local or regional pain centers, and should only be done by experienced anesthesiologists. For the test, pick this choice if offered.

- Medical therapy includes nonsteroidal antiinflammatory drugs (NSAIDs), steroids, propranolol (Inderal), and nifedipine (Adalat, Procardia) have all been used, but are generally of limited utility.

- Surgical sympathectomy may be used for advanced stages, and is most effective in patients who respond well to regional nerve block.

- Physical therapy may be effective and slow the progression of motor symptoms. Early intervention after an inciting event, which may lead to this disorder, is particularly important as it may prevent this disease or significantly slow the progression.

Mental Retardation

Symptoms

Subaverage mental functioning. Mild cases are sometimes overlooked until later in schooling. Characteristics include poor academic performance and inability to keep up with peer group. Moderate to severe cases are often found soon after birth, and may exhibit other genetic abnormalities that lead to diagnosis.

Diagnosis

Often low cognitive function coupled with low adaptive skills in two or more of the following: communication, self-care, home living, social skills, community interaction, self-direction, health and safety, and functional academics.

Classically characterized by low IQ (see Table 1.4);

Diagnosis is often idiopathic, but look for preventable causes such as transient hypoxia and phenylketonuria (PKU). Do genetic testing for common

TABLE 1.4 Severity of retardation by IQ score

Severity	IQ range
Mild	55–69
Moderate	40–54
Severe	25–39
Profound	0–24

syndromes such as Down syndrome and fragile X. This may be useful for future pregnancies.

Treatment

- If preventable, prevent it. This may be done by eliminating phenylalanine in the diet in PKU (must be done early). In non-preventable types, supportive care is the standard. Often caregiver counseling and training must be done to adjust to living with patient. If severe or profound, parents may elect to place child in an assisted living facility. Educational needs should be addressed as many patients benefit from special education tailored to their level of function. This is legally required by public school systems.

Paraplegia/Quadriplegia

Symptoms

Often accompanying trauma, symptoms include complete or partial motor dysfunction of the skeletal musculature. Sensory impairment usually accompanies these symptoms, but not always. Autonomic dysfunction more often in quadriplegia and may involve temperature dysregulation. Quadriplegia may also involve muscles of respiration, including the diaphragm that can require immediate support.

Diagnosis

Evident on exam that constitutes its diagnosis.
Imaging: MRI of the spine may show complete or partial transection in cases of trauma. Local edema of the cord and surrounding tissues is usual.

CT/plain radiograph may be useful to show tumor or bony abnormality in subacute or progressive symptoms.

Treatment

- Depends on the etiology. Trauma victims may benefit from immediate use of corticosteroids to reduce cord edema. Neurosurgeon should be consulted for all cases including less acute presentation or demonstrable tumor.

- After initial injury, physical therapy and rehabilitation play a vital role in re-educating the patient on limb movement and accessory muscle use. Some mobility of affected muscle may be seen with rehabilitation, but the course is usually prolonged. Patients with spinal cord transections usually never fully recover, but partial recovery and learned use of accessory muscles often return some functional capacity.

Q 1.3

Which medication below is acceptable and effective in the treatment of status epilepticus?

A. Phenobarbital.
B. Lorazepam (Ativan).
C. Thiamine/glucose alone.
D. Ethosuximide (Zarontin).
E. Carbamazepine (Tegretol).

Seizure Disorder

Many different etiologies exist including febrile, epileptic, infectious, hypoxic, metabolic, diabetic, conversion, cerebrovascular accident (CVA), vascular malformations, and idiopathic.

Symptoms

Generalized tonic/clonic seizures are the classic "grand mal" seizure that involves symmetric shaking of upper and lower extremities with transient disruption of consciousness (see Table 1.5). Of note, they do **not** involve hip thrusting (can be used to distinguish from conversion/malingering).

Partial seizures involve one specific place of the cortex and thus affect isolated parts of the body. By definition, it presents with preservation of consciousness. Classic presentation is of "Jacksonian March," which is seizure activity moving from one part of the body to another in a stepwise

TABLE 1.5 Stages of seizure

Stage	Symptoms
Preictal	Often associated with auditory, visual, or olfactory hallucinations (commonly familiar smell tips patient off to oncoming seizure)
Ictal	Seizure activity
Postictal	May range from sleepiness and lethargy to asymptomatic. Usually not cognitively impaired

fashion as activity in the brain moves across the cortex. May be associated with Todd's paralysis, which involves transient postictal paralysis of the affected limb.

Other forms exist such as partial–generalized (progression from partial to generalized), absence (usually seen in pediatric population involving rapid interruption in consciousness without postictal state), conversion (pseudo-seizure), and drop seizures (often in children and involve generalized transient paralysis).

Diagnosis

Labs: Check screening BMP, CBC, glucose, drug screen, and TSH for possible derangements and etiology.

Imaging: CT/MRI can be useful if trauma, lesion, or tumors are suspected etiologies.

EEG: Considered standard for diagnosis, but often falsely negative because it is done in interictal period. Video-monitored EEG with sleep deprivation may increase sensitivity of test.

Treatment

- Many anticonvulsants exist and often require periodic medication levels to monitor effective ranges. Start with monotherapy and add more if needed. Almost all are contraindicated in pregnancy, but weigh the risks/benefits.

- Status epilepticus (30 minutes of uninterrupted tonic/clonic seizure)—Airway, breathing, circulation (measures constituting CPR) (ABCs) followed by lorazepam (Ativan), thiamine, and glucose are classic treatment options. Add phenytoin (Dilantin) if seizure continues.

- Generalized tonic/clonic—Phenytoin (Dilantin), carbamazepine (Tegretol), or valproate (Depakene).

- Absence—Classically ethosuximide (Zarontin).

- Partial—Clinically effective single or combinations of above medications.

- Conversion—Psychiatry referral.

- **Surgery:** Stereotactic seizure focus ablation has showed effectiveness, but is reserved for medically refractory cases.

Cerebral Palsy

Symptoms

Early presentation of spastic movement disorders and paralysis. Often associated with severe functional and cognitive impairment. Take a good history of maternal pregnancy and exposures to toxoplasmosis. Other (Hep B, coxsackie, varicella), rubella, cytomegalovirus, herpes simplex, HIV, syphilis (TORCHES) infection, and toxins (including EtOH). Once thought to be caused by acute hypoxia at birth, but this theory is being disproved by recent research.

Diagnosis

Labs: Genetic analysis and screening are indicated and applicable to possible future pregnancies.

Imaging: MRI is appropriate to look for possible structural causes, but commonly shows normal findings.

EEG is appropriate since seizure disorder is common with cerebral palsy (CP).

Treatment

- Supportive and tailored to individual needs. Often surrogate caretakers are needed, sometimes on 24 h basis.
- Physical therapy is a mainstay to improve and maintain muscular ability. This can include specialized movement education programs that educate the patient on movement.
- Nutritional support and special diets in severe cases.
- Education is often in special education category, but CP patients may have average or better intelligence.
- Anticonvulsant therapy is often indicated to control commonly accompanying seizure disorder.
- Muscle relaxants such as baclofen (Kemstro) may be of some use. Botulinum toxin (Botox) IM injections have also been used to control spastic movement.

Trigeminal Neuralgia (Tic douloureux)

Symptoms

Sharp often stabbing paroxysmal facial pain that lasts seconds to minutes. Usually unilateral and occurs in distribution of the trigeminal nerve (V_1–V_3). Often in the elderly and may be exacerbated by trigger points.

Diagnosis

Physical exam: Extreme tenderness to palpation of the affected areas of the face.

Imaging: MRI may be used to rule out neoplasm in cerebellopontine angle causing similar symptoms.

Treatment

- Start with **carbamazepine (Tegretol)**; response is commonly considered diagnostic. May wane in efficacy over period of years and cause sedation as a side effect.

- Gabapentin (Neurontin), baclofen (Kemstro), phenytoin (Dilantin), valproate (Depakene), pimozide (Orap), and clonazepam (Klonipine) alone or in combination can be tried. Some antiepileptic drugs, such as lamotrigine (Lamictal) and topiramate (Topamax), have been reported to be useful. Oxcarbazepine (Trileptal), a derivative of carbamazepine, may also be effective.
- Do not forget that some of these drugs need periodic blood level monitoring.
- **Surgery:** Several surgeries exist and are effective for medically refractory cases: microvascular decompression, radiofrequency rhizotomy, glycerol rhizolysis, balloon decompression, gamma knife radiosurgery, linear accelerator radiosurgery, peripheral nerve block, and peripheral neurectomy.

Bell's Palsy

Symptoms

Unilateral facial nerve paralysis. History may reveal acute URI or head infection or history of herpes zoster of the face.

Diagnosis

Commonly a clinical diagnosis.
Physical exam: Local swelling, ipsilateral numbness, paralysis, loss of taste, and loss of corneal reflex.
Imaging: MRI to image posterior fossa may be indicated to rule out tumor or central infarcts. Usually not needed.
  EMG is very useful to confirm diagnosis.

Treatment

- Since patients often have difficulty blinking and wetting the affected eye, patching is recommended. Monthly inspections for abrasions are indicated throughout recovery course. Artificial tears may be useful as well.
- Surgery is only considered in prolonged cases.
- Vast majority are self-limiting, but recovery is often over many months.

Myasthenia Gravis

The autoimmune attack and resultant dysfunction of peripheral acetylcholine receptors.

Symptoms

Presentation often involves ptosis, difficulty chewing, and abnormal smile although the hallmark of disease is **muscular fatigability** (usually presenting after exercise). Extraocular muscles are often affected, which produces diplopia. Dysarthria, dysphagia, and neck muscle pain are also seen. Myasthenia gravis (MG) may eventually progress to respiratory compromise.

Diagnosis

Screening labs: Consider antinuclear antibody (ANA), TSH, rheumatoid factor, and vitamin B_{12} for screening of respective disorders.

Edrophonium (Tensilon) test: Administration of edrophonium (an anticholinesterase inhibitor with short half-life) to the diseased patient produces acute, transient reversal of symptoms.

EMG produces characteristic stepwise results.

Acetylcholine receptor antibodies (AChR-ab) can be detected in most affected patients, but their level does not correlate with clinical severity.

Imaging: MRI and CT are useful to rule out the commonly associated **thymoma**.

Treatment

- Pyridostigmine (Mestinon) is the classic treatment of choice. Dosing ranges from q. 4–6 h to q.d. depending on disease severity. Side effects are GI upset/diarrhea, salivation, and bronchial secretions (which are parasympathetic). Neostigmine (Prostigmine) can be used parenterally if in an emergency. Atropine is the antidote to this class.

- Steroids also have a role although dosage varies widely, and duration of therapy is often prolonged. Side effects are many, so weigh the risks/benefits.

- Azathioprine (Imuran) and cyclosporine may also be used for immunosuppressant therapy, and may be useful to decrease the dose of steroids.

- Plasmapheresis may be used in the severely ill hospitalized patient after other modalities fail.

- **Surgery:** Thymectomy in patients with severe generalized form or thymoma is indicated.

Guillain–Barré Syndrome

Symptoms

An ascending symmetric paralysis usually beginning with the lower extremities. History may reveal recent GI infection, cold/flu-like symptoms, surgery, or immunization. Acute, seemingly unrelated, illness usually results and paralysis begins days to weeks later. Presenting complaints are often of weakness on walking, foot drop, and mildly decreased sensation. This progresses up the body, usually sparing the sphincters. Proximal muscles are affected first, but respiratory compromise occurs in severe cases.

Diagnosis

Physical exam: Loss of deep tendon reflexes and complete paralysis of proximal muscles of affected limbs. Sensation may also be impaired.

LP shows increased CSF protein and IgG later in course.

EMG shows slowed conduction velocities, indicative of demyelination.

Treatment

- Disease is usually self-limited, with maximal peak of symptoms in second and third weeks.

- Plasmapheresis (plasma exchange) is the classic treatment, but must be started early in the disease course to be effective.

- Intravenous immunoglobulin (IVIG) infusion in hospitalized patients may be useful, and is an equivalent alternative to plasmapheresis.

- **Steroids must be avoided because they make the disease worse.**

- This disease is indication for hospital admission, and the patient must be monitored closely for the need for mechanical ventilation. Monitor development of bed sores and need to prevent deep vein thrombosis (DVT).

Subarachnoid Hemorrhage

Symptoms

Classically starts with a "thunder-clap" headache that is described as the **worst headache in the patient's life.** Further symptoms vary by the location of the bleed, but anterior circulation bleeds produce focal neurologic deficit and hemiparesis. If in the posterior circulation, they produce alteration of consciousness, imbalance, nausea, vomiting, delirium, seizure, or coma.

Diagnosis

Physical exam: Conjugate eye deviation, ophthalmoplegia, irregular breathing, papilledema, retinal hemorrhage, or pinpoint pupil(s). Tachycardia, arrhythmia, or hypertension are commonly detected as well. Over the course of 24–48 h, fever and nuchal rigidity may develop. Sequlae may occur in the less acute setting and go undetected, in which case symptoms often partially abate although some degree of neurologic impairment usually persists.

Imaging: CT is the best way to visualize hemorrhages in the brain; this is usually done with thin sections (3 mm) to detect possible small hemorrhages. CT should be done before LP is attempted to avoid possible herniation. MRI is less useful to detect acute bleeds, but may be used if CT is negative, or to look for ischemic changes.

LP may be done if CT is negative or clinical picture is still suggestive of subarachnoid hemorrhage (SAH). LP should be uniformly bloody (as opposed to traumatic tap) and may be under increased pressure. After a course of hours, xanthochromia should be found.

Cerebral angiography may be used to guide treatment and search for more extensive disease.

ECG and continuous cardiac monitoring is indicated because of high rates of arrhythmias.

Treatment

- Largely supportive. Place patient in a quiet, dark room with cardiac monitoring. Give stool softeners to prevent straining, and control headache with acetaminophen/codeine. Manage the airway with mechanical ventilation if needed. Give mannitol (Osmitrol) to decrease cerebral edema if present. Monitor fluid status.

- Nimodipine (Nimotop) should be given to treat cerebral vasospasm.

- Manage the blood pressure to keep mean arterial pressure (MAP) <125. Esmolol (Brevibloc) or enalapril (Vasotec) are good choices for this.

- **Surgery:** May be an option for accessible bleeds, and includes radiosurgery, endovascular obliteration, and AV malformation obliteration. All depending on neurosurgical evaluation of the case (see Table 1.6).

TABLE 1.6 Distinguishing features of subdural and epidural hematomas

	Subdural	Epidural
Etiology/associations	Rupture of bridging veins; may occur chronically	Rupture of artery; middle meningeal; look for "lucid interval" after the accident; skull fracture often evident
Prototypical age group	Elderly	Often young, after trauma
Evaluation	CT/MRI	CT/MRI
Treatment	Surgery can be lifesaving if large; supportive care and monitoring if small–moderate	Burr hole placement for decompression can be lifesaving

Q 1.4

A 17-year-old male baseball player is taking batting practice when he is struck in the side of the head by an errant pitch. He is briefly stunned, but is able to recover in a matter of minutes. His coach places him on the sidelines where he recovered and then returned to practice. After practice, he was noted to have severe pain on the traumatized side of his head and vomiting, after which he had prolonged loss of consciousness (LOC). He was then brought to the ER via EMS. What is the most likely mechanism of injury?

A. Laceration of the middle meningeal artery.
B. Rupture of bridging veins in the dura.
C. Acute cerebral edema development.
D. Occult foreign body penetration into the calvarium.
E. Seizure activity.

Transient Ischemic Attack

Symptoms

Transient but often sudden-onset neurologic symptoms lasting <**24 h**. Depending on the anterior or posterior circulation, may produce focal motor loss, slurred speech, blurred vision, diplopia, **amaurosis fugax** (ipsilateral unilateral visual loss characterized to resemble a shade being drawn over the eye), tinnitus, alteration of consciousness, headache, drop attacks, loss of sensation, or ataxia. Symptoms may mimic those of a stroke, but are transient. History of characteristic symptoms and presence of risk factors for atherosclerosis, hypertension, cardiac arrhythmia, endocarditis, or embolic producing disorder.

Diagnosis

Labs: Coagulation profile including INR, CBC, electrolytes. Consider protein C/S, factor V Leiden, antithrombin, if coagulation profile is abnormal.
Imaging: CT is the test of choice to evaluate for bleeding; however, it is not the test of choice for diagnosis. Diffusion-weighted MRI is much more sensitive to find small infarcts if present. MRA may be used if posterior circulation is suspected to be the source.
Cardiac evaluation: ECG, Holter monitoring, and transthoracic echocardiogram are appropriate to evaluate for arrhythmias or possible sources of embolization.
Carotid evaluation: Carotid angiography is the gold standard for imaging the carotid arteries; however, it is invasive and fairly impractical. **Duplex ultrasonography** is practically the best test to evaluate the carotid arteries and will give an accurate percentage of stenosis.

Treatment

- Depending on the results of the above investigation. If cardiac embolization, arrhythmia, or abnormality, treatment is aimed at treating the underlying disorder.

TABLE 1.7 Treatment of carotid stenosis based on percent stenosis present

Stenosis	Treatment
<50%	Medical management
50%–69%	Individual evaluation based on risk factors, ulceration of plaque, and symptoms
>70%	Surgical candidate

- In many cases, rupture of atherosclerotic plaques in the carotids is the etiology and should be treated with attention to the degree of stenosis (see Table 1.7).

- Medical management may include anticoagulant therapy or antiplatelet therapy.

- Anticoagulation should be started with heparin or low molecular weight heparin, enoxaparin (Lovenox), then warfarin (Coumadin).

- Antiplatelet options include aspirin, clopidogrel (Plavix), or dipyridamole (Persantine). Combinations of these including Aggrenox (dipyridamole/ASA) may be more effective than either agent alone. Ticlopidine (Ticlid) is an older drug once used, but has fallen out of favor because of side effects (agranulocytosis).

- **Surgery:** Carotid endarterectomy carries a risk based on the skill and experience of the surgeon, as well as the degree of disease in the patient. Certain centers perform more per year than others, and research has shown a clinically significant difference in effectiveness and morbidity/mortality to the patient. The extent of the patient's disease and the risk of the procedure must be taken into account. Generally acceptable guidelines include morbidity/mortality risk of <3% for asymptomatic, 5% for recurrent transient ischemic attacks (TIAs), 7% for stroke patients, and 10% for patients with recurrent stenosis.

- Remember to control risk factors of disease. This may include tight glycemic control, dietary/medical control of hyperlipidemia, control of hypertension, and reduction of tobacco and alcohol use.

Ischemic Stroke

Resulting from either cerebrovascular disease or cerebral embolism/thrombus blocking blood flow. Often occurring in distribution of the middle cerebral arteries.

Symptoms

A variety of neurologic symptoms may be seen commonly including those seen in TIA. Classically, contralateral hemiplegia, hemianesthesia, and

NEUROLOGY

hemianopias. May involve almost any neurologic sign from very subtle stepwise loss of function to evolving dementia to sudden coma or death.

Diagnosis

Physical exam: Increased temperature, change in mental status, focal neurologic changes such as paralysis or focal anesthesia.

Labs: Coagulation profile including INR, CBC, electrolytes. Consider protein C/S, factor V Leiden, antithrombin, if coagulation profile is abnormal.

Imaging: Noncontrast CT is the standard first choice to rule out bleeding. MRI remains the best test of diagnosis. MRA or arteriography may be useful in certain situations.

Carotid evaluation may be useful in the long term to find possible reversible cause, but not useful in the acute setting. As in TIA, carotid duplex ultrasound is the standard.

Treatment

- Treatment of ischemic stroke should start with the ABCs with particular attention to cardiac rhythm. Then be sure to give oxygen and fluids and perform basic lab tests. Give aspirin as early as possible, but only after intracranial hemorrhage is excluded with imaging.

- Anticoagulation is controversial and under investigation. Giving heparin/warfarin must be done under strict guidelines and only after intercranial hemorrhage is definitively ruled out.

- Antithrombotics such as tPA (Activase) or streptokinase are ultimately too complex for most test makers to ask about. Rules are extensive and these drugs should only be used on ideal, investigated candidates with symptom onset to drug time ≤3 h.

- Blood pressure should only be controlled if significantly elevated. Hypertension is a protective mechanism of the body and should be allowed, but monitored even at hypertensive emergency levels.

- After the stroke control risk factors such as emboli source, hyperlipidemia, hypertension, smoking, diet, and exercise.

- Rehabilitation is the main treatment of stroke. Significant function may be restored to affected areas by retraining with physical therapy and occupational therapy.

Malignant Intracranial Neoplasm

May include astrocytoma, medulloblastoma, oligodendroglioma, glioblastoma multiforme, glioma, schwannoma, ependymoma, meningioma, and craniopharyngioma.

Symptoms

In the broad sense, symptoms may be localizing or general and result from brain tissue effects localized to the lesion that may be peripheral, central, or specific. Mass effect may also develop, leading to generalized alteration of consciousness, seizure disorder, endocrine/electrolyte abnormalities, ocular problems, or herniation syndromes. Often focal effects evolve slower than stroke or infectious causes, and may involve compensation mechanisms in the brain.

Diagnosis

Labs: Initial screening with lab tests is important and should include electrolytes and renal function to evaluate for possible SIADH or other endocrine problems. CSF studies are rarely useful and should only be considered after CT is done to avoid herniation.

Imaging: CT to evaluate for mass effect, herniation, or acute bleeding. MRI is more accurate and may show lesions in better detail.

Treatment

- Treatment depends largely on the type of malignancy.
- Discrete lesions may be amenable to neurosurgery, radiation, or chemotherapy.

Q 1.5

A 21-year-old Asian woman comes to your office with complaints of worsening migraine headaches and requests therapy. She has tried many medications in the past and now seems to be a good candidate for ergot abortive therapy. What screening laboratory tests are mandated before beginning this medication?

A. CBC.
B. Bone marrow biopsy.
C. Electrolyte evaluation.
D. Vitamin B_{12} and folate levels.
E. β-hCG.

Migraine

Symptoms

Classic type begins with aura that may consist of a smell or visual effect (commonly flashing lights or scotomata). Common type generally lacks this aura. Both are generally unilateral with severe pain, photophobia, phonophobia, nausea, vomiting, and may involve focal neurologic deficit. Does not involve alteration of consciousness or seizure.

Diagnosis

Based mainly on typical history although exclusion with screening using lab tests (CBC, BMP) and possibly brain imaging may be considered.

Treatment

- **Prophyalaxis:** Topoisomerase (Topamax) and β-blockers such as propranolol (Inderal) have been used with some success. Amitriptyline (Elavil) or other tricyclic antidepressants (TCAs) may also be useful. Valproate (Depakene) and verapamil have also been tried with varied success.

- **Abortive:** The triptan class has shown excellent success and includes sumatriptan (Imitrex), rizatriptan (Maxalt), naratriptan (Amerge), zolmitriptan (Zomig), and others. Ergots including dihydroergotamine (Migranal) and ergotamine/caffeine (Cafergot) may also be used, but are absolutely contraindicated in pregnancy. Other combinations of the above drugs with acetaminophen or NSAIDs exist.

- **Analgesics:** Acetaminophen, NSAIDs may be very effective but may also not provide enough relief.

- Do not give opiates for migraine. Abuse potential is much too high.

- Several natural remedies have also been tried, but studies are lacking and conclusive evidence is scarce. These include such herbs as feverfew and butterbur.

Headache

See Table 1.8.

Delirium

Symptoms

Very similar presentation to dementia. Differences include usually more rapid onset of global (as opposed to recent) memory loss. Sundowning that may include hallucinations, illusions, and delusions may coexist. Arousal level and attention span are impaired.

Diagnosis

Based on history and physical exam. There should be a demonstrable reason for the delirium and that, by definition, is reversible.

Labs: Vitamin B_{12}/folate, thyroid function, electrolyte level, endocrine workup, VDRL, brain imaging, BUN/creatinine, and liver function should all be investigated as possible sources. Check CBC, UA/urine culture.

Imaging: Chest x-ray to investigate for infectious cause.

Consider "pseudodementia" and screen for depression.

Treatment

- Treat the underlying cause. Reversal can be dramatic.

TABLE 1.8 Common headaches

	Cluster	Tension	Caffeine withdrawal
Symptoms	Usually unilateral with association with periorbital and temporal areas; may involve tearing of the eye, nasal symptoms, facial sweating, ptosis, or miosis; patients are frequently man; pace during acute attacks	Bilateral and radiating from the posterior neck to frontal area; often worse in the PM or after exhausting day	Bilateral and stabbing; occurs in patients with high caffeine intake or recent attempt at reducing/quitting
Associations	More common in men; characteristically waxes and wanes in frequency over period of months	Associated with muscle spasm or tightness on exam	Caffeine-related
Treatment	High-flow oxygen with non-rebreather mask, verapamil for prophylaxis, systemic steroids, indomethacin (Indocin), or a triptan for abortive effect	NSAIDs or Tylenol; massage can be very effective	Long absence of caffeine to break addiction; some commercial analgesics contain caffeine (Excedrin) and thus are "very effective" at treating this headache

NSAIDs, nonsteroidal antiinflammatory drugs.

Syncope

Symptoms

By definition, syncope involves loss of consciousness and is often associated with a fall. Associated symptoms may include aura if cause is seizure, lightheadedness, vertigo, sweating, feeling of flushing/heat, tachycardia, fibrillations, chest pain, coughing, nausea, vomiting, micturition, or visual disturbance. History may indicate locking of the knees, sudden stress, rising quickly from seated/lying position, history of suspicious cause, turning head abruptly, wearing tight collars, or malingering.

Diagnosis

Largely based on history and physical. Assess volume status clinically and obtain postural blood pressures.

Labs: Glucose level, BUN/creatinine, electrolytes, and CBC. Consider cardiac ischemic enzymes in the high-risk patient.

Imaging: Generally not indicated unless trauma, mass effect, or intracranial tumor is suspected.

ECG/Holter monitor may be helpful to investigate possible ischemia and arrhythmias.

Echocardiology may be useful for structural abnormalities or steal syndrome.

EEG to investigate possible seizures.

Head-up tilt-table testing may be of use to elicit vasovagal response.

Carotid sinus massage: Can be dangerous and cause cardiac arrhythmias or asystole. For test purposes, do not use this as a screening test and only consider with cardiac monitoring and support personnel.

Treatment

- Depends on the cause.

- Hydrate aggressively to eliminate this possibility.

- **Vasovagal (neurocardiogenic syncope) reaction:** Behavioral modification and warning sign recognition. Breathing exercises have shown success in some people.

- Anticonvulsants for seizure disorder (see that section).

- Referral and treatment of cardiac anomaly may be indicated.

Tremor

See Table 1.9.

TABLE 1.9 Common tremors

Tremor type	Symptoms	Assoications/diagnosis	Treatment
Resting	Fine tremor usually of the hands	Parkinson's, Wilson's	Physical measures such as weights or conscious control methods
Intention	Oscillation intensifies on movement toward a target	Cerebellar outflow diseases such as multiple sclerosis	Treat underlying disease; otherwise not effective
Physiologic	Usually mild and may occur with rest or movement	Some degree is normal; otherwise strongly associated with anxiety/stress	Treat the cause or remove the stress; infrequent benzodiazepines in low doses; propranolol (Inderal) or primidone (Mysoline) may be effective for acute stressful states
Essential (benign hereditary)	Noticed with skilled tasks; affects hands, head, and voice	Hereditary; often seen in elderly	Benzodiazepines in low doses; propranolol (Inderal) or primidone (Mysoline) may be effective; physical measures such as weights or conscious control methods

Insomnia

Symptoms

Trouble falling asleep, staying asleep, or early morning awakening. History may reveal poor sleep habits, use stimulants/caffeine in excessive amount or time. Patients may report irregular sleep hours or travel, and may have external arousals such as young children.

Diagnosis

A good history and sleep diary are very useful. Interview specifically for caffeine, nicotine, alcohol, decongestant, prescription, or illicit drug use.
Labs: Obtain a TSH.
   Screen for depression.
   Sleep testing only in advanced, refractory cases.

Treatment

- Behavioral modifications to include regular sleep schedule, regular bedtime routine, sleep conducive environment, relaxation techniques, regular exercise, avoidance of stimulants and diuretics.

- Pharmacologic options include nonaddictive medications such as zolpidem (Ambien), zaleplon (Sonata), and eszopiclone (Lunesta). Other options include benzodiazepines including temazepam (Restoril), flurazepam (Dalmaine), triazolam (Halcion), estazolam (Prosom), lorazepam (Ativan), and clonazepam (Klonopin). When prescribing these medications, addiction potential is very high from both drug effect and psychologic dependence.

- Other medications include diphenhydramine (Benadryl) and TCAs such as amitriptyline (Elavil) and trazodone (Desyrel) mainly for their side effect of drowsiness.

- Valerian, melatonin, warm milk, and turkey are herbal and cultural alternatives, but none, to date, have been conclusively proved by consistent research to benefit insomnia patients.

Coma

Symptoms

Profound inability to arouse through any means including painful stimuli. Primitive neurologic reflexes may be present upon stimuli and include decorticate/decerebrate posturing. Often, history is unknown; but if witnesses are present, may reveal underlying disorder. Breathing may be irregular if metabolic derangement is present, for example, Cheyne–Stokes respiration.

TABLE 1.10 Glasgow coma scale

Eye	Verbal	Motor
No spontaneous	No verbal	No motor response
Response to pain	Unintelligible sounds	Extension to pain
Response to verbal	Inappropriate speech	Flexion to pain
Spontaneous	Confused	Withdrawal from pain
	Oriented	Localizing to pain
		Obeys commands
4	5	6

Scored 3–15: ≥13 Mild brain injury; 9–12 Moderate brain injury; ≤8 "Intubate".

Diagnosis

Physical exam: Evaluate Glasgow coma score, breathing pattern, and breath odor. Evaluate pupil reactivity and appearance (see Table 1.10).

Labs: Glucose level, arterial blood gas (ABG), drug screen (including EtOH), ammonia level, CBC, BMP, coagulation panel, liver function and transaminases (AST/ALT), blood cultures, D-dimer, and calcium. Consider gastric lavage if poisoning is on the differential.

Imaging: Obtain Acute CT and evaluate for possible bleed/herniation. MRI may also be useful, but is much slower. Do not forget get a chest x-ray.

LP is indicated if CT/retinal exam is not indicative of increased ICP.

EEG may be performed if all other tests are negative, and may give clue to nonconvulsive status epilepticus.

Treatment

- Treat the underlying cause. Use the mnemonic AEIOU TIPPS: **A**lcohol, **E**pilepsy/**E**lectrolytes, **I**nsulin, **O**piates, **U**remia, **T**rauma, **I**nfection, **P**oison, **P**sych, **S**troke.

- Minimal treatment usually includes ABCs, thiamine (before glucose), oxygen, temperature control, and fluids (with dextrose depending on glucose level).

- Do not give reversal drugs such as naloxone (Narcan) or flumazenil (Romazicon) unless you know the cause.

- Control shock if present.

Brain Death

Diagnosis

Exclude etiologies that may mimic conditions such as neuromuscular blockade, toxins, metabolic derangement, hypothermia, and hypotension.

Remember "nobody's dead until they're warm and dead" that is, warm all patients to exclude possibility of hypothermia.

Inform or make reasonable attempt to contact next of kin.

Tests of Brain Death

Oculocephalic/oculovestibular reflex: When turning head rapidly from side to side, patient does not exhibit "doll's eyes" as a normal person would.

Reactivity of pupils to light is negative.

Gag reflex is negative.

Caloric response reflex: Flushing the ears with cold water does not produce nystagmus.

Apnea test: Stopping mechanical ventilation for at least 8 min and monitoring respiratory movement. $PaCO_2$ must increase >20 mmHg from pretest baseline or rise above 55 mmHg for adequate test.

EEG shows electrical silence.

Four-vessel cerebral angiography shows no blood flow.

The special tests above should be done at least twice 2 h apart; if both batteries are positive, the person is brain dead.

Answers

1.1 B. The presentation suggests bacterial meningitis, which is the most emergent life-threatening infection in this case. Empiric therapy in this age-group should be ampicillin for coverage of group B strep and listeria as well as ceftriaxone (Rocephin) for *Streptococcus pneumoniae*.

1.2 D. This patient has the classic clinical triad of normal pressure hydrocephalus including incontinence, gait disturbance, and early dementia. The diagnosis should be confirmed, but therapy generally consists of ventriculoperitoneal (VP) shunt placement.

1.3 B. In status epilepticus treatment is aimed at acute cessation of seizure and not at maintenance control. For this, lowering the seizure threshold as soon as possible with a fast-acting benzodiazepine is the first-line strategy. If not effective, phenytoin or fosphenytoin may be used.

1.4 A. Laceration of middle meningeal artery is classically the cause of epidural hematoma formation. Because the bleeding is not instant and may take minutes to hours to form a significant hematoma, a "lucid interval" is sometimes observed as in this question. Other answers may occur, but would not explain this interval.

1.5 E. Ergot-derivative medications are effective migraine abortive medications, but carry an absolute contraindication in pregnancy.

Schizophrenia	40
Psychotic Disorders	42
Panic Attacks	42
Generalized Anxiety Disorder	43
Phobias	44
Obsessive-Compulsive Disorder	44
Posttraumatic Stress Disorder	45
Adjustment Disorder	46
Bereavement	46
Major Depressive Episodes/Disorders	47
Bipolar Disorders	48
Somatoform Disorders	50
Anorexia Nervosa	51
Bulimia Nervosa	51
Behavioral Disorders	52
Attention Deficit/Attention Deficit Hyperactivity Disorder	52
Autistic Disorder	54
Dementia	55
Postconcussive Syndrome	56
Alcohol Withdrawal	57
Chemical/Drug Abuse/Dependence	58
Personality Disorders	58
Tardive Dyskinesia	58
Akathisia, Drug-Induced	60

Schizophrenia

Symptoms/Diagnosis

Types of disease

1. Paranoid type
2. Disorganized type
3. Catatonic type
4. Undifferentiated type
5. Residual type.

History often reveals more males than females in their teenage to young 20s, with lower socioeconomic status, smoking, and family history. Suicide rate is as high as 10%.

Criteria and Key Features

See Table 2.1.

1. Psychotic symptoms present for at least **1 month**, including at least two of the following:
   - Hallucinations
   - Delusions
   - Disorganized speech
   - Disorganized or catatonic behavior
   - Negative symptoms.

Plus

2. Impairment of social or occupational functioning
3. Symptoms not primarily due to a mood disorder or schizoaffective disorder
4. Symptoms not due to a medical, neurological, or substance-induced disorder
5. Continuous signs of illness lasting ≥**6 months**.

TABLE 2.1 Symptoms of schizophrenia

Positive symptoms*	Negative symptoms†
Delusions	Flat affect
Hallucinations (often auditory)	Decreased speech
Bizarre behavior	Apathy
Thought disorder	Anhedonia
Poor attention	

*Better prognosis and better response to therapy.
†Worse prognosis and less response to therapy.

Treatment/Side Effects

- Admit to hospital if the patient is a threat to self or others. Generally, this may be done, legally, with a 48–72 h "involuntary hold." This may be extended with a court order, but the case must be brought before a court.
- Neuroleptics (antipsychotics) are the drug class of choice. Divide the starting dose until steady state is reached, ~4–5 days depending on half-life.
- *Atypical neuroleptics.* risperidone (Risperdal), olanzapine (Zyprexa), quetiapine (Seroquel), and ziprasidone (Zeldox, Geodon).
- These are the first-line drugs for schizophrenia, largely due to better side effect profile than typical agents.
- They show decreased incidence of extrapyramidal symptoms and anticholinergic effects, although they do have higher incidence of weight gain, DM type II, and QT prolongation.

Typical Neuroleptics

- High potency—haloperidol (Haldol) and fluphenazine (Prolixin).
- Low potency—chlorpromazine (Thorazine) and thioridazine (Mellaril).
- Side effects of neuroleptics are especially important and very often tested (see Table 2.2).

Neuroleptic malignant syndrome—may occur anytime during therapy; may be life-threatening; characterized by severe muscle rigidity, **fever**, altered mental status, and autonomic instability. Laboratories show elevated WBC, creatine phosphokinase (CPK), and aspartate aminotransferase/alanine

TABLE 2.2 Extrapyramidal side effects

Effect	Typical time course	Signs/symptoms	Treatment
Acute dystonia	10–14 days	Torticollis (writhing of neck), oculogyric movements, unusual tongue or facial muscle movements	Consider change to low-potency agent or decrease current dose; add benztropine (Cogentin) or trihexyphenidyl (Artane)
Akathisia	10–14 days	Feelings of extreme restlessness Walking or pacing	Addition of benztropine or β-blocker; benzodiazepines such as diazepam if refractory
Drug-induced parkinsonism	Months	Cogwheel stiffness in muscles, drooling, mask-like facies, shuffling gait	Anticholinergics such as benztropine (Cogentin), trihexyphenidyl (Artane), antihistamine, or lowering the dose of current treatment
Tardive dyskinesia	Years	Involuntary movements of tongue, lips (lip smacking), sucking, eye blinking, and grimacing	Discontinue the neuroleptics; otherwise, no treatment

aminotransferase (AST/ALT). Treatment involves admission (possibly to ICU), supportive care, discontinuing neuroleptics, giving dantrolene (Dantrium), amantadine (Symmetrel), or bromocriptine (Parlodel).

Anticholinergic side effects—dry mouth, dry eyes, urinary retention, and constipation.

Other common side effects include signs of increased prolactin such as gynecomastia, lactation, impotence, menstrual dysfunction, and libido change, as well as sedation, weight gain, orthostatic hypotension, cardiac effects, retinitis pigmentosa, photosensitivity, and cholestatic jaundice.

Clozapine (Clozaril)—unique atypical agent reserved for refractory cases; unique side effect profile with low or no excess prolactin, extrapyramidal, or neuroleptic malignant syndrome problems. Side effects include agranulocytosis, eosinophilia, leukopenia, and seizures. These make **frequent CBCs** mandatory.

Q 2.1

A 26-year-old Native American female with known past medical history of schizophrenia disorder is brought to the ER with decreased mental status, fever, sweating, and uncontrolled posturing of her back. Her home health nurse states that she has been fairly stable on medications including risperidone (Risperdal) and oral contraceptive pills and was found in her bed only this morning with these symptoms. Her vital signs show BP 165/100, heart rate (HR) 122, temperature 39.1°C (102.3°F), and respiratory rate (RR) 20. The patient is unresponsive to questioning but responds to pain with localization. She appears acutely agitated and demonstrates uncontrolled posturing and extension of her back. Initial labs are drawn and you are awaiting results. What is the next step in management?

A. Discontinue risperidone, commence IV fluids and dantrolene (Dantrium).
B. Discontinue risperidone, order for blood cultures then start on ceftriaxone (Rocephin).
C. Discontinue risperidone, commence lorazepam (Ativan), and physical restraints.
D. Haloperidol (Haldol) and IV fluids.
E. Give extra dose of risperidone immediately.

Psychotic Disorders

See Table 2.3.

Panic Attacks

Symptoms/Diagnosis

Recurrent, unexpected attacks with peak intensity within 10 min, and four or more of the following symptoms: palpitations, sweating, trembling, shortness of breath, feeling of choking, chest pain, nausea, dizziness or lightheadedness, depersonalization, fear of losing control or going crazy, fear of dying, paresthesias, or chills/hot flashes. Panic attacks are often accompanied by agoraphobia. The patient often adapts by avoiding situations of anticipated attack triggers. Interattack anxiety of the next attack is classic and often prominent.

TABLE 2.3 The schizophrenia spectrum

Disorder	Time course	Signs/diagnosis	Treatment
Brief psychotic disorder	1 day–1 month	Criteria for schizophrenia are met, except for time course; often preceded by emotional event/stress; patient returns to normal after event ends	Hospitalize if harmful to self or others, brief course of neuroleptic may help, lorazepam (Ativan) or short-acting benzodiazepine as indicated
Schizophreniform disorder	1–6 months	Criteria for schizophrenia are met, except for time course	Hospitalize if harmful to self or others, start course of neuroleptic, treat mood disturbances as needed
Schizoaffective disorder	>6 months	Symptoms meet criteria for schizophrenia and mood disorder; mood symptoms must be present for significant portion of the illness (although psychotic symptoms are present without them)	Hospitalize if harmful to self or others, start course of neuroleptic for psychotic symptoms; start antidepressant (SSRI, TCA, etc.) for mood symptoms; start mood stabilizer if bipolar symptoms are present

SSRI, selective serotonin reuptake inhibitor; TCA, tricyclic antidepressant.

Treatment

- Cognitive behavioral therapy (CBT), relaxation, and breathing techniques can be very effective.

- Propranolol (Inderal) may be used as "Dumbo's feather," and may be taken 30–45 min before anticipated situation leading to attack (i.e., public speaking).

- Selective serotonin reuptake inhibitors (SSRIs) (paroxetine, sertraline, etc.), tricyclic antidepressants (TCAs) (imipramine, amitriptyline), or rarely monoamine oxidase inhibitors (MAOIs) are the first-line medications, although they must be scheduled and not taken PRN.

- Benzodiazepines [alprazolam (Xanax), clonazepam (Klonopin)] may be useful as scheduled or PRN medication. However, they are addictive and may oversedate if used improperly.

- Buspirone (BuSpar) is *not* effective for panic disorder.

Generalized Anxiety Disorder

Symptoms/Diagnosis

Criteria include

Excessive anxiety or worry on most days during at least a 6-month period with at least three of the following:

- Restlessness
- Easy fatigability

- Difficulty concentrating
- Irritability
- Muscle tension
- Sleep disturbance.

Treatment

- Combine medications with psychotherapy (including CBT and insight-oriented psychotherapy) for best results.
- Venlafaxine (Effexor) and buspirone (BuSpar) are first-line drugs, but both take weeks to work.
- Other SSRIs may also be tried and are first line. Time course to action is 2–4 weeks.
- Benzodiazepines are faster, but considered second line because of side effects and addictive potential. If used, plan to taper after several weeks of therapy; this is commonly done while awaiting one of the above agents to take effect.

Phobias

Symptoms/Diagnosis

Unreasonable and excessive anxiety or fear response to particular situation or object. Response or anticipation of response may provoke panic attack. This response, or anticipation of response, interferes significantly with the individual's life. Duration of symptoms ≥6 months.

Treatment

- CBT is the mainstay of treatment and includes exposure and desensitization combined with relaxation and deep breathing techniques.
- β-Blockers and benzodiazepines may be effective adjuncts to CBT.

Obsessive-Compulsive Disorder

Symptoms/Diagnosis

Recurrent, persistent, intrusive, but conscious, compulsions or obsessions that negatively impact the patient's life. These are thoughts, images, impulses, or bizarre behaviors the patient experiences without apparent reason, which are conscious and purposeful. Repetitive behavior is common and may range from fairly logical, such as hand washing, to bizarre, such as touching a wall a certain way before leaving the room. The patients recognize them as intrusive and negative and a function of their own mind, and may try to compensate and suppress them. Behaviors often take a significant amount of time, typically >1 h/day.

Treatment

- Combination of medication and CBT is most effective.
- CBT should consist of thought stopping, desensitization, or flooding techniques.
- Medications include clomipramine (Anafranil) and SSRIs (may require high dosage).

Q 2.2

A 43-year-old Caucasian female comes to your primary care clinic for evaluation of stress and pervasive thoughts following a recent small plane crash 2 weeks ago. She states that her husband who was flying the aircraft suffered a broken leg and she had been diagnosed with mild soft tissue injury of the neck ("whiplash"). She states that the symptoms began after the crash and consist of obsessive type thoughts, with times of "reexperiencing" the event. Her previous psychiatric and medical history is noncontributory. What is the most likely diagnosis?

A. Panic attack disorder.
B. Adjustment disorder with psychotic features.
C. Posttraumatic stress disorder.
D. Acute stress disorder.
E. Bereavement.

Posttraumatic Stress Disorder

Symptoms/Diagnosis

Symptoms including feelings of guilt, poor impulse control, aggression, personality change, and depression occur after a significantly stressful event such as combat, rape. The patient persistently reexperiences the event through intrusive thoughts, nightmares, "daymares," and flashbacks. Persistent feelings of detachment, anhedonia, amnesia, restricted or blunted affect, and feelings of avoidance of similar or related events are present. A general state of increased arousal persists after the event, and may contribute to other symptoms such as insomnia and exaggerated startle response. Symptoms collectively cause impaired occupational and social functioning, which have significant impact on the patient's life. For posttraumatic stress disorder (PTSD), by definition, symptoms occur >1 month after the event.

Acute stress disorder—includes the above features of PTSD with onset <1 month from the time of event and lasting for 2–4 weeks.

Treatment

- Psychotherapy, behavioral therapy, support groups, and family therapy are effective and should be used with medications.

- SSRIs [most effectively sertraline (Zoloft)] are first-line medications. TCAs and MAOIs may be used as alternatives.
- Propranolol, lithium, anticonvulsants, and buspirone (BuSpar) may be effective if antidepressants fail.

Adjustment Disorder

Symptoms/Diagnosis

Symptoms similar to depression including thoughts of hopelessness, depressed mood, anhedonia, sleep disturbance, eating disturbance, amotivation, possible thoughts of suicide, and temporary obsession with triggering event or stressor. Symptoms occur within 3 months of inciting event/stressor and last <6 months.

Treatment

- Psychotherapy and talk therapy are first-line therapies. In most patients, expressing feelings surrounding inciting event begins them on the road to recovery.

Medications

- SSRIs are classically effective, but take 3–4 weeks to show effect. TCAs are second-line drugs due to possible toxicity and side effects, and they are also thought to be less effective.
- Electroconvulsive therapy (ECT) is not indicated for adjustment disorder.

Bereavement

Symptoms/Diagnosis

Associated most commonly with death or significant loss of a loved one. Symptoms tend to be classified into several stages. The classic five stages of grief are (1) denial, (2) anger, (3) bargaining, (4) depression, and (5) acceptance. Some sources organize these into stages including shock, preoccupation, and resolution. These begin within 2 months and may last >1 year. Despite time course, this is a temporary condition.

Treatment

- Psychotherapy and talk therapy are first-line therapies. In most patients, expressing feelings surrounding their loved ones (or their death) starts them on the road to recovery.

Medications

- SSRIs are classically effective, but take 3–4 weeks to show effect. TCAs are second-line drugs due to possible toxicity and side effects.
- ECT is not indicated for bereavement.

Major Depressive Episodes/Disorders

Symptoms/Diagnosis

Characterized by depressed mood, coupled with several other symptoms such as anhedonia, sleep disturbance, eating disturbance, loss of energy, feelings of guilt/worthlessness, lack of hope, loss of libido, and possible thoughts of suicide. Several clinical tools exist to aid in diagnosis, including a well-known pneumonic: SIGECAPS (Sleep, Interest, Guilt, Energy, Concentration, Appetite, Psychomotor status, Suicidal ideation).

These symptoms occur for >**2 weeks**, and cannot be associated with bereavement.

Variants exist and are listed in Table 2.4.

Dysthymia is very similar, but is a milder form. It may include less intense symptoms and be present for more days than not more than a period of **2 years**.

TABLE 2.4 Major depression variants

Psychotic features	Hallucinations, delusions
Chronic	Lasting 2 years and more severe than dysthymia
Catatonic features	At least two of the following: 1. Motor immobility or stupor 2. Excessive purposeless movement 3. Extreme negativism or mutism 4. Bizarre posturing, stereotyped movement, or grimacing 5. Echolalia or echopraxia
Melancholic features	Excessive anhedonia and at least three of the following: 1. Depressed mood 2. Worse in the AM 3. Early AM wakening 4. Psychomotor slowing 5. Significant weight loss 6. Excessive guilt
Atypical features	At least two of the following: 1. Significant weight gain from excessive diet 2. Hypersomnia 3. "Heavy" feeling in extremities 4. Chronic fear of rejection with resultant social isolationism
Postpartum	Onset within 4 weeks of delivery
Seasonal pattern	Recurrence during darker (late fall, winter, early spring) months. More than 2 years, symptoms have occurred twice

Treatment

- Screen for suicidal or homicidal ideation. If present, have patient "contract for safety" and write it down. Hospitalize if necessary.

Medications

- SSRIs are first-line therapy, but generally take 3–4 weeks to show effect. None have been shown superior to any other in efficacy, but selection is based on coexisting symptoms. For example, sertraline (Zoloft) is used more widely for depressive symptoms, paroxetine (Paxil) for anxiety. Common side effects include insomnia, sexual dysfunction, gastrointestinal upset, and agitation.

- TCAs are second-line medications and also take 3–4 weeks for being effective. Side effects are generally worse in the first month and include anticholinergic effects, sedation, and **cardiovascular effects** in overdose. TCAs are thought to be a poor choice for potentially suicidal patients given the toxic cardiovascular effects in overdose.

- MAOIs are rarely used. Side effects can be severe and include orthostatic hypotension and hypertensive "tyramine crisis" if patient does not strictly follow the accompanying diet of low-tyramine foods.

- Atypical agents include bupropion (Wellbutrin), venlafaxine (Effexor), nefazodone (Serzone), and mirtazapine (Remeron). These agents may be better in refractory cases or pregnancy, but also have unique side effects.

- Phototherapy may be effective for seasonal affective disorder.

- Use of medication with counseling is often more effective than either alone.

- Electroconvulsive Therapy (ECT) is effective, but used only after mood stabilizers and other therapies have failed.

Bipolar Disorders

Symptoms/Diagnosis

Bipolar I—major depressive episodes mixed with periods of mania. Classically presents with patients who spend money excessively, are hypersexual, have grandiose thoughts/schemes, and do not sleep.

Bipolar II—major depressive episodes mixed with hypomanic periods.

Mania—mood disturbance involving irritability, inflated self-esteem/grandiosity, decreased sleep, talkativeness, flight of ideas, distractibility, increased goal-directed behavior, and excessive involvement in pleasurable activities with a high potential for harm (i.e., sexual indiscretion).

Hypomania—the same basic elements of mood as mania, but less intense and for a lesser period.

Treatment

- Screen for suicidal or homicidal ideation. If present, have patient "contract for safety" and write it down. Admit if necessary.
- CBT in combination with medications is most effective.
- SSRIs may be used, but do so in conjunction with a mood stabilizer to avoid precipitation of manic episodes.

Mood stabilizers

- Lithium (Eskalith, Lithonate) is a first-line therapy, but toxic levels may easily be reached. Before beginning, check TSH, BUN/creatinine, electrolytes, blood glucose level, and ECG. Then monitor lithium levels weekly for 2 months and every month thereafter. Signs of toxicity include tremor, polyuria, thirst (diabetes insipidus), edema, weight gain, nausea, diarrhea, hypothyroidism, rash, elevated WBC, and T-wave flattening on ECG. Interactions include nonsteroidal antiinflammatory drugs (NSAIDs), ACE inhibitors, and diuretics. Hemodialyze if toxic levels are reached.
- Carbamazepine (Tegretol) is used as a second-line therapy. Pretreatment evaluation includes liver function tests (LFTs), ECG, CBC, electrolytes, and BUN/creatinine. Monitor levels for first month. Side effects include agranulocytosis, aplastic anemia, leukopenia, hepatitis, Stevens–Johnson syndrome, ataxia, confusion, and tremor.
- Valproic acid (Depakene) is quickly becoming a favorite secondary due to low side effect and toxicity profile. More effective for "**rapid cyclers**" than either lithium or carbamazepine. Check CBC, platelets, and PT/PTT for the first month of therapy. Side effects include: gastrointestinal distress including nausea/vomiting, sedation, mild elevations of LFTs, thrombocytopenia, and elevation of ammonia.
- Gabapentin (Neurontin) is a newer agent used for both neuropathic pain syndromes and mood stabilization. Little pretreatment evaluation is needed and only includes renal function (BUN/creatinine). Side effects include somnolence, fatigue, ataxia, nausea/vomiting, dizziness, and weight change.
- Other newer agents include lamotrigine (Lamictal), topiramate (Topamax), tiagabine (Gabitril), and oxcarbazepine (Trileptal). These agents have all been used widely for other disorders such as seizures or pain syndromes, and have recently been added to mood stabilization regimens. Side effects have been lower than traditional mood stabilizers, but efficacy is less proven.

Q 2.3

A 36-year-old Asian American female comes to your primary care office to discuss referral to a plastic surgeon for her fourth rhinoplasty. She has a long history of repeat cosmetic procedures on multiple areas of her body and complains of not being able to find a plastic surgeon that "understands what I want." She is dressed in baggy clothing on presentation and is shy to show you her face. Her body mass index (BMI) is 21. What is the most appropriate treatment course?

A. Referral to a reputable plastic surgeon.
B. Explanation of normal appearance of nose and counseling of no need for revising previous surgery.
C. Referral to psychological counseling and beginning an SSRI.
D. Start quetiapine (Seroquel) after initial laboratory evaluation.
E. Involuntary admission to the local hospital psychiatric ward to prevent harm being done to herself.

Somatoform Disorders

See Table 2.5.

TABLE 2.5 Somatiform disorders

Disorder	Key elements	Treatment
Somatization disorder	Onset before the age of 30 Many varied physical complaints Not explained by organic disease or severity of illness	Psychotherapy to address emotional issues underlying problem Regular doctor visits
Conversion disorder	Symptoms of neurologic or muscular origin (i.e., blindness, seizure) Not intentionally produced Not organic in origin Related to stressful event	Symptoms typically remit on their own after weeks–months Insight-oriented or behavioral therapy Anxiolytics and relaxation techniques may help
Hypochondriasis	Preoccupation with fear of having a serious medical condition Not reassured by negative test results Duration >6 months	Group therapy Regular doctor visits
Body dysmorphic disorder	Preoccupation with imagined defect in body appearance	Individual or group counseling, CBT, or SSRIs and clomipramine (Anafranil) are effective
Factitious disorder	Intentional production of physical or psychological symptoms to assume the sick role. Munchausen syndrome (symptoms in self) Munchausen's by proxy syndrome (symptoms/signs in patient's child)	Try to recognize early No specific treatment exists
Malingering	Staging of symptoms for secondary gain (i.e., money, time off work)	No specific treatment exists Criminal prosecution if indicated

CBT, cognitive behavioral therapy; SSRIs, selective serotonin reuptake inhibitors.

Anorexia Nervosa

Symptoms/Diagnosis

Usually female patients with distorted sense of self-appearance in regard to weight and body fat appearance. Often refuses to maintain weight >85% of ideal body weight, and feels intense fear of gaining weight. Denial of seriousness of current low weight and desires to lose more. **Amenorrhea for at least three cycles** in menstruating women is common; classically, female student living in upper class or higher socioeconomic class with good grades and exceptional will to excel.

Treatment

- Psychotherapies including psychodynamic psychotherapy, family therapy, behavioral therapy, and group therapy.
- Since major depression is common, SSRIs may be appropriate.
- Bupropion (Wellbutrin) is contraindicated because of the risk of seizures.
- Admission is indicated for seriously emaciated patients or those with severe, acute weight loss.
- Close monitoring, possibly inpatient, of oral calorie intake.
- Replace electrolytes as needed.

Bulimia Nervosa

Symptoms/Diagnosis

The patient engages in binging/purging cycles characterized as excessive eating, then vomiting or laxative use. Use of compensatory behavior for calorie intake is common, and may include laxative use, excessive exercise, diuretic use, or vomiting. These episodes occur on an average of **two times per week for at least 3 months**. Unlike anorexia patients, bulimia patients tend to be average or above average weight. Physical exam findings include poor dentition, finger/finger nail abnormalities caused by acid effect from vomiting.

Treatment

- CBT is most helpful.
- SSRIs, particularly fluoxetine (Prozac), is effective.
- TCAs are also used, including imipramine (Tofranil) and desipramine (Norpramin).
- Bupropion (Wellbutrin) is contraindicated because of the risk of seizures.

Q 2.4

What is the commonly seen adult form of conduct disorder?

A. Oppositional defiant disorder.
B. Antisocial personality disorder.
C. Histrionic personality disorder.
D. Narcissistic personality disorder.
E. Borderline personality disorder.

Behavioral Disorders

See Table 2.6.

Attention Deficit/Attention Deficit Hyperactivity Disorder

Symptoms/Diagnosis

Attention deficit disorder (ADD) and attention deficit hyperactivity disorder (ADHD) are two separate diagnoses.

Attention deficit has at least six of the following characteristics:

- Carelessness
- Inattention
- Does not listen
- Lack of task completion
- Disorganized

TABLE 2.6 Behavioral disorders

Disorder	Symptoms/diagnosis	Treatment
Conduct disorder	Child who is severely defiant and almost constantly in trouble; displays **cruelty to animals, lack of remorse, and enjoys destroying property**; often lies and violates the law. Adult form is termed **antisocial personality disorder**	Cognitive behavioral therapy, individual therapy, group and family counseling; intense behavioral modification techniques are needed; various mood stabilizers, antidepressants, propranolol (Inderal), neuroleptics, and atypical antidepressants have been tried with varied success
Oppositional defiant disorder	Milder form of behavioral disorder to include behavior that is stubborn, negativistic, provocative, and at time hostile; however, these kids are not lying, cheating criminals	Behavioral modification techniques such as token economies and reward systems; generally, medication is not needed, unless other disorders exist

- Dislike for goal-oriented tasks and homework
- Often loses things
- Distractibility
- Forgetfulness.

Add to these at least six of the following hyperactive problems for ADHD:

- Fidgeting in seat
- Often unable to stay seated
- Often runs or climbs at inappropriate times
- Difficulty with quiet play
- Often "on the go"
- Talkativeness
- Often answers questions before they are complete
- Difficulty awaiting their turn
- Often interrupts or intrudes on others.

These symptoms must be present in **two or more settings** (i.e., school and home), and some degree of these symptoms is present **before the age of 7 years**.

Treatment

- ADD/ADHD patients tend to do better in a structured, consistent environment. It is essential that everyone in the authority uses the same set of rules so that the child learns barriers.
- Token economies have shown good efficacy.

Medications

- Stimulant medications are the most effective class. These include methylphenidate (Ritalin, Ritalin SR, Concerta, Metadate) and amphetamine-dextroamphetamine (Adderall). Start with methylphenidate and titrate dosage to effect. Only short-acting amphetamine-dextroamphetamine is approved for children <6 years of age. Adverse effects include insomnia, decreased appetite, stomach pain, headache, **emergence or worsening of tics**, **decreased growth velocity** (although end growth appears unaffected), tachycardia, blood pressure elevation, rebound or deterioration of ADHD behaviors when medication wears off, emotional lability, irritability, social withdrawal, and flattened affect.
- Atomoxetine (Strattera) is a nonstimulant medication that selectively inhibits norepinephrine reuptake and has shown good efficacy.
- Consider "drug holidays" on the weekends or during the summer school break.

- Other medications can be used, such as bupropion (Wellbutrin), but only with the consent of the psychiatrist.
- Consider that these are controlled, addictive substances. Look for secondary gain motives in parents who are asking to increase dose/obtain more of these medications.

Autistic Disorder

Symptoms/Diagnosis

A disorder characterized by otherwise normal children seeming to "shut down" and stop communicating. Characteristics include three groups of impairment:

1. Impairment in social interaction including failure to use nonverbal gestures, failure to develop peer relationships, lack of seeking to share enjoyment or achievements, and lack of social reciprocity.

2. Qualitative impairment in communication: delay or lack of development of spoken language; in individuals with adequate speech, a marked impairment of initiating or sustaining conversation; repetitive use of language; lack of varied, spontaneous imaginative play; or social imitative behavior.

3. Restricted, repetitive, and stereotyped patterns of behavior: preoccupation of stereotyped behavior in intensity or focus; inflexible adherence to specific, nonfunctional routines; repetitive motor mannerisms; and preoccupation with parts of objects.

Add to these delays or abnormal functioning in social interaction, language as used in communication, or symbolic or imaginative play. These occur before the **age of 3 years**.

Treatment

- There is no cure for autism. However, specialized school programs and behavioral programs exist and have shown good efficacy, especially if begun early. Responsive patients may eventually compensate very well for their disorder and become very highly functional.

Medications

- Various classes including SSRIs, TCAs, stimulants, bupropion, and so on, have been used for various symptoms with varied success. These are basically only for specific symptoms and do not treat the overlying autism disorder.

Q 2.5

An 89-year-old male geriatric home patient is brought to the ER for evaluation of recent onset of fever and worsening dementia symptoms. He has previously been diagnosed with Alzheimer's disease and is mildly demented at baseline but his nursing home staff commented that these symptoms have become much worse lately, with recent predilection toward violence. His past medical history includes paralysis with loss of urinary control for which he normally is able to self-catheterize periodically. His other medical problems include controlled hypertension, type II diabetes mellitus, hypothyroidism, and early macular degeneration. What is the best characterization of this patient's mental state?

A. Worsening Alzheimer's dementia.
B. New onset vascular dementia.
C. Delirium likely due to noncompliance with medication.
D. Delirium likely due to occult urinary tract infection.
E. Typical "sundowning" phenomenon seen with Alzheimer's disease.

Dementia

Symptoms/Diagnosis

Onset of dementia is usually insidious, but may be stepwise (vascular), sudden, related to other medical conditions, related to drug effects/abuse, related to other brain disease (Parkinson's, Pick's, Alzheimer's), or often idiopathic. Symptoms always include some degree of memory impairment along with aphasia (language disturbance), apraxia (motor impairment), agnosia (identification disturbance), or executive brain functioning problems. Delirium must be ruled out. Patients are often unaware of these declines, and they may be confused about their current situation.

Several clinical dementia scales exist, but most common is the Mini-Mental Status Exam, which includes cognitive function testing. Score >24 is generally considered normal, but takes education level into account.

Labs/Imaging: CBC with differential, Chem-7, hepatic function panel, TSH level, urinalysis, drug screen, vitamin B_{12}/folate levels, and rapid plasma reagin (RPR) or VDRL. Consider obtaining heavy metal screen, lumbar puncture, ECG, chest x-ray, EEG, and MRI for possible infarcts. These will eliminate the possibility of delirium.

Treatment

- Make sure you are not dealing with delirium; and if so, treat it.

- Minimize medications that may contribute anticholinergic effects.

- See Chapter 1 for the treatment of Alzheimer's type dementia. Medications include donepezil (Aricept), rivastigmine (Exelon), and memantine (Namenda).

- If vascular dementia suspected, control blood pressure, give aspirin, and control risk factors [consider carotid endarterectomy (CEA)].

For Agitation

- Acute therapy includes haloperidol (Haldol) and lorazepam (Ativan). These are quick acting, but dose should be appropriate for renal function and age. Sedative effects often last much longer in the elderly. Additional options include buspirone (BuSpar), trazodone (Desyrel), risperidone (Risperdal), olanzapine (Zyprexa), and divalproex (Depakene).
- SSRIs may be used for concurrent depression, but TCAs are avoided because of anticholinergic effects.
- Social support for the family is essential and often involves assigning medical power of attorney to a relative, support groups, and close monitoring.
- Ensure the patient's home safety.

Postconcussive Syndrome

Symptoms/Diagnosis

Symptoms may include headache, dizziness, fatigue, irritability, anxiety, insomnia, loss of concentration and memory, and noise sensitivity. These are nonspecific and may exist in some background prevalence in the general population—hence the controversy on this topic. If postconcussive syndrome (PCS), mild concussion, or traumatic brain injury (TBI) has occurred in the recent past, symptoms may last up to 3 months in some patients but rarely longer. CT/MRI should have been done at the time of TBI evaluation; but if not previously done, do an MRI for better images of the brain. Neuropsychological testing has shown only a very small difference in PCS patients and is not considered clinically useful. Seizures and vomiting are *not* a part of PCS and should be evaluated.

Treatment

- Exclude structural brain injury.
- Reassure the patient and provide education.
- Treat symptoms such as headaches and insomnia.

Q 2.6

A 48-year-old African American male with previous known alcoholism is admitted to the surgery service of your hospital for scheduled knee replacement. After the uncomplicated procedure he was reported to do well but was being kept an extra day by the surgeon because she wanted to make sure the new device she used was working correctly. On the last night of his stay, you are consulted for evaluation of onset of hallucinations in the patient who thinks that ants are crawling inside his skin. On exam he is restrained, diaphoretic, and acutely agitated. What is the most effective treatment for this patient's condition?

A. Lorazepam (Ativan) acutely.
B. Consultation to the psychiatric service.
C. Broad-spectrum antibiotics and laboratory studies to determine source of infection.
D. Urine drug screen.
E. Haloperidol (Haldol).

Alcohol Withdrawal

Symptoms/Diagnosis

See Table 2.7.

Treatment

- Patients should be assessed for risk of serious withdrawal. If high risk or if risk is unknown, patient should be placed in the ICU for close monitoring.

- A clinical assessment tool such as the CIWA (Clinical Institute Withdrawal Assessment for Alcohol) scale should be used for routine objective monitoring. The same person should judge this score each time the evaluation is done.

TABLE 2.7 Spectrum of alcohol withdrawal

Syndrome	Clinical symptoms	Onset after last drink	Duration
Minor withdrawal	Tremulousness, mild anxiety, headache, diaphoresis, palpitations, anorexia, gastrointestinal upset, tachycardia	6–36 h	Up to 2 weeks
Seizures	Generalized, tonic–clonic seizures, rarely status epilepticus	6–48 h	Usually seconds to minutes
Alcoholic hallucinosis	Auditory > visual, tactile	12–48 h	<6 days
Delirium tremens (DTs)	Delirium, tachycardia, hypertension, agitation, fever, diaphoresis	2–5 days	<3 days

- IV fluids should be started, with the replacement of likely fluid deficit. Multivitamins and electrolyte replacement should be started concurrently. Classically, **thiamine** is the vitamin mostly needing replacement in alcoholics. **Always give thiamine before glucose** to prevent eliciting Wernicke's encephalopathy or Korsakoff's syndrome. Often a "banana bag" can suffice for repletion.

Medications

- **Benzodiazepines:** For acute control, lorazepam (Ativan) is most effective because of rapid onset in IV/IM form and short half-life. Diazepam (Valium) may also be given acutely, but has a somewhat longer half-life. For prophylactic administration in the high-risk (nonvomiting) patient, chlordiazepoxide (Librium) or oxazepam (Serax) may be scheduled by mouth (PO).

- Barbiturates (phenobarbital) or propofol (Diprivan) may be used if the patient is refractory to high-dose benzodiazepines. If these are necessary, prepare for intubation.

- Haloperidol (Haldol) and other antipsychotics are not recommended because of their tendency to lower the seizure threshold, as well as their lack of cross-tolerance with alcohol.

- Schedule an alcohol cessation program at the end of treatment.

Chemical/Drug Abuse/Dependence

See Table 2.8.

Personality Disorders

See Tables 2.9–2.11.

Tardive Dyskinesia

Symptoms/Diagnosis

Involuntary movements of the mouth, tongue, head, fingers, toes, and other body parts. It is related to therapy with antipsychotic medications (except clozapine), which have a 3% per year risk of producing this condition. Disease is irreversible once begun, but most cases are mild because of early recognition. The development of tardive dyskinesia may progress after the offending agent is stopped.

TABLE 2.8 Common illicit drug profiles

Illicit drug	Intoxication	Withdrawal syndrome	Treatment
Opioids (heroin, Rx pain medications)	CNS depression, pupillary constriction, respiratory depression, constipation	Yes	Naloxone (Narcan) acutely
Amphetamines (crystal, speed, crank)	Psychomotor agitation, tachycardia, pupillary dilation, paranoia, sudden death	Yes	Haloperidol (Haldol) or other antipsychotics; benzodiazepines acutely as needed
Phencyclidine hydrochloride (PCP)	Belligerence, psychosis, violence, vertical/horizontal nystagmus	Yes	Benzodiazepines acutely; haloperidol may be useful to calm patients
Lysergic acid diethylamide (LSD)	Hallucinations, delusions, pupillary dilation	No	Benzodiazepines acutely
Marijuana	Euphoria, impaired judgment, dry mouth, increased appetite, conjunctival injection, paranoia	No	Isolation from drug
Cocaine	Euphoria, insomnia, impulsive behavior, arrhythmia, cerebral infarct, paranoid ideation, weight loss	Yes	Benzodiazepines and antipsychotics acutely; clonidine, amantadine (Symmetrel), or carbamazepine (Tegretol) may decrease cravings

TABLE 2.9 Cluster A personality disorders (weird)

Type	Features	Treatment
Paranoid	Suspiciousness, fear of exploitation, harm, bearer of grudges, reactionary	Psychotherapy
Schizoid	Social detachment, restricted effect, solitary by choice, lack of friends; similar to negative symptoms usually linked to schizophrenia	Individual psychotherapy
Schizotypal	Odd beliefs and magical thinking, paranoia, suspiciousness; strange behavior; similar to positive symptoms usually linked to schizophrenia	Psychotherapy; antipsychotics may be useful for excessive delusional states

TABLE 2.10 Cluster B personality disorders (wild)

Type	Features	Treatment
Antisocial	Deceitfulness, criminality, exhibits disregard and violation of rights of others Lack of remorse for behavior. Associated with **conduct disorder** as a child	Inpatient group therapy if available
Borderline	Fear of abandonment, intense personal relationships, imagined traumatic behavior, splitting, self-mutilation	Psychotherapy; SSRIs for depressive, anxiety symptoms
Histrionic	Excessive emotionality and attention-seeking. Need to be center of attention; often hypersexual behavior	Insight-oriented psychotherapy
Narcissistic	Egotistical, delusions of grandeur, sense of entitlement, lacks empathy; superiority complex	Psychotherapy

SSRIs, selective serotonin reuptake inhibitors.

TABLE 2.11 Cluster C personality disorders (whacky)

Type	Features	Treatment
Avoidant	Social inhibition, excessively sensitive to criticism, feelings of inadequacy prevail; inferiority complex	Individual or group psychotherapy, assertiveness training, desensitization training; SSRIs are often helpful
Dependent	Submissive, clinging behavior. Pervasive need to be cared for; difficulty making decisions	Insight-oriented psychotherapy, group and behavioral therapies; family therapy
Obsessive–compulsive	Preoccupation with orderliness, cleanliness, perfectionism; reluctance to delegate tasks. Rigid	Long-term individual therapy

SSRIs, selective serotonin reuptake inhibitors.

Treatment

- Stop the offending neuroleptic.
- Replace the medication with clozapine (Clozaril) if continued therapy is needed.
- No other drug class has been shown to be effective.

Akathisia, Drug-Induced

Akathisia is a condition characterized as a strong inner feeling of restlessness, and is manifested by difficulty remaining still and the need to walk or pace. This is a side effect of neuroleptic drug therapy.

Treatment

- This condition may respond to the addition of an anticholinergic agent or β-blocker.
- Propranolol (Inderal) is the β-blocker of choice.
- Benzodiazepines such as diazepam (Valium) are used for refractory cases.

Answers

2.1 A. This patient is exhibiting four cardinal signs of neuroleptic malignant syndrome, namely autonomic instability, altered mental status, fever, and history of neuroleptic use. This is a medical emergency and requires prompt treatment to reduce morbidity and mortality in this patient. This includes discontinuation of neuroleptic therapy, supportive care (intubation if necessary), and medications aimed at reducing effects of the disorder which include dantrolene (Dantrium), amantadine (Symmetrel), or bromocriptine (Parlodel).

2.2 D. This patient has experienced an acute event causing psychological trauma, leading to significant symptoms. The time course, however, is the key to diagnosing her condition as acute stress disorder (being <1 month in duration). If symptoms persist for >1 month, posttraumatic stress disorder may be apparent.

2.3 C. This patient likely has body dysmorphic disorder, exhibiting a strong history of previous cosmetic surgeries without satisfaction. Treatment may be by multiple modalities but often involves group or individual counseling, CBT, and beginning a SSRI or clomipramine (Anafranil).

2.4 B. Antisocial personality disorder patients commonly have had the symptoms of conduct disorder in their childhood. Conversely, those child patients with conduct disorder commonly grow up to suffer from antisocial personality disorder as adults.

2.5 D. This patient is likely exhibiting delirium evidenced by relatively acute worsening of mental state accompanied by fever. This should make the physician look for signs of infection that may be responsible for his medical decline. The best source of infection in this patient would be his urinary system since he is normally responsible for self-catheterization. Medication noncompliance may also be a source of delirium but residence in a skilled nursing facility coupled with presence of fever in this patient make this less likely.

2.6 A. This known alcoholic is likely in acute withdrawal as seen in his classic symptoms. Treatment acutely often requires short to mid-acting benzodiazepines such as lorazepam (Ativan) to control symptoms. This is of excellent use because these medications also offer control of possible seizure activity and sedation. Strategies of subacute and chronic control of alcohol withdrawal syndrome vary greatly but often employ variations of the benzodiazepine class.

3 Ophthalmology

Ophthalmic Manifestations of Diabetes	63
Macular Degeneration	64
Retinal Detachments, Defects, and Disorders	65
Glaucoma	66
Cataracts	68
Visual Disturbances	68
Visual Field Defects	68
Conjunctivitis	70
Disorders of the Eyelid/Lachrymal System	70
Orbital Cellulitis	72
Strabismus	73
Nystagmus	73
Pterygium	74
Corneal Abrasion	74

Ophthalmic Manifestations of Diabetes

Symptoms

May present as gradual visual loss, difficulty in reading, blurred vision, halos around lights, or dark spots in visual field. Neovascularization can be a leading cause of vision loss; evidence is seen on exam.

Diagnosis

On retinal exam, may observe "dot and blot" hemorrhages, which are caused by retinal vessel microaneurysms, or "cotton wool" spots, which occur from microinfarcts resulting in decreased retinal perfusion. Retinal edema may also be seen and if longstanding can lead to "hard exudates" seen on exam.
Imaging: Fluorescein angiography may be used to further evaluate the disease.

Treatment

- Diabetic patients should be referred for ophthalmologic exam annually. Otherwise good control of glucose levels and blood pressure is very effective.
- Panretinal laser photocoagulation may be helpful in proliferative retinopathy with neovascularization.
- Treatment of nonproliferative retinopathy consists of laser photo-coagulation to affected area.
- For retinal hemorrhage, vitrectomy may be indicated.

Q 3.1

A 78-year-old carpenter comes to your clinic with progressive long-term visual loss. He states that his vision has been declining for years and that he notices it mostly when he measures straight lines for his woodwork. His past medical history includes obesity, smoking cigars, psoriasis, depression, and gastroesophageal reflux disease (GERD). On exam, you note several drusen deposits on the retina with one to two hemorrhagic areas of the macula in each eye. Amsler chart testing confirms your suspicion. Modification of what risk factor below may slow the progression of this disease?

A. Stopping smoking.
B. Vitamin supplementation.
C. Control of GERD.
D. Control of psoriasis.
E. Increasing surrounding light while working.

Macular Degeneration

Symptoms

Painless visual loss often accompanied by visual distortion when looking at straight lines. Risk factors include:

- Age
- Caucasian race
- Smoking
- Hypertension
- Vascular disease
- Fatty diet
- UV light exposure.

Diagnosis

Retinal exam shows pigmentary or hemorrhagic disturbance in the macular region accompanied by "drusen" deposits.

Amsler's chart of gridlines is often used to diagnose. Patient will see distorted lines. Fluorescein angiography also shows a neovascular membrane beneath the retina.

Treatment

- Prevention with antioxidant use (vitamins A, C, E, zinc, and beta carotene) may prevent some degree of disease.

- **Dry type**: Laser photocoagulation may be useful although neovascularization is a significant complication. For others, assistive visual aides are the only treatment.

- **Wet type**: Treatment may benefit some patients and includes intravitreous injection of a VEGF inhibitor [e.g., ranibizumab (Lucentis), bevacizumab (Avastin)], thermal laser photocoagulation, photodynamic therapy, and macular translocation surgery.

- Both types benefit from risk factor control as a means of prevention.

Retinal Detachments, Defects, and Disorders

See Table 3.1.

TABLE 3.1 Common retinal disorders

Disorder	Description	Associations/diagnosis	Treatment
Central retinal artery occlusion	Blockage of the central retinal artery producing unilateral blindness	Sudden, painless onset; caused commonly by atherosclerosis, emboli, or **temporal arteritis;** exam shows "cherry red" spot on retina	Treatment must be immediate and consists of acetazolamide, **manual massage** to closed eyelid, or anterior chamber paracentesis; all to reduce intraocular pressure acutely; also important to protect the other eye by treating temporal arteritis (if present) with systemic steroids
Central retinal vein occlusion	Blockage of the central retinal vein producing gradual blindness/vision defects	Gradual, painless vision loss; commonly in elderly with glaucoma, DM, HTN; exam often shows retinal hemorrhages in single quadrant of retina; neovascularization is apparent; fluorescein angiography can diagnose	No good treatment available
Retinal detachment	Separation of neural retina from the underlying retinal pigment epithelium	Associated with trauma, but is painless vision loss; floaters and flashes or curtain falling is classic; direct visualization is key	Immediate referral to ophthalmologist is key; retinal reattachment or laser surgery may correct vision loss

DM, diabetes mellitus; HTN, hypertension.

Glaucoma

State of increased intraocular pressure (IOP) producing long-term or short-term visual problems.

Symptoms

Open-angle glaucoma: 90% of glaucoma cases; painless; pressure 20–30 mmHg. Produces gradual loss of visual fields. Risk factors include Black race, age >60 years, diabetes mellitus (DM), hypertension (HTN), myopia, and family history.

Closed-angle glaucoma: Rare type that is often tested, but almost never seen. Sudden, painful unilateral vision changes. Halos around lights, red eye, nausea/vomiting, and vision loss are common.

Screening: The US Preventive Services Task Force (USPSTF) found no evidence supporting a screening schedule for normal adults. The American Academy of Ophthalmology recommends yearly screening after age 20 at varying intervals. Since the test is quick and easy, at least screening of high-risk groups is a reasonable approach.

Diagnosis

Screen by tonometry to assess IOP. Visual field testing and gonioscopy are also useful. Further imaging may include optical coherence tomography to measure neurofiber layer thickness.

Open-angle glaucoma: Exam reveals optic nerve changes with increased cup-to-disk ratio (see Figure 3.1).

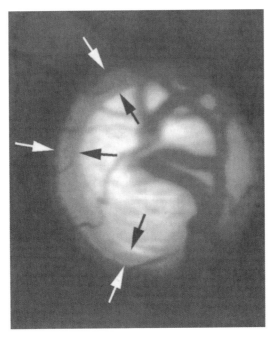

FIGURE 3.1 Retinal exam in open-angle glaucoma. Note increased cup size (*black arrows*) as compared to optic disk (*white arrows*).

Wolff's Headache and Other Head Pain. Seventh edition. Edited by Silberstein SD, Lipton RB, Dalessio DJ. Copyright 2001. Oxford University Press.

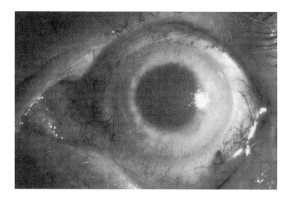

FIGURE 3.2 Acute angle-closure glaucoma. Note typical characteristics of the eye including edematous cornea, "steamy" dull appearance of light reflex, middilated, somewhat irregularly shaped pupil, and injected conjunctiva.

Wolff's Headache and Other Head Pain. Seventh edition. Edited by Silberstein SD, Lipton RB, Dalessio DJ. Copyright 2001. Oxford University Press.

Closed-angle glaucoma: Exam reveals fixed, dilated pupil with IOP >30 mmHg. Palpation of globus with closed eyelid reveals noticeably hard eye. Retina reveals **cupping of the optic disk** (see Figure 3.2).

Treatment

- **Open-angle glaucoma:** Start with medical treatment and progress to surgery after concurrent use of three agents fail. Classes of medications include miotics (pilocarpine, physostigmine, neostigmine), carbonic anhydrase inhibitors (acetazolamide), α_2-selective adrenergic agonist (apraclonidine), β-blockers (timolol), prostaglandins (latanoprost), and osmotic diuretics (mannitol, glycerin).

- **Closed-angle glaucoma:** Immediate referral to ophthalmology. Treat in the meanwhile with **pilocarpine, acetazolamide, timolol, and mannitol or glycerin**. Surgery may be warranted.

Q 3.2

An 83-year-old Latino woman comes to your clinic for a routine eye exam. Her vital signs are normal, but you notice her uncorrected vision is poor. She states she is able to read, drive, and volunteer in the local hospital with the aid of glasses and states, "Its no problem, honey, I can still get around fine." On exam, you note opacification of the lenses of both eyes. What is the next step in the management of this patient?

A. Reduction of intraocular pressure with acetazolamide and referral to ophthalmology.
B. Gentle closed-lid massage of the eyes.
C. Fluorescein angiography to confirm diagnosis.
D. No treatment is necessary at this point.
E. Referral for artificial lens implantation.

Cataracts

Symptoms

Painless, progressive loss of vision usually presenting at older age, but may be congenital. Risk factors include old age, female gender, estrogen exposure, DM, and trauma (lightening strikes).

Diagnosis

Physical exam: Loss or absence of red reflex or grossly opacified lens on exam. Slit lamp exam is indicated for diagnosis.

Treatment

- Surgery is the mainstay and is one of the most commonly performed surgeries in the United States. Replacement of the opacified lens with artificial implants dramatically corrects the problem. Surgery may, however, be postponed until significant disturbance in lifestyle is reported.

Visual Disturbances

See Table 3.2.

Treatment

- Corrective devices such as glasses or contacts are usually very effective. New surgeries such as laser in situ keratomileusis (LASIK) or photorefractive keratectomy (PRK) are gaining popularity and are becoming very safe. Others include radial keratotomy (RK) and astigmatic keratotomy (AK) for mild myopia and astigmatism, respectively.

Visual Field Defects

See Table 3.3 and Figure 3.3.

TABLE 3.2 Definitions of visual disturbances

Term	Definition
Myopia	Nearsightedness; focal point of incoming light is before it reaches the retina
Hyperopia	Farsightedness; focal point of incoming light is behind the retina
Presbyopia	Age-related loss of ability to accommodate
Astigmatism	When the cornea is steeper in one meridian than the other or the globe is irregularly shaped. Thus, light is not properly focused on the retina
Diplopia	Double vision, that is, seeing two images of a particular object. When diplopia exists after covering one eye, it is either malingering or corneal related. When it resolves when one eye is covered, it is likely neurological

TABLE 3.3 Visual field defects

Visual field	Defect	Location	Investigation
	Bitemporal (heteronymous) hemianopsia	Optic chiasm	MRI or CT to look for tumor
	Left homonymous hemianopsia	Right optic tract	MRI
	Right upper quadrant anopsia	Optic radiations in the left temporal lobe	MRI
	Right lower quadrant anopsia	Optic radiations in the left parietal lobe	MRI
	Right homonymous hemianopsia with macular sparing	Left occipital lobe from posterior cerebral artery occlusion	MRI/MRA

Note: White areas of visual field chart represent clear vision; black areas represent lack of vision.

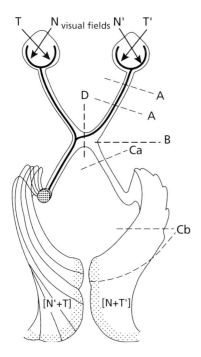

FIGURE 3.3 Areas of neural lesions and corresponding consequent visual disturbances. (A) Total blindness, right eye; (B) nasal hemianopsia of right eye; (C) left homonymous, hemianopsia, (a) with macular splitting, (b) with either macular splitting or macular sparing; (D) bitemporal (heteronymous) hemianopsia. N and N', nasal visual fields; T and T', temporal visual fields.

Conjunctivitis

Common etiologies include viruses, bacteria, or mechanical irritation.

Symptoms

Redness, pain, irritation, tearing, and watering of affected conjunctiva. Prominent features are almost always irritation and watering. Patients report waking up with "crusted" eye. If viral, history of similar symptoms in casual contact and/or spread from contralateral eye. If bacterial, suspect *Neisseria gonorrhoeae/Chlamydia* in a neonate or sexually active adult. Mechanical may be produced by foreign body, wind, snow reflection, allergies, dust, or smoke.

Diagnosis

Physical exam: Hyperemia and lachrymation of the affected eye. Vision and cornea are normal (unless foreign body is present). Slit lamp and glaucoma testing may be needed if history suggests foreign body or glaucoma. If present in neonate after silver nitrate eye drops is used (<24 h of life), most likely chemical conjunctivitis. Otherwise, largely a clinical decision.

Treatment

Neonate

- *N. gonorrhoeae/Chlamydia* (always treat mother and treat for both) → Ceftriaxone (Rocephin) and erythromycin.

Suppurative Nongonococcal, Nonchlamydial

- Bacitracin-polymyxin B ophthalmic ointment/drops.

Bacterial Contact Lens Wearers (*Pseudomonas*)

- Tobramycin (Tobrex) or gentamicin (Genoptic) **plus** piperacillin or ticarcillin eye drops q.15–60 min around the clock × 1–3 days.

Viral

- Herpes simplex I or II—trifluridine (Viroptic) eye drops.
- Unknown viral—Supportive care with cool artificial tear drops may help. Vasoconstrictors such as naphazoline (Naphcon) may help.

Allergic

- Artificial tear drops, vasoconstrictors, and antihistamines such as azelastine (Optivar) and epinastine (Elestat). Other antiallergy systemic medications as indicated.

Disorders of the Eyelid/Lachrymal System

See Table 3.4 and Figure 3.4.

TABLE 3.4 Common disorders of the eyelid and lachrymal system

Disorder	Associations/diagnosis	Treatment
Dacryostenosis (nasolacrymal duct obstruction)	Common in the newborn period; can be congenital or acquired; exam shows overflow tearing and mild erythema of lachrymal opening	Gentle fingertip **massage** BID is usually enough treatment, but should resolve by 6 months; if not dilation and probe may be needed
Blepharitis	Presents with lid edema, pain, loss of eyelashes, and conjunctival irritation; may occur with seborrheic dermatitis; usually *Staphylococcus aureus*	Bacitracin-polymyxin B ointment and warm compresses; monitor for common resistance
Hordeolum (stye)	Usually Staphylococcal infection on single eyelid gland or eyelash follicle; often seen after blepharitis	**Warm compresses.** Will quickly form a small abscess that can then be squeezed or incised; if internal, PO Nafcillin/Oxacillin; topical antibiotics usually ineffective

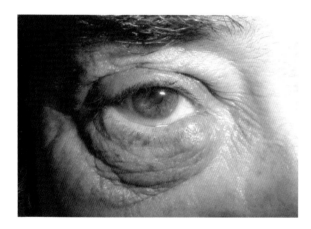

FIGURE 3.4 Hordeolum (stye) on medial lower eyelid.

Courtesy: Charlie Goldberg, M.D., University of California, San Diego School of Medicine, San Diego VA Medical Center.

Q 3.3

A 5-week-old female is brought to your outpatient clinic for evaluation of tearing of the right eye. The mother states she has an increased discharge and crusting of the eye although the area does not seem tender and the patient is not having a fever. On exam, the eye is not found to be infected, but clear discharge and a moderate amount of mucous is present. What is the next step in the management of this patient?

A. Bacitracin-polymyxin B ophthalmic ointment.
B. Trifluridine (Viroptic) eye drops.
C. Naphazoline (Naphcon).
D. Fingertip massage to medial canthus.
E. Fluorescein investigation for corneal abrasion.

Q 3.4

A 13-year-old boy comes to your clinic with a history of left eye redness and pain. The boy's mother states he has had recurrent sinus infections and has just gotten over one a few days ago. He complains of pain and swelling of the left eye and surrounding tissues, and states he has had some blurring of his vision lately. His mother also reports that he has a fever and that he has missed several days of school secondary to this illness. On exam, you note lid swelling and erythema, hyperemia of the conjunctiva, tenderness to ocular movement, and proptosis. What is the best diagnostic test to confirm the most likely diagnosis?

A. MRI of the orbits.
B. CT scan of the orbits.
C. Plain skull x-rays including Waters' view.
D. Lumbar puncture.
E. Tonometry.

Q 3.5

What is the most serious complication seen with this disease?

A. Brain abscess.
B. Retinal ischemia.
C. Meningitis.
D. Central retinal artery occlusion.
E. Trochlear nerve compression and neuritis.

Orbital Cellulitis

Ophthalmologic emergency.

Symptoms

Severe pain around eye, swelling, proptosis, impaired mobility of the eye, conjunctival hyperemia and edema, fever, and malaise. History of sinusitis, dental infection, or procedure, or trauma may reveal inciting event.

The key point is to tell whether the examination is of preseptal or orbital cellulitis. Orbital cellulitis has features including proptosis, painful or impaired ocular motility, decreased visual acuity, or decreased color vision. Preseptal cellulitis does not have these features.

Diagnosis

Physical exam: Increased temperature, eyelid swelling, erythema, painful or impaired ocular motility, decreased visual acuity, decreased color vision, and proptosis.
Imaging: Stat CT scan. Features of orbital cellulitis include diffuse orbital infiltrate, proptosis with or without sinus opacity, or orbital abscess.
Labs: Make sure to take local conjunctival cultures as well as blood and nasal discharge cultures.

Treatment

- Antibiotics IV to include cefuroxime (Ceftin), cefoxitin (Mefoxin), and cefotetan (Cefotan).
- Possible surgical drainage if not resolved or improved in 36 h.
- Monitor closely for signs of spread to CNS and optic neuritis.
- Ophthalmology consult.

Strabismus

Esotropia: The strabismus in which the visual axes converge.
Exotropia: The strabismus in which the visual axes diverge.

Symptoms

Misalignment of one eye in relation to the other. Often observed in otherwise normal newborns. Usually the misalignment shows no specific favored direction.

Diagnosis

Physical exam: Disconjugate gaze.

Treatment

- Treatment is generally needed only if strabismus persists beyond 4 months of age.
- Referral to ophthalmology is in order, but therapy likely to consist of corrective lenses, orthoptic training, and possibly surgery.
- If untreated may lead to amblyopia, which is the condition of one-eye dominance and affected eye visual disturbance and blindness. At the point of amblyopia, patching of the normal eye may be used to suppress the two unmatched images and thus force the affected eye into normal sight.

Nystagmus

A physical exam finding that shows rhythmic movements of the eyes, usually in unison.

Possible causes include alcohol intoxication, illegal drug use, vestibular apparatus disease, vertigo, Meniere's disease, water or fluid in outer or middle ear, or primary neurological disorder such as multiple sclerosis, stroke, or tumor.

Diagnosis

The vestibular system of each ear may be tested by installation of varying temperature water into the external ear canals. The direction of the resultant horizontal nystagmus (in the normal-functioning patient) will be the same as in the mnemonic **COWS** → **C**old **O**pposite, **W**arm **S**ame. Keep in mind "direction" indicates the direction of the short beat.

Imaging: MRI may be of value to find the neurologic cause.

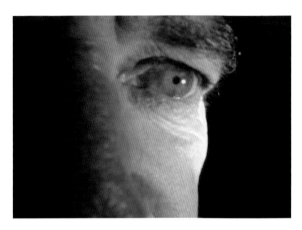

FIGURE 3.5 Pterygium of left medial aspect of eye. Note lesion starting to encroach on iris.

Courtesy: Charlie Goldberg, M.D., University of California, San Diego School of Medicine, San Diego VA Medical Center.

Treatment

- Treat the underlying cause. In vertigo (see Chapter 1), scopolamine (Scopace) or meclizine (Antivert) may be useful.

Pterygium

A triangular elevated mass arising from the conjunctiva that invades the cornea. This may impede vision if invasion is extensive enough to involve the pupil. It may be related to sunlight, wind, previous chemical insult, or heat exposure. Usually not painful, but may be unsightly and uncomfortable (see Figure 3.5).

Treatment

Consists of referral to ophthalmologist and likely surgery. Medical treatment is ineffective.

Corneal Abrasion

Symptoms

Excruciating and extreme eye pain. Often feeling of foreign body is present even if none actually exists in the eye. Other signs are excessive tearing, hyperemia, and photophobia. Likely history of mechanism of foreign body in eye or trauma.

Diagnosis

Fluorescein staining with Wood's lamp exam is very useful in making diagnosis. If positive, do slit lamp exam to show the defect in better detail. Make sure to examine closely with lid eversion to look for foreign bodies.

Treatment

- Topical anesthetic is certainly warranted. Consider irrigation of the eyes for at least 15 min if history suggests chemical or metal foreign body. Give erythromycin, tobramycin (Tobrex), or bacitracin-polymyxin B eye drops for antibacterial coverage.

- Systemic opioids for pain relief.

- Avoid contact lens use.

- The cornea is one of the fastest healing tissues of the body. Symptoms should significantly improve in 48 h.

Answers

3.1 A. This patient likely has macular degeneration with several risk factors present in his history. Modification of these risk factors may improve disease course. Of the answers given, stopping smoking will likely produce the greatest improvement in the disease.

3.2 D. This patient likely is suffering from worsening cataracts; however, she is not complaining of significant impairment in lifestyle. Thus, education about lens replacement, but deferral of surgery, is indicated until the patient feels she is significantly impacted by this problem.

3.3 D. This patient presents with classic features of dacryostenosis. Early treatment consists of fingertip massage of the medial canthus, which commonly relieves the obstruction.

3.4 B. This patient exhibits classic signs of orbital cellulitis. The best next diagnostic step is to investigate with a CT scan of the orbits. Lumbar puncture may be indicated if orbital cellulitis is diagnosed, but not at this time.

3.5 C. Meningitis is the most immediate life-threatening complication. This may develop very rapidly from extension of the infection into the optic tract and into the brain. Brain abscess is another complication, but will generally take some time to develop.

4   Ear, Nose, and Throat

Mastoiditis	77
Otitis Media	79
Cholesteatoma	80
Labrynthitis	80
Vertiginous Disorders	81
Tinnitus	81
Hearing Loss	82
Peritonsillar Abscess (Quinsy)	83
Allergic Rhinitis	84
Nasal Malformations	85
Epistaxis	85
Sinusitis	86
Dental Caries	87
Temporomandibular Joint Syndrome	88
Laryngeal Carcinoma	88
Cancer of the Lip, Oral Cavity, and Pharynx	89

Mastoiditis

Symptoms

Ear pain, postauricular or supraauricular swelling, erythema, pain, hearing loss, fever, and headache are most common. Often after acute otitis media (AOM), but chronic symptoms may exist.

Diagnosis

Physical exam: Erythematous, bulging, and possibly suppurative tympanic membrane (TM). Palpable mass, swelling, and tender area either above or behind the ear.

Labs: CBC may show leukocytosis.

Imaging: Plain mastoid films may reveal clouding of mastoid air cells. CT shows air cells in better detail and may show loss of septation between them.

Treatment

- Treat AOM before complications can develop. Empiric antibiotic choice is the same as that for AOM.
- Myringotomy with placement of pressure equalization (PE) tube with culture of the fluid. Tailor antibiotic regimen to cultures.
- Mastoidectomy is reserved for refractory or complicated cases (CNS involvement).

Q 4.1

A 6-year-old boy presents to your office for evaluation of ear pain that began the night before presentation. He has had three prior ear infections in the past 6 months. His temperature today is 37.3°C (99.1°F), and he has a mildly erythematous right TM with an air fluid level distinguishable. There is somewhat decreased TM mobility, but landmarks are clear and identifiable. What is the next step in management?

A. Nonsteroidal antiinflammatory drugs (NSAIDs) or aural benzocaine (Auralgan) for pain and follow up after several days.
B. Amoxicillin for 3 days.
C. Amoxicillin/clauvulanate (Augmentin) for 14–21 days.
D. Trimethoprim/sulfamethoxazole (TMP/SMX) (Bactrim, Septra) for 7 days.
E. Referral to ENT for tympanostomy tube placement.

Q 4.2

At the scheduled follow-up appointment, the mother mentions that her son's teacher has indicated he has recently had very poor grades in all subjects although he had previously done well. Does this change your initial management plan?

A. Yes, the patient should receive antibiotic therapy for an extended period of time.
B. Yes, the patient should be tried on a second-line antibiotic for an extended course.
C. Yes, the patient should be referred to ENT for possible tympanostomy tube placement.
D. Only if the patient has clinically failed to improve.
E. No, research shows no benefit given this clinical presentation.

Otitis Media

Symptoms

Ear pain, otorrhea, fever, ear fullness, decreased or loss of hearing—often after upper respiratory infection or rhinitis. Nonmodifiable risk factors include low socioeconomic factors, young age, native American or Eskimo ethnicity, or family history. Modifiable risk factors include exposure to tobacco smoke, pacifier use, "bottle propping" when bottle feeding, and sleep position.

Diagnosis

Physical exam: Erythematous, inflamed TM. TM may be bulging, be retracted, show air fluid level (indicating middle ear effusion), be resistant to pneumatic movement, or show rupture. Pus may be present in external canal. Fever is often present. A joint committee of the American Academy of Pediatrics (AAP) and the American Academy of Family Physicians (AAFP) determined the need for three clinical criteria. These include history of acute presentation with typical symptoms, signs/symptoms of acute middle ear inflammation, and presence of middle ear effusion. Thus, the diagnosis is clinical.

Treatment

- Remember, monitoring without antibiotics is an option. Especially in the older child or adult when diagnosis is not clear.

- Control pain with NSAIDs, Tylenol, or topical analgesics like benzocaine (Auralgan).

- Treat with antibiotics in young children if diagnosis is certain or in children <6 months old even if not. Recommendations are for amoxicillin or amoxicillin/clavulanate (Augmentin) for 7–10 days. Use ceftriaxone (Rocephin) for 3 days as an alternative.

- Control modifiable risk factors.

- Consider tympanostomy in

  - children who have structural damage to the TM or middle ear.

  - children who have otitis media of 4 months duration with persistent hearing loss or other signs/symptoms.

  - children with recurrent or persistent otitis media who are at risk of speech, language, or learning problems, regardless of hearing status.

- Close follow-up for 48–72 h is strongly recommended.

Cholesteatoma

Growth of desquamated, stratified, squamous epithelium within the middle ear space.

Symptoms

Sensorineural hearing loss, vertigo, disequilibrium, facial paralysis (from pressure on the facial nerve); if left untreated may progress to meningitis, brain abscess, or sepsis.

Diagnosis

Physical exam: Otoscopy may reveal tumor-like structure in the posterior/superior quadrant of the visible TM.
Imaging: CT scan may be helpful, but MRI with visualization of the middle ear is best.

Treatment

- Surgical excision is the standard.

Labrynthitis

Symptoms

Most commonly vertigo, which may be accompanied by dizziness, hearing loss, nausea/vomiting, tinnitus, and ataxia. Causes vary, so history may reveal trauma, recent viral infection, alcohol use, drug/medication use, or vasculitis.

Diagnosis

Physical exam: Nystagmus, hemotympanum, or ear infection. Romberg test for balance, and Weber and Rinne test (to distinguish sensorineural from conductive hearing loss).
Imaging: MRI is best for possible cranial nerve involvement. Thin-cut CT of cerebellum can help evaluate the etiology of vertigo.

Treatment

- Sensory deprivation in a quiet, dark room during acute attacks.
- Avoid dietary sodium.
- A relatively long (2–3 weeks) but tapering course of systemic steroids is often helpful in acute phase.
- Meclizine (Antivert), diphenhydramine (Benedryl), dimenhydrinate (Dramamine), or scopolamine (Scopace) helps counteract vertigo by anticholinergic actions. However, all cause drowsiness as side effect, and care must be taken in the elderly. Prochlorperazine (Compazine), promethazine (Phenergan), metoclopramide (Reglan), and ondansetron (Zofran) are very effective for nausea and vomiting. Benzodiazepines may also be used for sedation.

Q 4.3

A 93-year-old African American male comes to your clinic with complaints of vertigo and consequent nausea and vomiting for the past 2 days. He has had a cold with nasal and chest congestion for the past 2 weeks and was treated symptomatically with ibuprofen and acetaminophen. What medication below should be avoided in this patient's treatment course?

A. Meclizine (Antivert).
B. Prednisone.
C. Metoclopramide (Reglan).
D. Clonazepam (Klonopin).
E. Amoxicillin/clavulanate (Augmentin).

Vertiginous Disorders

Symptoms

Vertigo, dizziness, lightheadedness. These may be accompanied by ear pain, blurry vision, tinnitus, or nausea/vomiting. Many etiologies exist, but a strong history of when the symptoms are worse and when they started is the key.

Diagnosis

Physical exam: Nystagmus is common. Neurologic signs such as focal deficits, agnosia, or ataxia may be present.

Tests include caloric stimulation test, Romberg test, and Dix–Hallpike maneuver.

Imaging: MRI is best for imaging brain and cerebellum; thin-cut CT is useful in the evaluation of acute stroke in cerebellum.

Treatment

- Depends on disease and etiology.
- Various maneuvers (Epley, Brandt–Daroff, etc.) exist for the therapy of benign paroxysmal positional vertigo.
- Medications include the standard meclizine (Antivert), scopolamine (Scopace), dimenhydrinate (Dramamine), or diphenhydramine (Benedryl). However, all cause drowsiness as a side effect and care must be taken in the elderly. Prochlorperazine (Compazine), promethazine (Phenergan), metoclopramide (Reglan), and ondansetron (Zofran) are very effective for nausea and vomiting. Benzodiazepines may also be used for sedation.

Tinnitus

Symptoms

Perceived sound that is not associated with external source. This may be buzzing, ringing, whistling, roaring, or hissing. Types include continuous, intermittent, or pulsatile sound. Categories of etiology include vascular, neurogenic, eustachian tube dysfunction, or others. History may elicit the use of ototoxic drugs such as aminoglycosides, ACE inhibitors, or antimalarials, just to name a few. Obtain detailed history of tone, timing, characteristic, and quality to determine possible areas of dysfunction.

Diagnosis

Physical exam: Otoscopy is important; also look for neurologic symptoms, nystagmus, possible vascular disease, and other symptoms. No one physical exam provides diagnosis.

Imaging: Head imaging with MRI, CT, or angiography may be reasonable while looking for vascular or tumor origin based on history.
Audiometry is a must.

Treatment

- Treat the underlying cause if identified.
- Tinnitus retraining therapy, masking devices, biofeedback techniques, and cognitive behavioral therapy are also proven options.

Hearing Loss

Symptoms

Obvious hearing loss or deafness. History is very important and may reveal sudden or gradual decline associated with loud noises or ear trauma. Commonly starts with loss of high-frequency sound, which progresses. May also reveal ototoxic drugs (aminoglycosides, etc.) in the recent or remote past.

Diagnosis

Physical exam: Otoscopy important to evaluate for infection, tympanosclerosis, cerumen impaction, middle ear effusion (MEE), or TM perforation.

Weber test: Apply tuning fork to midline vertex of the head to check if sound is loudest in the deaf ear, if conductive hearing loss is present, if sound is loudest in normal ear, if sensorineural hearing loss is present.

Rinne test: Apply tuning fork to mastoid process of each ear, then next to the ear without touching the head. Time in seconds until the sound is not heard is recorded. Normally, air conduction hearing is two times longer than that with bone conduction. If bone conduction is longer than air conduction, conductive hearing loss is present. If air conduction is less than twice as long as bone conduction, sensorineural hearing loss is present.
Audiometry is a must (see Figure 4.1).

Imaging: Consider MRI and CT scan to evaluate for CNS lesion or cholesteatoma.

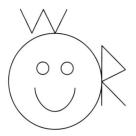

FIGURE 4.1 Simple figure to show placement positions of tuning fork for Weber and Rinne tests.

Treatment

- Treat etiology if simple and identified.
- Most conditions warrant referral to otorhinolaryngologist who will evaluate for treatment. Some conditions require surgery or targeted therapy. Do not miss the treatable causes such as acoustic tumor, cholesteotomas, acute rupture, otosclerosis, and others. Treatments also include hearing aids or cochlear implants.
- Refer to ENT as needed.

Peritonsillar Abscess (Quinsy)

Symptoms

Extreme sore throat, odynophagia, dysphagia, trismus, fever, "hot potato voice," or drooling or pooling of saliva in mouth.

Diagnosis

Physical exam: Erythematous posterior pharynx, unilaterally swollen tonsil, contralaterally displaced uvula, and cervical lymphadenopathy.
Labs: CBC reveals leukocytosis, culture any aspirated fluid.
Imaging: Ultrasound often shows fluid-filled cavity. CT scan also shows abscess pocket well.

Treatment

- Incision and drainage under operative conditions or needle aspiration have shown equal efficacy. Culture the fluid in either case. When performing the procedure, have capabilities for intubation ready if needed. Recurrence after drainage and antibiotic use is rare.
- If recurrence occurs, consider tonsillectomy.
- Classic antibiotic is penicillin. Start with IV or IM dosing, then switch to PO. Add metronidazole (Flagyl) if Gram-negative coverage is needed. Alternatives include cephalosporins. Tailor regimen to cultures if possible.

Allergic Rhinitis

Symptoms

Congestion, nasal stuffiness, rhinorrhea (usually clear), sneezing, and possibly watery, reddened eyes. Often seasonal, but may be triggered by known allergens.

Diagnosis

Physical exam: Red, runny, and possibly swollen turbinates. Blood may be present from local irritation. Look for associated nasal polyps.
Labs: Often unnecessary, but nasal washings show many eosinophils.

Patch skin testing or RAST (radioallergosorbent test) may be useful in finding the specific allergy. Often does not add anything to treatment.
Imaging: Radiographs may show opacity of nasal areas; CT for sinus evaluation is often unnecessary.

Treatment

- Avoid the allergen if known.
- Intranasal, oral, or ophthalmic medications as listed in Table 4.1.
- Allergy shot desensitization is useful in some, but requires referral to allergist.

TABLE 4.1 Common treatments for allergic rhinitis

Class	Examples
Antihistamines (H1 blockers)	Diphenhydramine (Benedryl) Hydroxyzine (Atarax)
Antihistamines (Second generation)	Loratadine (Claritin) Fexofenadine (Allegra) Cetirizine (Zyrtec)
Decongestants	Pseudoephedrine Phenylephrine nasal spray
Mast cell stabilizers	Cromolyn (Nasalcrom, gastrocrom) Olopatadine (Patonol) eye drops
Leukotriene antagonist	Montelukast (Singular)
Intranasal steroids	Fluticasone (Flonase) Mometasone (Nasonex) Budesonide (Rhinocort) Flunisolide (Nasalide, Nasarel)
Intranasal anticholinergic	Ipratropium (Atrovent nasal)
Direct vasoconstrictor	Oxymetazoline (Afrin) Warning: Do not use >5 days
Saline nasal spray	Saline water

Nasal Malformations

See Table 4.2.

Epistaxis

Symptoms

Blood loss from the nares signifies an anterior source such as Kiesselbach's plexus.

Blood loss from posterior nasal opening causing postnasal drip, hemoptysis, hematemesis, anemia, or melena is most often of a posterior nasal origin.

History may reveal cause including trauma, sensitivity to low humidity, coagulopathy, foreign body, or intranasal drug use.

Diagnosis

Physical exam: Standard otoscopy may reveal source. Pharyngeal exam may show blood, but not solely indicative of posterior bleeding.
Labs: CBC for hematocrit. Consider toxicology screen if drug use is suspected. PT/PTT/INR to evaluate for bleeding dyscrasias.
Imaging: Often unnecessary unless fracture or tumor is suspected. Plain radiographs or CT may be helpful for these.

Nasal endoscopy if source cannot be identified and bleeding is not controlled (which also makes the procedure difficult).

Treatment

- Apply direct pressure to the anterior nares (with or without packing) for 15–20 min. This stops majority of bleeds.
- *Anterior bleeds:* Phenylephrine nasal spray or oxymetazoline (Afrin) may vasoconstrict adequately. Anterior nares packing is also effective. Tampons are very useful for this and may be expanded by adding water after insertion.
- *Posterior bleeds:* Often otorhinolaryngologist is consulted. Placement of specialized inflatable packing balloons is ideal. A foley catheter balloon will suffice if packing balloon is not available. Insert through anterior nares and inflate for tamponade effect.
- Packing or balloon tamponade usually left in place for 1–3 days.
- Surgical cauterization with laser or electrocautery may be needed if bleeding uncontrolled and profuse.

TABLE 4.2 Common structural disorders of the nose

Disorder	Associations	Treatment
Nasal polyps	Asthma, nose picking, aspirin sensitivity	Surgery
Deviated nasal septum	Snoring, breathing problems	Surgery

Q 4.4

A 32-year-old Caucasian female comes to your clinic with complaints of recent low-grade fever, unilateral facial pain and fullness, unilateral eye watering, and nasal congestion. She reports a history of recurrent sinus infections and says her current symptoms started in a more indolent course, which then worsened approximately 2 days ago. What is the best test to confirm the diagnosis?

A. CT scan of the sinuses.
B. Plain radiography including Water's view.
C. MRI of the sinuses.
D. Ultrasound of the sinuses.
E. No imaging is warranted at this time.

Sinusitis

Acute: Disease <4 weeks duration.
Chronic: Disease >8–12 weeks duration.

Symptoms

Unilateral facial pain above or below the eyes, increased pain on leaning forward, maxillary toothache, purulent rhinorrhea, headache, or fever. History importantly may reveal "second sickening," meaning symptoms initially improved then worsened. Patient may also have a history of sinusitis.

Diagnosis

Physical exam: Swollen, erythematous turbinates with purulent discharge. Unilateral frontal or maxillary sinus tenderness. Maxillary tooth tenderness, facial erythema or swelling, visual changes, or change in mental status are of particular concern.

Imaging: Acute sinusitis often does not need imaging. Plain x-ray (either four-view standard or **Water's view**) in a chronic setting may reveal air-fluid levels, mucosal thickening, or opacification although these are of low specificity. Plain x-ray is limited, depending on which sinus is suspected of disease. Limited sinus CT scan may be helpful to determine possible anatomic etiology (tumor, polyp, abscess, etc.) in chronic setting. MRI shows better detail but is often unneeded.

Nasal endoscopy may be performed by a specialist, and cultures may be taken; this is the gold standard (see Figure 4.2).

Treatment

- Determine if viral or bacterial by clinical presentation. If mild disease, antibiotics likely not effective. If moderate to severe, antibiotics reasonable.

- High-dose **amoxicillin** commonly first line if no prior antibiotic use or amoxicillin-clavulanate (Augmentin) if there has been. Alternatives include TMP/SMX (Bactrim, Septra), cefdinar

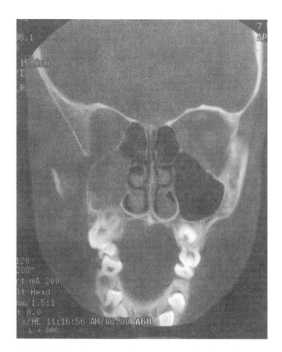

FIGURE 4.2 Coronal CT scan of the sinuses demonstrating normal left-sided anatomy and right maxillary sinus opacification.

Wolff's Headache and Other Head Pain. Seventh edition. Edited by Silberstein SD, Lipton RB, Dalessio DJ. Copyright 2001. Oxford University Press.

(Omnicef), azithromycin, or ceftriaxone (Rocephin). Duration is 10–14 days or up to 21 days with chronic presentation.

- Nasal decongestants are often helpful. Nasal steroids are controversial.
- Systemic decongestants such as pseudoephedrine (Sudafed) or mucolytics are anecdotally effective.
- Saline nasal spray often improves symptoms.
- Endoscopic sinus surgery if chronic, recurrent, refractory, or complicated.

Dental Caries

Symptoms

Dental pain is the most common symptom. May be seen by parent or care-giver as black dot on tooth. History often reveals young age, excess sugar consumption, no exposure to supplemental fluoride, or previous caries.

Diagnosis

Physical exam: Characteristic black or discolored area of tooth. Often tender to manipulation. Look for surrounding gum inflammation, swelling, erythema, or drainage, which may indicate abscess or gingivitis.

Treatment

- Prevention with tooth brushing after every meal, use of fluorinated water or toothpaste, and low-sugar diet.
- Refer to dentist.
- Filling with various amalgams and filling material is common and effective.

Temporomandibular Joint Syndrome

Symptoms

Pain, clicking, popping, locking, or catching with jaw movement. May progress to headache, facial, neck, or ear pain.

Diagnosis

Physical exam: Tenderness or audible symptoms on jaw range of motion. Erythema, swelling, ecchymosis, or deformity may reveal fracture.

Imaging: Single-contrast videoarthrography is helpful in demonstrating joint dynamics and disc movement; plain radiographs for bone structure. MRI is most helpful for the visualization of structures.

Treatment

- Dependant on etiology and dysfunction.
- General measures include jaw rest, analgesics, NSAIDs, local heat application, and soft diet. Stress reduction and therapy may help some with psychosomatic cause.
- Orthodontic guidance appliance may be indicated. Teeth guard at night may reduce tooth grinding problems.
- Surgical correction of fracture, slipped disc, or implantation may be needed if refractory.

Laryngeal Carcinoma

Symptoms

Persistent hoarseness, stridor, dysphagia, hemoptysis, weight loss, neck mass, or neck pain. History often reveals age >40 and smoking/drinking.

Diagnosis

Physical exam: Palpable mass in the neck, fullness of throat region, or regional lymphadenopathy.

Labs: Chem-7 for electrolyte abnormalities; hepatic function panel for possible metastatic liver disease.

Imaging: Laryngoscopy with biopsy is the gold standard. Biopsy reveals histology and may help in staging. CT or MRI for better visualization. These may be used to rule out metastasis in other areas. Order a bone scan and chest x-ray to rule out likely areas of metastasis.

Treatment

- Early disease may be treated with local excision, laser vocal cord-ectomy, and/or radiation. More advanced cases require laryngec-tomy with follow-up radiation. Metastatic disease often responds to chemotherapy.

- Stop smoking/drinking.

Cancer of the Lip, Oral Cavity, and Pharynx

Symptoms

Symptoms depend on site.

Lip cancer presents with ulceration or exophytic lesion with pain and bleeding. Local involvement of the mental nerve may lead to numbness or pain of chin area.

Oral cavity cancer presents with nonhealing mouth ulcers, loosening of teeth, ill-fitting dentures, dysphagia, odynophagia, weight loss, bleeding, or referred otalgia.

Pharyngeal cancer presents much later in the course with pain, bleeding, or a neck mass. Look for history of smoking and alcohol abuse.

Diagnosis

Physical exam: Palpable mass in the neck, lymphadenopathy, ulceration, or tumor in the oral cavity or pharynx.
Labs: Chem-7 for electrolyte abnormalities, hepatic function panel for possible metastatic liver disease, alkaline phosphatase for bone involvement. Fine needle aspiration of either the tumor in question or locally enlarged nodes is helpful to determine the histology. Direct biopsy is best if possible.
Imaging: CT scan and MRI are used widely for the staging and evaluation of local disease, as well as the evaluation of distant organ/tissue metastasis. Obtain a bone scan for screening for metastasis. PET or integrated PET-CT scanning is also useful and has high sensitivity and specificity.

Treatment

- Surgically excise early disease.

- Radiotherapy is often added to reduce chances of recurrence.

- Chemotherapy, although effective at controlling local disease, is controversial without metastatic spread.

- Consult oncology for treatment recommendations.

- Stop smoking/drinking.

Answers

4.1 A. This patient likely has a mild otitis media (OM) and concurrent middle ear effusion. This mild infection can safely be treated with analgesia and follow-up without antibiotic therapy.

4.2 C. The patient has now shown signs of being at risk for learning difficulties and thus qualifies for tympanostomy tubes, thus referral is indicated.

4.3 A. This patient is suffering from acute labynthitis. Meclizine (Antivert) works by anticholinergic action, which often causes typical side effects in the elderly. Other answers listed are either suitable for this disorder or are not a treatment indicated for labrynthitis.

4.4 E. This patient has classic symptoms of sinusitis by prior history of infection, current symptoms, and description of the "second sickening" syndrome. No imaging is therefore needed in this patient in order to decide management course.

Diseases of the Thyroid Gland	92
Malignant Lesions of the Thyroid Gland	92
Disorders of the Thyroid Gland	92
Hypothyroidism	92
Hyperthyroidism	95
Diabetes Mellitus	97
Diabetic Ketoacidosis	98
Disorders of Endocrine Glands	100
Hypoglycemia	100
Disorders of the Parathyroid Gland	101
Hyperparathyroidism	101
Endocrine Disorders	102
Diabetes Insipidus	102
Syndrome Inappropriate Antidiuretic Hormone (SIADH)	102
Disorders of the Adrenal Gland	103
Cushing's Syndrome	103
Addison's Disease (and Secondary Hypoadrenalism)	104
Hyperaldosteronism and Conn's Syndrome (Primary)	105
Pheochromocytoma	107
Malnutrition	108
Protein-Energy Malnutrition	108
Vitamin and Mineral Deficiencies	109
Other Metabolic/Immunity Disorders	111
Phenylketonuria	111
Disorders of Lipid Metabolism	112
Gout	113
Disorders of Mineral Metabolism	114
Electrolyte and Fluid Disorders	116
Hyponatremia	116
Hypernatremia	117
Hypokalemia	117
Hyperkalemia	118
Hypovolemia	118
Hypervolemia	119
Immunity Deficiency	120

Diseases of the Thyroid Gland

Malignant Lesions of the Thyroid Gland

There are several different types of thyroid cancer. The names and differences between them are as follows.

Papillary: Most common type (50%–80%) but is slow growing. Usually presents after lymphatic spread and is usually mixed lesion with follicular type. Histologically, has **psammoma bodies** that are pathognomonic.

Treatment: Surgery, either total thyroidectomy or lobectomy depending, on the stage. May also use radioactive iodine for ablation, but must suppress thyroid function with thyroxine afterward because these tumors are responsive to TSH.

Follicular: More aggressive spread (hematogenously instead of lymphatically), and incidence increases with age. Can metastasize to bone and cause pathologic fractures.

Treatment: Surgery and radioactive iodine as earlier. Also needs suppressive thyroxine for patients with metastases.

Anaplastic: Most aggressive type that is usually found after metastases. Death at diagnosis usually predicted in number of months. Fortunately, fairly rare ($<$10%).

Treatment: Usually palliative, but radiation and chemotherapy have been tried with some success.

Medullary: Also aggressive. Tends to invade locally and can involve recurrent laryngeal nerve causing vocal cord paralysis. Patient may present with a hoarse voice. Associated with rapid growth. Can produce paraneoplastic syndrome and high plasma calcitonin effect from **thyrocalcitonin**. When paired with pheochromocytoma and hyperparathyroidism, it is called **multiple endocrine neoplasia type II (MEN II)**.

Treatment: Surgery and screen relatives for MEN II.

Disorders of the Thyroid Gland

Hypothyroidism

Symptoms

Fatigue, **hyperlipidemia**, coarse hair, weight gain, depression, slow speech, **cold intolerance**, menstrual disturbance (usually increased), constipation, carpal tunnel syndrome, decreased reflexes, and anemia of chronic disease. Generally reflective of a whole body "slow down." The severe form of hypothyroidism is **myxedema coma**, characterized by altered mental status and hypothermia. The patient may or may not have a history of thyroid disturbance but often the state is precipitated by infection, myocardial ischemia, trauma, or stroke.

Diagnosis

Causes

Hashimoto's thyroiditis: Most common type. May have brief hyperthyroid stage, then burn out. Lymphocytes infiltrate the gland and **antimicrosomal antibodies** attack it. May be associated with other autoimmune diseases and usually occurs in women.

Iodine deficiency: Historically and internationally important. Lack of iodine is the cause. Virtually eliminated in the United States secondary to institution of iodized salt.

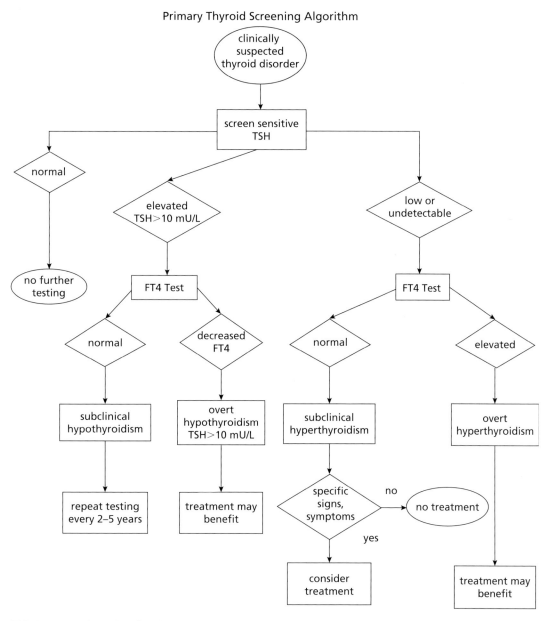

FIGURE 5.1 Algorithm for the approach to thyroid dysfunction.

Euthyroid syndrome—can be caused by any illness, but usually status post serious hospitalization. Characterized by normal TSH and low T_4 and T_3. Usually self-limited after treatment of underlying cause.

Medications

Multiple medications can cause hypothyroidism. Classics are amiodarone, lithium, warfarin, and rifampin. Do not forget radioactive iodine from the ablation of hyperthyroid state.

See Figure 5.1 for algorithm. Basically check TSH first, then evaluate for T_4. Look for TSH to be high and T_4 to be low.

If myxedema coma is suspected, obtain labs including screening electrolytes for hypoglycemia and hyponatremia, CBC for signs of infection, and TSH and T_4 levels. Cortisol level measurements are also indicated to assess the adrenal function for possible emergent state.

Treatment

- Give T_4 as levothyroxine. The following and slow increase in dose of levothyroxine should be q. 6–8 weeks until the patient is found to be clinically stable by repeated TSH monitoring. Some sources (and clinicians) advise to follow TSH levels, but the ultimate adjustment is still officially a clinical decision. This is due to the long time course required for TSH to actually change (up to 8 weeks).

- Mortality for myxedema coma is 20%–50%, so if found remember ABCs and then give IV levothyroxine and IV hydrocortisone. Correction of hypothermia, electrolyte abnormalities, and hypoglycemia as indicated. Close monitoring is mandatory.

Q 5.1

A 61-year-old Caucasian woman is brought to the ER by her daughter who states her mother has been complaining of fatigue and flu-like symptoms for the past 3 days. She is visiting her daughter from out of town for the past week and has no available medical history. She is now nonresponsive to questioning and is lethargic in appearance. Her vital signs are BP 102/56 mmHg, HR 48, temperature 96.5°F, respiration rate 14. She is responsive to pain and rolls her eyes to loud questioning and light stimuli. Her examination shows 2+ pitting edema of the legs. Initial screening labs show the following:

Na	130 mEq/L	Glucose	62 mg/dL
K	4.1 mEq/L	WBC	14.1×1000 cells/mm^3
Cl	102 mEq/L	Hemoglobin	14 g/dL
CO$_2$	26 mEq/L	Hematocrit	42%
BUN	19 mg/dL	Platelet	306,000/mm^3
Cr	0.9 mg/dL		

What are the other useful labs to do that may lead to the correct diagnosis?

A. D-dimer.
B. TSH, T_4, and cortisol level.
C. Ischemic cardiac markers.
D. Liver function tests.
E. Skip the labs and obtain stat head CT.

Q 5.2

After correcting the glucose and raising her body temperature to 98.0°F with warm blankets, the patient still has decreased mental status. An IV line is placed and normal saline (NS) is started. Her daughter now tells you she found an empty bottle of levothyroxine in her mother's purse and states she remembers she has had some sort of "gland problem." What is the correct management of myxedema coma?

A. NS IV fluids and supportive care.
B. Immediately start oral replacement of levothyroxine at double dose until the patient is stable.
C. IV levothyroxine, IV hydrocortisone, and ICU admission.
D. NS IV fluids, then oral propylthiouracil.
E. IV hydrocortisone and frequent repeat of labs.

Hyperthyroidism

Symptoms

Insomnia, palpitations, tachycardia, thinning hair, menstrual irregularities, diarrhea, hyperphagia, weight loss, anxiety, **heat intolerance**, **osteoporosis**, and **atrial fibrillation**. Graves' disease is also associated with exophthalmos (autoimmune-related hypertrophy of the ocular muscles) and pretibial myxedema (see Figure 5.2).

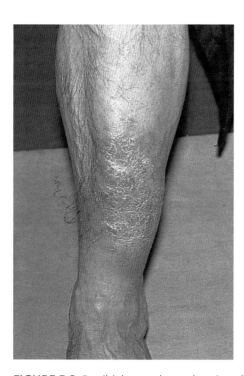

FIGURE 5.2 Pretibial myxedema showing characteristic raised, reddish plaques and nodules on the shins.

Clinical Dermatology. Fifth edition. MacKie, RM. Copyright 2003. Oxford University Press.

Diagnosis

Causes

Subacute thyroiditis (includes de Quervain's): Associated usually with viral infection/upper respiratory infection (URI). Transient hyperthyroid state leading to transient hypothyroid state, which may then resolve. Often has low radioiodine uptake on radioactive iodine uptake (RAIU) scan. May give nonsteroidal antiinflammatory drugs (NSAIDs) and other pain relief drugs for often tender thyroid, but patients usually recover without the need for long-term treatment.

Graves' disease: Most common form of hyperthyroidism. Caused by auto-activating antibodies to the TSH receptor. Action of these antibodies produces excess thyroid hormone, causing hyperthyroid state. Causes are multiple and diverse, molecular mimicry likely plays a role. If suspected, order thyroid function tests (TFTs) and thyroid-stimulating immunoglobulin for investigation.

Toxic adenoma and toxic multinodular goiter: Caused by mutation and hyperplasia of the thyroid hormone-producing follicular cells, resulting in hyperthyroid state.

See Figure 5.1 for algorithm. Basically check TSH first, then T_4. Look for TSH to be low and T_4 to be high. RAIU scan may be indicated for exact diagnosis.

Treatment

- **Two classic drugs:** Methimazole (Tapazole) and propylthiouracil (PTU). PTU is used with more severe disease, while methimazole is for more moderate disease. Methimazole is also available in single daily dose and is easier for compliance. Both drugs cross placental barrier and thus are ill advised in pregnancy. Use PTU preferentially if forced to make a choice, but also use the lowest effective dose. In all patients, use either drug for 6 months to 1 year, then stop and follow T_4 for remission. Also, 40%–60% of patients relapse and need further treatment.

- **Propranolol:** May be used to control symptoms such as tachycardia and palpitations.

  - *Side effects of therapy*: Granulocytopenia, aplastic anemia, mouth ulcers, skin rash, drug-induced lupus, and PTU-induced subclinical liver injury (usually transient).

- **Radioactive iodine (^{131}I), that is, radioactive ablation:** Commonly used AFTER trying above therapy. Contraindicated in pregnancy. High incidence of induced hypothyroid state with the need for levothyroxine therapy.

- **Surgery:** Can be used with cases refractive to classic drugs and in those who are not candidates for ablation (pregnancy). Side effects include both hypothyroidism and risk of hypoparathyroidism if too many parathyroids are accidentally taken.

Q 5.3

What are the two most common side effects of metformin (Glucophage) therapy?

A. Metabolic acidosis and depression.
B. Metabolic acidosis and GI disturbance.
C. Respiratory acidosis and uremia.
D. Increased transaminases and hyperventilation.
E. Increased transaminases and prolonged activated partial thromboplastin time (aPTT).

Diabetes Mellitus

Symptoms

Classic symptoms include polyuria, polydipsia, polyphagia, and weight loss. Clues can include repeated infections (especially yeasts), blurring of vision, nonhealing ulcers, usually on feet, and many other varied symptoms.

Types

See Table 5.1.

Diagnosis

American Diabetic Association recommendations

One of the following categories

- A **random** plasma glucose value ≥200 mg/dL with classic symptoms (polyuria, polydipsia, weight loss).

Or

- A **fasting** plasma glucose (FPG) ≥126 mg/dL. Fasting defined as NPO for 8 h or more.

Or

- Two-hour glucose tolerance test of ≥200 mg/dL after a 75 g of oral glucose load.

Each criterion above should be confirmed by repeat testing on a different day (in the absence of overt hyperglycemia).

TABLE 5.1 Comparison of type I and type II diabetes

Type I (insulin-dependent)	Type II (noninsulin-dependent)
β-Cell burnout of pancreas	Peripheral insulin resistance and inadequate pancreatic compensation
Usually insulin controlled	Usually diet or PO medication controlled (may progress to insulin dependence)
Diabetic ketoacidosis (DKA) is a life-threatening complication	Hyperglycemic hyperosmolar nonketotic state (HHNKS) is a life-threatening complication
Onset usually <30 years old	Onset often >30 years old
Not associated with obesity	Obesity common

Treatment

- Type I diabetic patients usually started directly on insulin. Use a combination of long-acting and short-acting insulin at first. The goal is to provide a somewhat constant basal insulin level with separate peaks to match meals (see Tables 5.2 and 5.3). Typically, a combination of NPH and regular insulin with AM and PM dose. Test makers will require tweaking of these regimens, so know them.

- Typical regimen involves estimated total daily insulin requirement (ETDIR) method (estimated at onset to be 0.5 U/kg). ETDIR divided into two-thirds is given in AM and one-third is given in PM. At each dosage time, give two-thirds long-acting and one-third short-acting insulin. Typically, have the patient take fingerstick blood glucose (FSBG) values at least four times per day (before breakfast, lunch, dinner, and bedtime) and PRN. Adjust insulin regimen accordingly.

- Type II diabetic patients are started on oral hypoglycemics **after** a **3-month** trial of lifestyle changes including diet and exercise. Best plan is to start with monotherapy and add additional agents if blood sugars are not well controlled. Goals are FPG <126 mg/dL and HbA1C <7. Weight reduction and increased lean body mass can sometimes lead to the cure of type II diabetes mellitus (see Tables 5.4 and 5.5).

Diabetic Ketoacidosis

Major life-threatening complication, usually with type I diabetes.

Diagnosis

Patients may present with polyuria, polydipsia, change in mental status, "fruity" acetone breath, Kussmaul respirations (rapid, deep breathing

TABLE 5.2 Long-acting insulin

Insulin	Onset (h)	Peak (h)	Duration (h)
NPH/Lente	1–4	8–12	12–20
Ultralente	3–5	10–16	18–24
Glargine/Lantus	1–2	? Flat	24

TABLE 5.3 Short-acting insulin

Insulin	Onset	Peak	Duration
Regular	0.5–1 h	2–4 h	4–8 h
Lispro/Aspartate Humolog/Novalog	5–15 min	1–2 h	3.5–5 h

TABLE 5.4 Oral medications for type II diabetes

	Sulfonylureas	Meglitinides	Biguanides	Thiazolidinediones	α-Glucosidase inhibitors
Target population	Recent type II DM diagnosis, diagnosis <5 years	Recent type II DM diagnosis	Obese, insulin-resistant	Obese, insulin-resistant	Elevated postprandial glucose
Advantages	Rapid fasting plasma glucose (FPG) reduction, cost	Short-acting, meal-adjusted dosing, decreased-risk hypoglycemia	No weight gain, decreased risk of hypo-glycemia	Decreased secretion of insulin, decreased-risk hypoglycemia	Decreased-risk hypoglycemia
Disadvantages	Weight gain, increased-risk hypoglycemia	High cost	GI side effects, high cost, metabolic (lactic) acidosis, not used with renal failure/ insufficiency	High cost, weight gain, slow onset of action, question of liver toxicity; likely negative cardiovascular effects including congestive heart failure (CHF)	High cost, GI side effects, i.e., flatulence

TABLE 5.5 Oral medications for type II diabetes

	Sulfonylureas	Meglitinides	Biguanides	Thiazolidinediones	α-Glucosidase inhibitors
Prototypic drugs	Glipizide (Glucotrol) Glyburide (Micronase, DiaBeta)	Repaglinide (Prandin)	Metformin (Glucophage)	Pioglitazone (Actos) Rosiglitazone (Avandia)	Acarbose (Precose) Miglitol (Glyset)
Mechanism of action	Stimulates pancreatic insulin release	Stimulates pancreatic insulin release (non-sulfonylurea)	Decreases hepatic glucose production; increases peripheral insulin sensitivity	Increases peripheral insulin sensitivity	Inhibits intestinal enzymes delaying glucose absorption

presumably to blow off excess acidic ketones), or no symptoms at all. Signs include

- Hyperglycemia
- Metabolic acidosis with **anion gap**
- Serum bicarbonate <15 mEq/L
- Serum or urine **ketones**

Treatment

- First treat ABCs, then establish diagnosis with CBC, BMP (to include glucose and BUN/creatinine), arterial blood gas (ABG) (to look for acidosis and type), and urine or plasma ketones. Panculture the patient and obtain chest x-ray CXR and ECG. Often diabetic ketoacidosis (DKA) is precipitated by infection.

- Give fluids (NS initially) via two large-bore IVs. This alone will decrease glucose and start patient in the right direction. May initially need 6–8 L fluid.

- Monitor electrolytes, BUN/creatinine and glucose, every 1–2 h.

- Start IV insulin drip after initial boluses of fluid.

- Replete electrolytes PRN. **Monitor potassium carefully**. Place on cardiac monitoring if indicated to monitor for arrhythmias.

- Switch fluids to 5% dextrose NS solution when FSBG values decrease to <250 mg/dL.

- Adjust insulin drip to maintain FSBGs between 150 and 250 mg/dL until anion gap normalizes.

- Initiate sliding-scale insulin therapy and stop insulin drip when the resolution of DKA is achieved. Overlap these two therapies by 2–3 h to ensure adequate insulin saturation.

- Bicarbonate therapy is only indicated for pH <7.0. Can worsen cerebral edema and potassium derangement, so only choose if in dire straits on examination.

Disorders of Endocrine Glands

Hypoglycemia

Symptoms

Patient presents with sweating, tremors, tachycardia, anxiety, headache, fatigue, visual changes, and in severe cases syncope, change in mental status, hemiplegia, or coma.

One of the first things to check when any patient presents in obtunded/coma state is FSBG.

Diagnosis

Roughly defined as FSBG <50 mg/dL. Symptoms as above. Relief from these symptoms by the ingestion of carbohydrates is often enough to diagnose.

State may be due to pathologic and nonpathologic issues. Most commonly caused by fasting hypoglycemia that can occur in normal individual. Other causes include factitious source of insulin, hypoglycemic medications, and insulin-secreting pancreatic tumors (insulinomas).

In all cases, check C-peptide level and insulin level, and repeated FSBG.

C-peptide level is low in factitious insulin administration and is diagnostic. Look for the test question dealing with a nurse with access to insulin and a flair for the dramatic.

A supervised fast of 24–72 h resulting in high levels of insulin despite low levels of plasma glucose is pathognomonic for insulinoma.

Treatment

Usually giving 5% dextrose in the ER is both diagnostic and curative. One or two ampoules of 50% of dextrose may also be used depending on presentation. Then, if tests for factious insulin administration show positive results, call psych; if insulinoma is suspected, do supervised fast. If positive, the tumor must be localized and excised. For normal individuals and children, give candy PRN.

Disorders of the Parathyroid Gland

Hyperparathyroidism

Seen in primary and secondary forms. Primary usually involves dysfunction of parathyroid glands themselves, while secondary involves kidney failure. When thinking of parathyroid disease always think of parathyroid hormone (PTH), phosphorus, and calcium.

Primary hyperparathyroidism: High calcium, high PTH, low phosphorus.
Secondary hyperparathyroidism: High calcium, high PTH, high phosphorus.

Symptoms

Fractures, osteoporosis, pancreatitis, kidney stones, and neurological and psychiatric disturbances. Generally illness due to bone breakdown to maintain unnaturally high blood calcium levels.

Diagnosis

Check electrolytes including magnesium, phosphorus, and Ionized calcium, and the main actor, PTH. Check kidney function. Expect plasma alkaline phosphatase to be elevated in bone turnover.

Expect PTH to be high in hyperparathyroidism and low in other forms of hypercalcemia. If other causes of hypercalcemia are suspected (such as ectopic secretion), check PTH-related peptide.

Treatment

Therapy is aimed at reducing the blood calcium. IV NS and furosemide are the mainstay of treatment. Bisphosphonates also protect bone from further resorption. Surgery is definitive treatment, but hypoparathyroidism is a common side effect. After removal, give calcium supplements to counter the sudden decrease of plasma calcium from the bones snapping it all back up after withdrawal of PTH.

Endocrine Disorders

Diabetes Insipidus

Lack of amount or effect of antidiuretic hormone (ADH). Two types:

Central diabetes insipidus (DI): Often idiopathic but linked to trauma (especially chest), neoplasm, sarcoid.

Nephrogenic DI: Medications are the most common cause including **lithium**, demeclocycline, methoxyflurane, colchicine.

Symptoms

Patient presents with severe polydipsia, polyuria. Urine volumes can be amazingly high (in the tens of liters per day).

Diagnosis

High plasma osmolarity and low urine osmolarity in both central and nephrogenic forms.

Water deprivation test is gold standard and can tell the difference between the two types. The patient is restricted from water ingestion in a controlled environment until dehydration is achieved (usually judged by hypernatremia). Then, IV vasopressin (ADH) is administered. In the central DI patient, urine osmolarity increases in proper response. In the nephrogenic DI patient, urine osmolarity will change (since the kidneys do not respond correctly).

Treatment

- **Central DI:** Exogenous vasopressin (DDAVP) is the treatment of choice.

- **Nephrogenic DI:** Thiazide diuretics are the treatment of choice because of a paradoxical effect.

Syndrome Inappropriate Antidiuretic Hormone (SIADH)

Excess ADH in blood produces hyponatremia, decreased serum osmolarity, and increased urine osmolarity, often seen as **normovolemic hyponatremia**. Can be from many different causes including medications such as morphine and oxytocin. Also from malignancy, classically small cell of the lung. Trauma (especially chest), postoperative status, lung infections, and many others.

Diagnosis

Labs: Hyponatremia, decreased serum osmolarity, increased urine osmolarity. Elucidation of a cause often suggests this diagnosis, but since this disorder is caused by such a wide range of problems, often the etiology is hard to find.

Treatment

Water restriction is the mainstay of treatment in most cases. Demeclocycline (Declomycin) can also be used in refractory cases. Be warned not to correct the hyponatremia too quickly as the classic complication of central pontine myelinolysis is possible.

Disorders of the Adrenal Gland

Cushing's Syndrome

Caused by too much **Cortisol**.

Adrenocorticotropic hormone (ACTH)-dependant causes:

- Cushing's *disease* (pituitary hypersecretion of ACTH)
- Paraneoplastic secretion of ACTH by distant tumor
- Paraneoplastic secretion of corticotropin-releasing hormone (CRH) by distant tumors causing pituitary hypersecretion of ACTH
- Iatrogenic or factitious Cushing's syndrome due to administration of exogenous ACTH

ACTH-independent causes:

- Iatrogenic or factitious administration of exogenous glucocorticoids
- Adrenocortical adenomas or carcinomas

Symptoms

Classic **"moon" facies**, **buffalo hump**, central truncal obesity, striae, osteoporosis, and DM. Other associations include psychiatric problems, easy bruising, poor wound healing, and menstrual irregularities or viralism in women (see Figure 5.3).

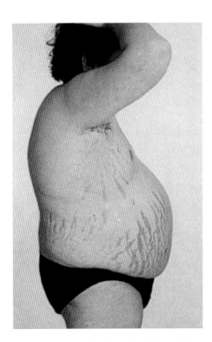

FIGURE 5.3 Classic "Cushingoid" appearance.

Oxford Handbook of Clinical Medicine. Sixth edition, Longmore M, et al. Copyright 2004. Oxford University Press.

Diagnosis

Because of normal daily variations of cortisol in the serum, it is hard to measure these concentrations and be accurate (although AM, PM, and 24-h totals are elevated if measured).

Urinary cortisol level is the best assay. Normal value is 20–100 µg/24 h; Cushing's patients >**120 µg/24 h.**

Dexamethasone suppression test: Distinguishes increased cortisolism caused by pituitary abnormality versus other forms of Cushing's syndrome. Administration of 1 mg dexamethasone PO at 11AM to 12 PM should suppress cortisol in the normal patient in the morning the next day. In Cushing's syndrome from a nonpituitary source, cortisol will continue to have elevated levels. In Cushing's syndrome from a pituitary source (the disease), the urinary cortisol level should decrease, since ACTH from the pituitary is subject to feedback inhibition by cortisol (in this case, exogenous glucocorticoid). Thus, the reaction to change proves that the elevated levels are pituitary in nature.

Imaging: CT/MRI (MRI is best) to visualize pituitary or adrenal tumors. Try to visualize any other source you may suspect of being the culprit, for example, small cell of the lung.

Treatment

- **Surgery:** Wherever it may be. If the pituitary is the culprit, a transphenoidal resection; if ectopic, remove it; if adrenal, remove them (be careful of the side effects of losing the adrenals, though).
- Then **replace** with adrenocorticoids for cortisol replacement.
- If from exogenous steroids, reduce/stop them.

Addison's Disease (and Secondary Hypoadrenalism)

Technically, Addison's disease is only from hypofunctioning of the adrenals (primary hyposecretion). But symptoms and discussion can be similar in secondary adrenal insufficiency from other causes such as pituitary hypofunction (see Figure 5.4).

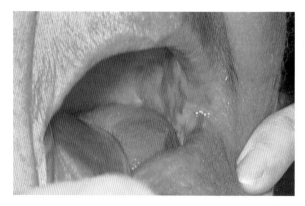

FIGURE 5.4 Intraoral hyperpigmentation of buccal mucosa in a patient with Addison's disease.

Clinical Dermatology. Fifth edition. MacKie RM. Copyright 2003. Oxford University Press.

TABLE 5.6 Lab derangements

Blood chemistries	Hematology
Low Na	Elevated hematocrit
High K	Low WBC count
Low fasting glucose	Relative lymphocytosis
Low plasma bicarbonate	Increased eosinophils
Elevated BUN	

Symptoms

Hyperpigmentation of skin (pathognomonic for Addision's secondary to high ACTH), postural hypotension, dehydration, anorexia, nausea/vomiting, diarrhea. Can lead to the complication of Addisonian crisis, which can lead to death.

Diagnosis

Cosyntropin stimulation test (a.k.a. ACTH stimulation test): Administration of exogenous cosyntropin (Cortrosyn) will elevate levels of cortisol in normal individuals. In Addison's, the levels will remain unchanged. This is diagnostic (see Table 5.6).

Treatment

- **Acute setting:** Addisonian crisis needs stat administration of **hydrocortisone** to save the patient's life. Often tested as unexplained hypotension in hospitalized patient. Hydrocortisone 100 mg IV × 1. Remember your ABCs to manage the rest, such as hypotension. Also monitor and manipulate electrolytes as needed.
- **Chronic setting:** Mineralocorticoid replacement is the mainstay. **Hydrocortisone** in two divided doses. **Fludrocortisone** in one daily dose. Monitor coexisting conditions such as diabetes and thyroid problems, and correct as needed.

Hyperaldosteronism and Conn's Syndrome (Primary)

Syndrome from excess secretion of aldosterone most likely produced by an adrenal cortex adenoma. Look for low renin levels.

Secondary hyperadosteronism is more common and related to renovascular hypertension and edematous disorders such as heart failure, cirrhosis, and nephrotic syndrome.

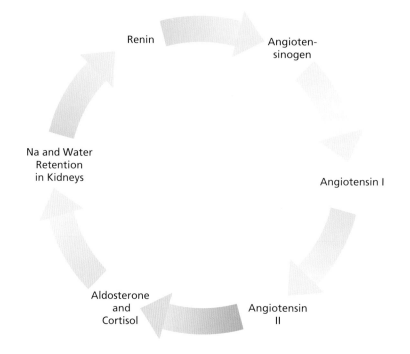

FIGURE 5.5 Renin–angiotensin cycle.

Symptoms

Symptoms include electrolyte disturbances, personality disturbances, fatigue, weakness, cramps, headache, palpitations, hyperglycemia, or most commonly **moderate hypertension** (see Figure 5.5).

Diagnosis

Electrolyte disturbances such as hypernatremia, hypokalemia, metabolic alkalosis.

Check renin levels. May be high or low depending on primary or secondary cause.

Check aldosterone levels.

CT the abdomen looking for adenomas.

Treatment

- Trial of **spironolactone** for 5–8 weeks can both treat and help diagnose.
- Surgery is definitive.

Q 5.4

A 35-year-old male comes to your office complaining of episodes of headaches and sweating for the past 5 weeks. He states he has not had previous health problems but does endorse chest palpitations, profuse sweating, headaches, and dyspnea precipitated by exertion. Vital signs reveal mild tachycardia and hypertension to 158/98 mmHg. The patient seems tired and nervous on interview.

What lab tests will most likely lead to the diagnosis?

A. Serum glucose and basic metabolic panel.
B. Serum cortisol level.
C. Serum adrenaline level.
D. Urinalysis for protein.
E. A 24-h urine collection for catecholamines.

Pheochromocytoma

Usually a catecholamine-producing tumor that produces norepinephrine and epinephrine.

Associated with other disorders including MEN II, and von Hippel–Lindau disease.

Symptoms

Classically **fluctuant hypertension**, tachycardia, palpitations. Follow the rule of five Hs:

- Headache

- Hypertension

- Hyperhidrosis

- Hyperglycemia

- Hypermetabolism

Diagnosis

Labs: The 24-h urine collection for catecholamines (metanephrines) is increased.

Imaging: CT is useful but only in finding tumors >1/2 inch diameter. MRI is useful since pheochromocytomas have distinctive appearance.

Scintigraphy: Uses ^{131}I-MIBG and can better localize extraadrenal tumors. Newer and not as practical as above.

Treatment

- Volume expansion as needed, then a combination of α- and β-blockers can be used. Use prazosin and phenoxybenzamine for α-blockade and propranolol for β-blockade.

- Then **surgery**, usually laproscopic, is the treatment of choice.

Malnutrition

Protein-Energy Malnutrition

Two forms:

Marasmus: Lack of both **calories** and **protein**. Caused by starvation state.

Kwashiorkor: Lack of **protein** with adequate calories (usually in carbohydrate form). Often seen in the Third World countries when young children stop breastfeeding (see Figures 5.6 and 5.7).

Symptoms

Children with marasmus tend to appear thin, short in stature, lethargic, and undernourished.

Children with kwashiorkor appear edematous, ascetic, with thin arms and legs. Often with "flaky paint" dermatosis, short in stature, and enlarged fatty liver.

Diagnosis

Various vitamin deficiencies accompany both forms. Kwashiorkor patients tend to have low albumin, essential amino acids, and glucose. Electrolyte abnormalities often exist including hypokalemia, hypocalcemia, hypophosphatemia, and hypomagnesemia.

Treatment

First replace fluid and electrolytes. Commonly done over 24–48-h period. Then replace macronutrients including lipid, protein, and carbohydrate using

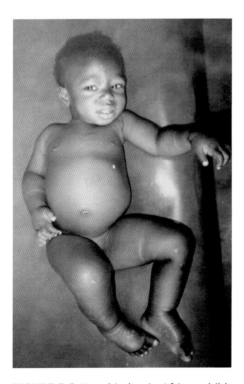

FIGURE 5.6 Kwashiorkor in African child.

With Permission, Courtesy of Tom D. Thacher, M.D.

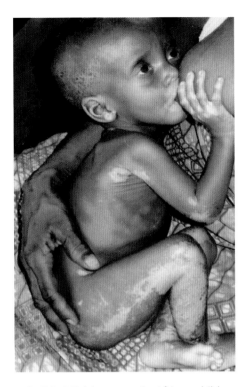

FIGURE 5.7 Marasmus in African child.

With Permission, Courtesy of Tom D. Thacher, M.D.

PO forms. This process can take up to 12 weeks, but is associated with better prognosis with earlier intervention.

Vitamin and Mineral Deficiencies

See Tables 5.7 and 5.8.

TABLE 5.7 Common vitamin deficiencies

Vitamin	Associations/signs	Treatment
A*	Night blindness, dry eyes, scaly rash, increased infections	PO or IM replacement
D*	Rickets, osteomalacia, hypocalcemia; low $25(OH)D_3$, $1,25(OH)_2D_3$, and PO_4^{3-} levels	PO replacement
E*	Hemolytic anemia, peripheral neuropathy, ataxia	PO replacement
K*	Hemorrhage, increased PT time (INR)	PO replacement for nonemergency, IM/SC for emergency (phytonadione is generic name)
B_1 (thiamine)	Wet beriberi (high-output cardiac failure) Dry beriberi (peripheral neuropathy) Wernicke and Korsakoff syndromes	PO for mild cases IM, IV for moderate/severe or unknown (always give thiamine before glucose)

(continued)

TABLE 5.7 Common vitamin deficiencies

Vitamin	Associations/signs	Treatment
B_2 (riboflavin)	Angular stomatitis, dermatitis, cheilosis. Difficult to diagnose based on hx/pe alone	PO replacement can be both diagnostic and curative; IM also available
B_3 (niacin)	Pellagra (3 Ds—dementia, dermatitis, diarrhea), stomatitis, glossitis	Niacinamide instead of niacin to avoid side effect; start PO and use IM/SC if needed may also use niacin, but watch for SEs.
B_6 (pyridoxine)	Medicine: Hydralazine, Isoniazid, penicillamine, OCPs. Seborrheic dermatitis, anemia (normo/microcytic) peripheral neuropathy, glossitis, cheilosis, lymphopenea, and convulsions in infants	Correct the underlying cause of medication; PO replacement in adults and IM/IV in infants
B_{12} (cobalamin)	Macrocytic anemia plus neurologic symptoms; look for pernicious anemia, infection with *Diphyllobothrium latum* (fish tapeworm)	PO or IM/SC replacement
Folate	Macrocytic anemia without neurologic symptoms. Occurs much quicker than vitamin B_{12} in alcoholics. Look for pregnancy and neural tube defects in infants	PO replacement
C	Scurvy (bleeding gums, opening of old wounds, petechiae), poor wound healing, bone pain; associated with "tea and toast" diet seen in elderly	PO replacement

*Indicates lipid-soluble vitamins.

TABLE 5.8 Common mineral deficiencies

Mineral	Associations/signs	Treatment
Iron	Microcytic anemia; most common mineral deficiency in the world. May see pica; order iron panel for better look at status; **ferritin** is best test to evaluate	PO $FeSO_4$ supplements if mild/moderate; IV iron for severe cases; give stool softener for common SE of constipation
Iodine	Diffuse goiter, cretinism, hypothyroidism	Iodine supplement (usually supplied in iodized salt in the developed world) at ~10 times normal maintenance dose ×2–3 weeks
Zinc	Slow wound healing, anorexia, slowed growth, delayed sexual maturation, dermatitis, impaired taste, alopecia	PO replacement
Copper	Rare; associated with malnourished states, infantile diarrhea, diet limited in milk, sprue, prolonged total parenteral nutrition (TPN) use	PO replacement
Selenium	Rare; cardiomyopathy, myalgias	Selenomethionine supplement PO
Chromium	Rare; glucose intolerance, peripheral neuropathy. Associated with TPN use	PO replacement

Other Metabolic/Immunity Disorders

Phenylketonuria

Congenital lack of phenylalanine hydroxylase resulting in toxic levels of phenylalanine.

Symptoms

Mental retardation is evident often after the infant stage and is most often severe. Seizures and abnormal electroencephalograms (EEGs) develop later. May also tend to have lighter skin, hair, and eyes. **"Mousy odor"** can also accompany.

Diagnosis

Phenylketonuria (PKU) screen routinely done on every child born in the United States within 72 h. Child is fed normal diet of milk; and if PKU is present, phenylalanine levels will rise in the blood and become detectable. In infants with the family history of PKU and normal screen, check urine after 4–6 weeks and periodically until 1 year of age. Screening tests must be confirmed by further testing if positive.

Treatment

Restriction of phenylalanine in the diet is paramount. This prevents retardation. Lofenalac is the formula of choice and is widely available in the United States. Other foods with limited phenylalanine are becoming more widely available, and food makers have started placing warnings on food that contains phenylalanine (such as artificial sweeteners, dairy).

Q 5.5

A 61-year-old male comes to your office for the follow up of recent maintenance laboratory work from a previous visit. His previous labs indicated hypertriglyceridemia with low high-density lipoprotein (HDL). You decide to start him on nicotinic acid therapy for these derangements. What is the most common side effect and what may be done to lessen the effect?

A. Dysphagia that may be treated with small meals at first, then titrating to larger ones.
B. Fatigue that may be avoided by slow titration to increased dosage of drug.
C. Muscle soreness, which may be treated with increased PO hydration when starting drug.
D. Flushing of skin, which may be treated with concurrent NSAID use and slow titration of drug dose.
E. "Blue vision" that only may be treated with discontinuation of drug.

Disorders of Lipid Metabolism

Third Report of the National Cholesterol Education Program (NCEP) Expert Panel on Detection, Evaluation, and Treatment of High Blood Cholesterol in Adults (Adult Treatment Panel III, or ATP III)

Major risk factors (Exclusive of LDL Cholesterol) that modify LDL goals (see Tables 5.9–5.13):

- Cigarette smoking
- Hypertension (BP ≥140/90 mmHg or on antihypertensive medication)
- Low HDL cholesterol (<40 mg/dL). (HDL cholesterol ≥60 mg/dL counts as a "negative" risk factor; its presence removes one risk factor from the total count.)

TABLE 5.9 Goals and levels of initiation of therapies for lipid disorders

Risk category	LDL goal	LDL level at which to initiate therapeutic lifestyle changes (TLCs)	LDL level at which to consider drug therapy
Coronary heart disease (CHD) or CHD risk equivalents	<100 mg/dL	≥100 mg/dL	≥130 mg/dL (100–129 mg/dL: drug optional)
2+ risk factors	<130 mg/dL	≥130 mg/dL	≥130 mg/dL ≥160 mg/dL
0–1 risk factor	<160 mg/dL	≥160 mg/dL	≥190 mg/dL (160–189 mg/dL: LDL-lowering drug optional)

TABLE 5.10 Range of HDL cholesterol

HDL-cholesterol levels	
Less than 40 mg/dL	A major risk factor for heart disease
40–59 mg/dL	The higher your HDL, the better
60 mg/dL and above	An HDL of 60 mg/dL and above is considered protective against heart disease

TABLE 5.11 Range of triglyceride levels

Triglyceride levels	
Less than 150 mg/dL	Normal
150–199 mg/dL	Borderline-high
200–499 mg/dL	High
500 mg/dL or above	Very high

TABLE 5.12 Range of LDL cholesterol level

LDL-Cholesterol levels	
Less than 100 mg/dL	Optimal
100–129 mg/dL	Near optimal/above optimal
130–159 mg/dL	Borderline high
160–189 mg/dL	High
190 mg/dL and above	Very high

TABLE 5.13 Hyperlipidemia medications

Drug class	Agents and daily doses	Side effects	Contraindications
HMG CoA reductase inhibitors (statins)	Lovastatin, pravastatin, simvastatin, fluvastatin, atorvastatin	Myopathy increased liver enzymes	Absolute • Active or chronic liver disease • myopathy Relative • Concomitant use of certain drugs such as azole antifungals, etc.
Bile acid sequestrants	Cholestyramine, colestipol, colesevelam	Gastrointestinal (GI) distress Constipation Decreased absorption of other drugs	Absolute • dysbeta-lipoproteinemia • TG > 400 mg/dL Relative • TG > 200 mg/dL
Nicotinic acid	Immediate release (crystalline) nicotinic acid, extended-release nicotinic acid (Niaspan), sustained-release nicotinic acid	Flushing Hyperglycemia Hyperuricemia (or gout) Upper GI distress Hepatotoxicity	Absolute • Chronic liver disease • Severe gout Relative • Diabetes • Hyperuricemia • Peptic ulcer disease
Fibric acids	Gemfibrozil, fenofibrate, clofibrate	Dyspepsia Gallstones Myopathy	Absolute • Severe renal disease • Severe hepatic disease

- Family history of premature coronary heart disease (CHD) (CHD in male first-degree relative <55 years; CHD in female first-degree relative <65 years)
- Age (men ≥45 years; women ≥55 years).

Gout

Acute or chronic arthritis caused by inflammatory urate crystals deposited in joint synovial fluid. Primary form is associated with overproduction or underexcretion of uric acid. Acute attacks are associated with some medications including hydrochlorthiazide, aspirin, and allopurinol.

Symptoms

"Podagra," an inflammatory presentation of the great toe metatarsophalangeal (MTP) joint is classically the first place of presentation. Otherwise, seen as mono- or pauci-articular arthritis. Associated with obesity, excess EtOH use, and purine (protein)-rich diet.

Diagnosis

Gold standard is **aspiration and examination of synovial fluid** in polarized light. Gout has negative birefringent crystals, pseudogout (a related crystalline arthritis) has positive birefringent crystals.

Imaging: Classically shows "punched out" lesions with preserved joint space. May also show tophi presence.

Check blood urate levels to support the diagnosis, but not specific enough to rule it out.

Uric acid excretion test: A 24-h urine collection. If gout confirmed by joint aspiration and uric acid secretion is:

<800 mg/day on unrestricted diet or <600 mg/day on purine-free diet → patient is **underexcreter**.

>800 mg/day on unrestricted diet or >600 mg/day on purine-free diet → patient is **overproducer**.

Treatment

- **General measures:** Patients need to increase fluid intake dramatically, abstain from EtOH use, reduce protein in their diet, and loose weight.

- **Acute attack:** Colchicine in acute attacks is classic, but controversial secondary to side effects including severe abdominal pain, nausea/vomiting (N/V), and diarrhea. If used, colchicine must be given in the first 24 h of onset of attack to abort it. NSAIDs (not ASA) are also used with great efficacy. Indomethacin (Indocin) is a favorite. Oral or intraarticular steroids have been shown to relieve symptoms. In severe cases, use narcotics for pain relief.

- **Chronic prophylaxis:** Colchicine can be given to ward off attacks, but side effects generally prevent this. Classic prophylactic medications are:
  - **Allopurinol** for overproducers
  - **Probenecid** of underexcreters.

Disorders of Mineral Metabolism

See Tables 5.14–5.16.

TABLE 5.14 Calcium

	Hypo	Hyper
Associations	Tetany, muscle cramps, QT prolongation, psychosis	"Bones, stones, groans, psychotic overtones" for fractures/osteopenia, nephrolithiasis, abdominal pain/pancreatitis, depression/mental status changes
Etiology	Parathyroid removal (often mistaken for thyroidectomy) pancreatitis, short bowel syndrome, decreased vitamin D intake, low magnesium	C—Calcium excess H—**Hyperparathyroid**/hyperthyroid I—Thiazide diuretics M—Metastases/milk alkali syndrome P—Paget's disease A—Addison's disease N—Neoplasm Z—Zollinger–Elleson syndrome E—Excess vitamin D E—Excess vitamin A S—Sarcoid
Treatment	Correct calcium for Albumen Measure ionized calcium IV or PO replacement	IV fluids and Lasix to increase excretion. Treat underlying cause calcitonin, bisphosphonates including zoledronic acid (Zometa) or pamidronate (Aredia), may be useful depending on the level of abnormality. Dialysis if severe

TABLE 5.15 Magnesium

	Hypo	Hyper
Associations	Tetany/increased DTRs, arrhythmias, constipation, other electrolytes (especially K classically hard to correct)	Too much $MgSO_4$ given to woman in labor! Decreased DTRs, CNS depression, respiratory failure
Etiology	Diarrhea/vomiting, celiac disease, renal failure	Too much $MgSO_4$ given to woman in labor! Renal failure
Treatment	IV/PO replacement (watch over correction.)	IV calcium, insulin and glucose, Lasix, dialysis if severe

TABLE 5.16 Phosphorus

	Hypo	Hyper
Associations	General muscle weakness, diaphragmatic weakness	Metastasis, hypocalcemia
Etiology	DKA	Renal failure, parenteral overadministration
Treatment	PO or IV if severe	Calcium carbonate

Electrolyte and Fluid Disorders

Hyponatremia

Low plasma sodium level.

Symptoms

Commonly asymptomatic, especially if it has existed for long term. Mental status change. Confusion, muscle cramps, lethargy, and seizures can occur acutely.

Diagnosis

Measurement of plasma sodium. Remember to correct for glucose level.
   Plasma osmolarity then will help divide further.

Hypertonic hyponatremia: Due to increased osmols from glucose or hypertonic infusion of glucose, mannitol, or glycine.

Isotonic hyponatremia: Due to pseudohyponatremia from osmols present because of hyperlipidemia, hyperproteinemia, or isotonic infusions of glucose, mannitol, or glycine.

Hypotonic hyponatremia: Further consideration of volume status needed (biggest and most tested group).

_Hypo_volemic hypotonic hyponatremia: Get FENa labs

$$FENa = \frac{UNa(PCr)}{PNa(UCr)} \times 100$$

UNa = Urine Sodium,
UCr = Urine Creatinine,
PNa = Plasma Sodium,
PCr = Plasma Creatinine

See Table 5.17.

Etiologies: Dehydration, diarrhea/vomiting, diuretics, nephropathies, partial urinary tract obstruction, or adrenal insufficiency.

_Eu_volemic hypotonic hyponatremia:

Etiologies: Syndrome inappropriate antidiuretic hormone (SIADH), psychogenic polydipsia, hypothyroidism, or beer potomania.

_Hyper_volemic hypotonic hyponatremia (edematous states):

Etiologies: Congestive heart failure (CHF), liver disease, nephrotic syndrome, or advanced renal failure.

TABLE 5.17 Results of Fractional Excretion of Sodium (FENa) calculation

FENa	
<1%	Prerenal
>2%	Intrinsic renal

Treatment

- If mental status changes are extreme, consider "hot salts" (3% NaCl solution) over 6 h. Otherwise, try to correct the underlying cause (stop infusions, lower lipids, etc.). In hypotonic hyponatremia, consider volume status. Treatments are aimed at correcting plasma Na to normal, but be careful to not correct over 12 mEq/L per day to avoid the dreaded **central pontine myelinolysis**.
- **Hypovolemic hypotonic hyponatremia:** Fluid restriction to <1 L/day and administration of isotonic saline.
- **Euvolemic hypotonic hyponatremia:** Fluid restrict only.
- **Hypervolemic hypotonic hyponatremia:** Fluid restrict and diuretics as needed.

Hypernatremia

Symptoms

Similar symptoms to hyponatremia: Mental status change, confusion, seizures, hyperreflexia.

Diagnosis

Often caused by dehydration, so check urine output and plasma osmolarity, BUN/creatinine.

Consider evaluation for DI (water deprivation test).

Treatment

- Treat the underlying cause.
- **Dehydration:** IV NS until rehydrated.
- Treat DI if present.
- Do not correct to fast to avoid **cerebral edema.**

Hypokalemia

Symptoms

Fatigue, muscle weakness, **cramps**, hyporeflexia, flaccid paralysis if severe.

Diagnosis

ECG: ECG shows **T-wave flattening** and possibly U-waves. May progress to ST depression, AV block, and cardiac arrest.
Labs: Plasma potassium, urine potassium, plasma pH

Urine potassium high (>20 mEq/L) → renal potassium losses

Lactic or ketoacidosis, hyperaldosteronism, Cushing's syndrome, hypomagnesemia, or medications (amphotericin, diuretics, gentamicin)

Urine potassium low (<20 mEq/L) → nonrenal potassium causes

Transcellular shift from insulin, β-blockers, alkalosis or GI losses from diarrhea, laxative abuse, vomiting, or nasogastric (NG) suctioning.

Treatment

Treat the underlying disorder. Remember to replace magnesium. Give IV KCl (often as K rider) and monitor closely, then switch to PO.

Hyperkalemia

Symptoms

Ventricular fibrillation, intestinal colic, areflexia, weakness, paralysis, parasthesias.

Diagnosis

Recheck blood draw. Order repeat K and electrolytes to include magnesium. **ECG: Peaked T-waves**, PR prolongation, wide QRS, **loss of P-waves** potentially progressive to sine waves, then to cardiac arrest.

Place on continuous cardiac monitoring.

Most common cause is spurious from the hemolysis caused by sitting in the vial too long. Nonspurious causes include renal failure, mineralocorticoid deficiency, cellular shifts from insulin deficiency, and tumor lysis. Medications are also major category and include effects from spironolactone, triamterene, angiotensin-converting enzyme inhibitors (ACEIs), heparin, pentamidine, amiloride, arginine, trimethoprim, NSAIDs, succinylcholine, digitalis effect, and β-blockers.

Treatment

- For mild derangement not evident clinically on ECG, may give PO treatment and correct underlying cause. Sodium polystyrene sulfonate (Kayexalate) PO/NG or retention enema.
- For clinically apparent derangement or ECG changes:
  - *Acutely:* Calcium gluconate to stabilize cardiac muscle.
  - Consider albuterol breathing treatment.
  - IV glucose + insulin to shift K into cells.
  - Furosemide IV to increase excretion.
  - Dialysis as last resort.
- Remember to replace magnesium if needed.

Hypovolemia

Symptoms

Poor skin turgor, dry mucous membranes, low urine output, concentrated urine, tachycardia. Children may have lack of tears, lethargy, and increased fussiness.

Diagnosis

Remains a clinical decision.
Labs: Urine specific gravity, BUN/creatinine. FENa <1%.

Treatment

IV fluids

- NS or Lactated Ringer (LR) by bolus and then maintenance for adults. See Tables 5.18 and 5.19 for guidance with children.
- Children
  - Bolus (LR or NS)
    Small children: 20 mL/kg (2% body wt)
    Adolescents: 10 mL/kg (1% body wt)
  - Deficit

    $$D_5 0.45 \, NS + 20 \, mEq/L \, K$$

    Based on estimate 5% mild, 10% moderate, 15% severe. Two different methods (see Table 5.18).

  - Maintenance calculation

    $$D_5 0.2 \, NS + 20 \, mEq/L \, K$$

    Holliday–Segar formula (see Table 5.19).

Hypervolemia

Symptoms

Depending on the reason: weight gain, edema, increasing belt or waistband size, jugular vein distention (JVD), rales/crackles in lungs, or hypertension.

Diagnosis

Clinical assessment
Labs: Urine specific gravity, BUN/creatinine.
Imaging: Chest x-ray showing pulmonary edema/effusion.

TABLE 5.18 Two differing strategies for fluid replacement

	Combined deficit and maintenance	Sequential deficit and maintenance
First 8 h after bolus	½ remaining deficit + $\frac{1}{3}$ daily maintenance	Remaining deficit (after bolus)
Next 16 h	½ remaining deficit + $\frac{2}{3}$ daily maintenance	Daily maintenance

TABLE 5.19 Holliday-Segar method for maintenance fluid replacement

Weight (kg)	kcal/day or ml/day	kcal/h or ml/h
0–10 kg	100/kg per day	4 ml/kg/h
11–20 kg	1000 + (50 ml/kg/day above 10)	40 + (2 ml/kg/h above 10)
>20 kg	1500 + (20 ml/kg/day above 20)	60 + (1 ml/kg/h above 20)

Treatment

Diuresis with furosemide (Lasix) or dialysis if severe.

Immunity Deficiency

See Table 5.20

TABLE 5.20 Inherited immune deficiencies

Disorder	Associations/diagnosis	Treatment
B-cell		
X-linked (Bruton's) agammaglobulinemia	B-cell deficiency in boys; *pseudomonas* infections in infancy; quantitative Ig levels (specific subclasses) are low	IV immunoglobulin (IVIG) and prophylactic antibiotics
IgA deficiency	Most common immunodeficiency; recurrent infections, URIs	None/unnecessary
T-cell		
DiGeorge syndrome (Thymic aplasia)	Tetany (from hypocalcemia) in first days of life. Dx with absolute lymphocyte count, mitogen stim response, and skin testing	Bone marrow transplant (BMT) and thymus transplant have showed success
Ataxia-telangiectasia	Oculocutaneous telangiectasias, progressive cerebellar ataxia; likely shortened life span to <30 years	IVIG and antibiotics may help acutely; ultimately no treatment
Combined		
Severe combined immunodeficiency (SCID)	Lack of both B- and T-cells. Chronic, severe, infections including fungal and others	BMT and stem cell transplant. IVIG. Prophylaxis for PCP. Gene therapy in future?
Wiskott–Aldrich syndrome	Eczema, thrombocytopenia, Increased IgE, IgA, decreased IgM, X-linked	BMT, splenectomy, continuous antibiotics, IVIG; prognosis poor with death before 15 years old if no BMT
Complement		
Hereditary angioneuroctic edema (C1 esterase deficiency)	Autosomal dominant; repeated episodes of possibly life-threatening angioedema commonly brought on by stress or minor trauma; diagnose with compliment levels	Daily danazol for prophylaxis
Terminal complement deficiency (low C5–C9)	*Neisseria* infections; gonococcal infections	Vaccinate against *Neisseria* and antibiotics as needed

Answers

5.1 B. The patient has a nonresponsive presentation with vitals indicating slowing of metabolic functioning, specifically hypotension; bradycardia; and hypothermia. Labs further show hyponatremia, hypoglycemia, and evidence of infection. Investigation should include the evaluation of thyroid status, especially in the setting of lack of medical history. Other labs listed may be reasonable, but would not lead to the correct suspected diagnosis.

5.2 C. Management of myxedema coma may be done by stabilization of the patient with ABC protocol, correction of electrolyte abnormality including hypoglycemia, and aggressive IV fluid replacement at the onset. Then IV thyroxine (T_4) or triiodothyroxine (T_3) should be given with IV hydrocortisone. The patient should then be monitored in an ICU setting until stable. Consideration of empiric antibiotics should be made if infection is thought to play a role in precipitation.

5.3 B. Metabolic (lactic) acidosis and GI disturbance including diarrhea are the two most common side effects of metformin, and are the common reasons for noncompliance of patients.

5.4 E. The diagnosis suggested in the question is pheochromocytoma, an adrenal tumor that episodically produces increased catecholamines with adrenaline-like effects. Episodic headaches, hyperhydrosis, and hypertension are three of the clinical "five Hs." The other two are hyperglycemia and hypermetabolism. The other given answers would not reveal the diagnosis, although they may yield some abnormalities.

5.5 D. Flushing is a well-known and common side effect of nicotinic acid therapy. This is so common that it should be anticipated when starting this medication and may be mediated by slow titration of drug dose and concurrent use of NSAIDs during beginning of therapy. The other choices are not side effects of nicotinic acid.

6   Hematology

Non-Solid Malignancies	123
Hodgkin's Lymphoma	123
Non-Hodgkin's Lymphoma	124
Multiple Myeloma	125
Leukemia	127
Anemias	129
Microcytic Anemias	129
Normocytic Anemias	129
Macrocytic Anemias	130
Sickle Cell Anemia	130
Septicemia	132
Polycythemia	133
Transfusion Reaction	133
Hypercoagulable States	134
Disseminated Intravascular Coagulation	135
Hemophilia	135
Idiopathic Thrombocytopenic Purpura	136
Thrombotic Thrombocytopenic Purpura and Hemolytic Uremic Syndrome	137

Non-Solid Malignancies

Hodgkin's Lymphoma

Four types comprising nodular sclerosis, mixed cellularity, lymphocyte depleted, and lymphocyte predominant.

Symptoms

Presentation varies widely and may include new-onset fever, night sweats, weight loss, fatigue, anorexia, or pruritus. Alcohol-induced pain in the areas of lymphoma. Patients may also notice prominent lymphadenopathy. Obtain a complete family history.

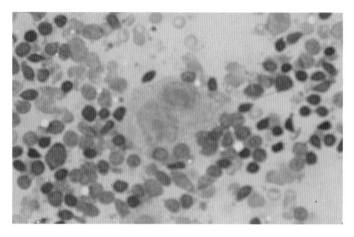

FIGURE 6.1 Giant Reed–Sternberg cell in the center with "spongy" chromatin pattern and "mirror" image nucleus.

With permission Nivaldo Medeiros, MD.

Diagnosis

Diagnosis made by biopsy of an enlarged lymph node. **Reed–Sternberg cells** are pathognomonic and have "owl eye" or "mirror" appearance under microscope.

Physical exam: Cervical or supraclavicular lymphadenopathy, weight loss, increased temperature. Hepatosplenomegaly may be prominent.

Labs: CBC with manual differential for lymphocytic abnormalities, normocytic anemia; CRP/ESR often increased; liver function tests (LFTs); and transaminases may indicate liver involvement.

Imaging: Chest x-ray, CT of chest, abdomen, and pelvic areas for staging. Ultrasound as well as MRI may be useful for staging. Gallium scan or PET scan may also be used. Stage using the Ann-Arbor staging system.

Obtain bone biopsy, especially for higher-stage disease (see Figure 6.1).

Treatment

- Radiation therapy, chemotherapy, or a combination of both is commonly effective. Radiation is the treatment for localized disease of early stage. Chemotherapy, consisting of quadruple cyclic cocktail of adriamycin, bleomycin, vinblastine, and dacarbazine (ABVD) is used for higher stages.

- Cell transplant may also be added for recurrent disease or to improve initial survival.

Non-Hodgkin's Lymphoma

A heterogeneous group of lymphomas characterized by the absence of Reed–Sternberg cells on biopsy. Non-Hodgkin's lymphoma (NHL) may present with similar symptoms including night sweats, weight loss, fever, fatigue, anorexia, and lymphadenopathy. It tends to spread in more unpredictable ways, however, and is harder to stage. Diagnosis is similar in that biopsy is the gold standard, with histologic grade being the most important. Treatment decisions should be made by an experienced oncologist, but often involves various cyclic regimens of chemotherapy and/or radiation.

Q 6.1

A 68-year-old Caucasian man comes to your office with complaints of recent lethargy, weakness, dyspnea, and back pain when standing. He has felt this way since you had treated him as an outpatient 2 months ago for nephrolithiasis. He also states he has felt as if his vision has been impaired lately describing it as if "looking through a car windshield in the rain." What is the next step in the diagnosis of the most likely condition?

A. Peripheral blood smear.
B. Reticulocyte count.
C. Alkaline phosphatase level.
D. Whole-body bone scan (scintiography).
E. Bone marrow biopsy.

Q 6.2

All of the following findings may be present in this patient EXCEPT:

A. Increased ESR.
B. A 25% plasma cell predominance on bone marrow biopsy.
C. Compression fracture of L_4 vertebra.
D. Normal alkaline phosphatase level.
E. Microcytic anemia.

Multiple Myeloma

Symptoms

Bone pain (backache common), lethargy, weakness, dyspnea, pallor, palpitations, recurrent infections, and common bleeding episodes. Associated conditions include carpal tunnel syndrome, macroglossia, diarrhea, symptoms of hyperviscosity (eye sight difficulties, headaches, etc.) or symptoms of hypercalcemia ("stones, bones, abdominal moans, and psychotic overtones").

Diagnosis

Physical exam: Bone tenderness, pathologic fractures, pallor, and increased temperature.
Labs: Serum and urine protein electrophoresis (**SPEP and UPEP**) are essential and show immunoglobulin M (IgM) M-spike and increased **Bence Jones proteins**, respectively. CBC may show normocytic anemia with Rouleaux

formations prominent, neutropenia, and thrombocytopenia. High ESR is common. Serum calcium and ionized calcium are often high (despite normal alkaline phosphatase). Renal function often shows increased BUN and creatinine, indicating renal failure.

Imaging: Obtain full-body radiographic scan (*not* scintiography) and look for "**punched out**" lesions. MRI may be helpful to visualize bone involvement.

Bone marrow biopsy characteristically shows **plasma cell predominance** (see Figure 6.2).

Diagnosis is made by the presence of the following criteria:

1. Monoclonal protein in SPEP or UPEP.

2. Plasma cell infiltration of the bone marrow.

3. Presence of end-organ damage felt related to the plasma cell proliferation (hypercalcemia, lytic bone lesions on x-ray, renal failure, etc.).

Treatment

- Chemotherapy is effective and regimens vary. These often include either melphalan (Alkeran) or cyclophosphamide. Thalidomide may be useful, although in combination with dexamethasone (Decadron).

- Stem cell transplant, especially in younger patients, has shown good effect but falls short of cure.

- Local radiation therapy is effective and is often used in the areas of pathologic fracture.

- Renal failure is treated with aggressive oral hydration. Hypercalcemia is treated with aggressive hydration and bisphosphonates such as pamidronate (Aredia).

- Anemia is treated with either transfusion or erythropoietin (Epogen).

- Monitor for infections and treat them early. Remember to vaccinate.

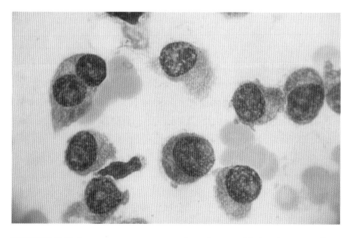

FIGURE 6.2 Bone marrow smear showing multiple plasma cells, one binucleate form.

With permission Nivaldo Medeiros, MD.

Q 6.3

A 37-year-old Latino auto mechanic comes to your office with complaints of recent fever, fatigue, sore throat, bruising, and spots on her extremities. She states she has worked in her father's garage for 15 years and commonly uses chemicals including benzene to clean machine parts. On physical exam, she has noticeable ecchymoses on all four extremities and sacral area. Her mouth reveals moderate pharyngeal wall erythema, gingival hypertrophy, but otherwise good dentition. What laboratory abnormalities are most likely in this patient?

A. Auer rods on peripheral blood smear.
B. Smudge cells on peripheral blood smear.
C. t(9,22) translocation on genetic analysis.
D. Infiltration of lymphocytes in bone marrow biopsy.
E. Increased leukocyte alkaline phosphatase levels.

Q 6.4

What therapy may be used for the most severe life-threatening complication of this condition?

A. Imatinib (Gleevec).
B. Platelet infusion.
C. Bone marrow transplant.
D. Fresh frozen plasma (FFP).
E. Dexamethasone IV.

Leukemia

See Table 6.1 and Figure 6.3.

TABLE 6.1 The leukemias

	Acute lymphocytic leukemia (ALL)	Acute myelogenous leukemia (AML)	Chronic lymphocytic leukemia (CLL)	Chronic myelogenous leukemia (CML)
Associations	Children; viral-like prodrome and refusal to walk. Bone pain, bruising, and fever	Adults; exposure to smoking, benzene, radiation, or may occur *de novo*. Bruising, fatigue, dyspnea, fever, petechiae	Older adults; slow progression of disease. Lymphadenopathy, fatigue, hepatosplenomegaly, easy bruising	Middle-aged adults; stable chronic phase that progresses to acute *"blast crisis."* Symptoms include fatigue, fever, malaise, weight loss, and night sweats. Blast crisis has fever, bone pain, weight loss, and splenomegaly

(continued)

TABLE 6.1 The leukemias

	Acute lymphocytic leukemia (ALL)	Acute myelogenous leukemia (AML)	Chronic lymphocytic leukemia (CLL)	Chronic myelogenous leukemia (CML)
Diagnosis	Lymphadenopathy and splenomegaly. CBC shows anemia, decreased platelets, and variable WBCs. Increased LDH, uric acid. Obtain bone marrow biopsy and LP for leukemic cells. CXR for mediastinal involvement	Gingival hypertrophy. Peripheral smear shows *Auer rods*. Decreased leukocyte alkaline phosphatase (LAP). *DIC* may be seen in coagulation studies. CBC shows anemia, decreased platelets, and marked leukocytosis	Lymphocytosis prominent with **"smudge cells"** on smear. CBC shows anemia, thrombocytopenia. Bone marrow biopsy shows infiltration with lymphocytes. LDH increased. Genetic analysis often helpful. Expression of CD5 and CD23 on cell surface is characteristic	CBC shows prominent leukocytosis and anemia. Decreased LAP, increased vitamin B_{12} levels. Genetic analysis for **Philadelphia chromosome, t(9,22)** is diagnostic
Treatment	Good prognosis; phases of chemo include remission induction, consolidation, and remission maintenance. Regimens vary and may be used with radiation	Treat DIC if present, cyclic chemotherapy is the treatment of choice. Supportive care as needed for side effects	Supportive care often used since disease has typical indolent course. Chlorambucil or fludarabine are the classic chemotherapy agents. Supportive care for complications or side effects. May eventually need splenectomy	Hydroxyurea and interferon-α are classic to suppress blast crisis in the chronic phase. Bone marrow transplant may also be successful. When in blast crisis, **imatinib (Gleevec),** a receptor tyrosine kinase (RTK) inhibitor is very effective

CXR, chest x-ray; DIC, disseminated intravascular coagulation; LDH, lactate dehydrogenase.

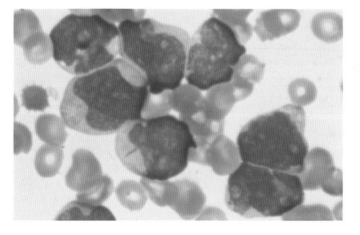

FIGURE 6.3 Blood smear acute myelogenous leukemia (AML). Several blasts and one of them showing rod-shaped structure in the cytoplasm known as Auer body.

With permission Nivaldo Medeiros, MD.

Anemias

Symptoms

Pallor, tachypnea, palpitations, fatigue, dyspnea on exertion, chest pain, pica, and poor exercise tolerance. History may be pertinent for chronic or acute blood loss, dietary deficiency/malnutrition, sensitivity to certain foods, exposure, or family history.

Microcytic Anemias

Iron deficiency anemia (IDA): May be caused by malabsorption, malnutrition, or, commonly, chronic blood loss. Look for sources of bleeding including the urine or GI tract. Exam may show spooning of nails or angular cheilosis around the mouth. Although Hemoccult stool testing is not intended for this purpose, it may be useful if positive. Serum ferritin (low in IDA) is the single most useful test in diagnosis; it is also an acute-phase reactant, so may be falsely elevated in the setting of illness. Obtain an iron panel including serum iron (low), total iron-binding capacity (high), and transferrin (high). Replace with oral iron.

Thalassemia: Autosomal recessively inherited group of abnormalities involving the formation of α- and β-hemoglobin chains. More common in those of Mediterranean descent; severity of illness related to the state of one or both genes being defective (although wide spectrum of severity exists). The test of choice is hemoglobin electrophoresis, which will reveal if disease is α- or β-thalessemia and heterozygous or homozygous. Peripheral smear shows target cells, nucleated RBCs, and diffuse basophilia. Skull x-ray shows "hair-on-end" appearance. Treat with transfusions as necessary and iron chelation therapy to prevent resultant iron overload.

Lead poisoning: Often seen in children due to chronic exposure. History may reveal residence in house with lead paint or parental occupational exposure to lead. Blood lead levels taken for screening usually are capillary and need to be confirmed by venous sample if positive. Peripheral smear shows characteristic "basophilic stippling." Serum erythrocyte protoporphyrin level is increased and should be cross-confirmed with blood lead level. Plain radiographs reveal metaphyseal "lead lines" in children chronically exposed. Treatment is chelation therapy with oral succimer (Chemet) or parental dimercaprol (BAL) + Ca EDTA (calcium edetate disodium). Monitor for seizures during chelation.

Normocytic Anemias

Acute blood loss: Produced by acute injury; recent blood loss will produce a normocytic anemia only after volume replacement or some time after recovery. Do not rely on blood studies to determine the amount of blood loss or threshold for transfusion in the acute setting.

Anemia of chronic disease: May be normo- or microcytic. Patient is often in chronically ill state, which may contribute to symptoms. Reticulocyte index (normal 0.5%–2.0%) is often inappropriately low, indicating decreased response to anemia. Erythropoietin (Epogen) may improve condition. Treat the underlying disease if possible. Iron is not helpful.

Glucose-6-phosphate dehydrogenase (G6PD) deficiency: An X-linked recessive trait affecting men. Patients may experience hemolysis and hemoglobinuria after exposure to certain oxidant-containing foods or medications. Triggers commonly include fava beans, antimalarials, sulfa compounds, antihelminths, and others. Several enzyme-linked screening tests exist including direct RBC enzyme assay. Newborns and infants may have excessive jaundice. Treat by stopping or avoiding the offending ingestion. Hydrate to increase urine output. For infants, consider phototherapy. Transfuse if necessary.

Macrocytic Anemias

Folate/vitamin B$_{12}$ deficiency: Commonly seen in chronic alcoholics, pregnant women, chronic gastritis, the elderly eating "tea and toast" diet, pernicious anemia, methotrexate, or phenytoin use, fish tapeworm infection (*Diphyllobothrium latum*), or patients with prior GI surgery. Often asymptomatic, but may show neurologic involvement such as paresthesias, ataxia, spasticity, or delirium. Peripheral smear shows large RBCs and hypersegmented neutrophils. Check serum levels of both. A Schilling test may delineate the etiology of B$_{12}$ deficiency. Replace vitamins orally if no absorption problems. Give vitamin B$_{12}$ shots every month if needed.

Sickle Cell Anemia

Symptoms

Sickle cell patients are asymptomatic until crisis. Vasoocclusive crisis is often very painful and occurs commonly in the hands and feet, but may occur anywhere in the body. **Cold weather, hypoxia, or infection** tend to be triggers.

Visceral sequestration caused by sickling within organs may be life-threatening. Splenic sequestration/infarction often occurs in younger patients and repeated events lead to autosplenectomy.

Acute chest syndrome (ACS) is life-threatening and has symptoms of severe chest pain, dyspnea, hypoxia, and air hunger.

Aplastic crisis occurs particularly associated with ***parvovirus B19*** infection, and is characterized by drop in hematocrit (Hct) and reticulocyte count.

Other complications are stasis ulcers, shortened fingers/toes (due to repeated infarction), pigment gallstones, and osteomyelitis (commonly *Salmonella* spp.).

Diagnosis

Labs: CBC for hemoglobin and hematocrit (Hct/Hb), which are typically low. Search during history for baseline values and compare to determine if patient is in acute crisis. Leukocytosis and thrombocytosis often present. Peripheral smear shows sickled cells and commonly "Howell–Jolly" bodies indicating splenic damage. Reticulocyte index often very elevated. "Sickledex" test is positive. Bilirubin high and haptoglobin low. Elevated lactate dehydrogenase (LDH). Hemoglobin electrophoresis will show increased Hb S and is the definitive test.
Imaging: Chest x-ray to evaluate for acute chest syndrome, CT/MRI if indicated to evaluate for cerebrovascular accident (CVA). Bone scan is mandatory if suspected osteomyelitis (see Figure 6.4).

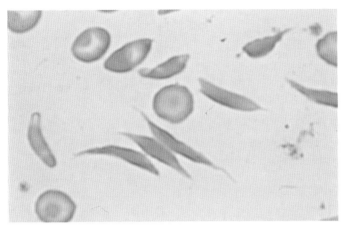

FIGURE 6.4 Erythrocytes exhibiting a definite sickle shape with pointed ends.

With permission Nivaldo Medeiros, MD.

Q 6.5

An 18-year-old African American male reports to the ER for fever, productive cough, myalgias, and chest congestion. He reports a past medical history of sickle cell disease with a long history of admissions to the hospital. He denies overt shortness of breath (SOB) or chest pain. You order an initial chest x-ray and laboratory. Imaging reveals an opacity indicative of pneumonia. What is the most likely organism causing this infection?

A. *S. aureus.*
B. *S. pneumoniae.*
C. *M. pneumoniae.*
D. *Listeria.*
E. *N. meningitis.*

Treatment

- Vaccinate known sicklers (*Haemophilus, Pneumococcus, Meningococcus*).

- Avoid triggers such as exposure to cold weather, dehydration, hypoxia, certain medications.

- Oral penicillin or amoxicillin recommended for children aged 2 months to 5 years. Continue until puberty if frequent crises or indications.

- Prevent crisis with folic acid supplement and hydroxyurea (Droxia).

- In acute crisis, give oxygen, aggressive IV hydration, and warmth.

- Treat acute crisis with nonsteroidal antiinflammatory drugs (NSAIDs), Tylenol, ketorolac (Toradol), or tramadol (Ultram) when possible. Elevation to narcotic analgesics such as morphine or meperidine (Demerol) may be needed.

- Transfuse if necessary.
  - Exchange transfusion may be needed in severe crisis or acute chest syndrome.
- Treat any infection aggressively and early. Educate the family to monitor for fever and respond quickly to avoid crisis.
- Monitor for narcotic pain dependence/seeking on presentation. This is often a fine line, but be aware many sicklers also have comorbid narcotic dependence.

Septicemia

Diagnosis

See Table 6.2.

Treatment

- Initiate ABCs as needed.
- For systemic inflammatory response syndrome (SIRS), treat the underlying cause, which may or may not be bacterial.
- Blood cultures should always be taken before beginning antibiotics.
- Start empiric broad-spectrum antibiotics. These may include gentamicin + third-generation cephalosporin [such as ceftriaxone (Rocephin)]. Add vancomycin if gram-positive organisms suspected or metronidazole (Flagyl) if anaerobic organisms suspected.
- Fluid resuscitation if shock is present. Add pressor agents such as dopamine or norepinephrine (Levophed) if needed.
- Consult surgery if septic focus is thought to be abscess. Will need immediate incision/drainage.

TABLE 6.2 Spectrum of systemic inflammation

Term	Criteria
Systemic inflammatory response syndrome (SIRS)	Elevated or decreased temperature
	Elevated heart rate >90 beats per minute
	Elevated respiratory rate >20 breaths per minute
	WBC count >12,000/mm^3 or <4000/mm^3 or >10% band form
	Two or more of the above need to be present for SIRS
Sepsis	SIRS + documented infection (typically bacterial)
Septic shock	Sepsis-induced hypotension and end-organ hypoperfusion

Polycythemia

Symptoms

Symptoms often stem from hyperviscosity and include headache, dyspnea, blurred vision, pruritus particularly to hot water, gout, and facial plethora. In polycythemia rubra vera, etiology is genetic, but secondary polycythemia may be from heavy smoking, high altitudes, or lung disease with chronic hypoxia.

Diagnosis

Physical exam: Facial plethora, retinal venous engorgement, and **splenomegaly**.
Labs: CBC showing increased red cell mass and Hct/Hb. WBCs and platelets are often increased above normal. Neutrophil alkaline phosphatase (NAP) level is increased as are vitamin B_{12} levels. Erythropoietin level is low. Uric acid often increased, contributing to gout comorbidity.

Treatment

- Serial phlebotomy is the mainstay of treatment. Goal is Hct <45%.
- Hydroxyurea (Hydrea) may reduce frequency of phlebotomies.
- Low-dose aspirin to reduce platelet function.
- Interferon-α is under investigation for this purpose and shows promise.

Transfusion Reaction

See Table 6.3.

TABLE 6.3 Spectrum of transfusion reaction

Reaction	Associations	Diagnosis	Treatment
Immediate	Chills, anxiety, fever, flushing, tachycardia, hypotension, or pain. Wrong blood type or Rh antigen in previously sensitized patient	Coombs test (positive), low haptoglobin, elevated serum bilirubin, urinalysis shows hemoglobinuria. Repeat type and cross of donated blood and recipient blood	Stop transfusion. Maintain BP and urine output (goal ≥100 cc/h). Use intravenous fluids (IVFs), furosemide (Lasix), and/or dopamine as needed
Delayed	2–14 days after transfusion. Symptoms of jaundice, anemia, and fever	Unexpected drop in Hct/Hb well after transfusion. Decreased haptoglobin. Hyperbilirubinemia	Supportive care. Usually is self-limited

(continued)

HEMATOLOGY

133

TABLE 6.3 Spectrum of transfusion reaction

Reaction	Associations	Diagnosis	Treatment
Allergic reaction	Due to unknown allergen in donor blood. Often occurs on short-term basis. Pruritus or urticaria may develop	No signs of hemolysis upon laboratory investigation	Antihistamine [diphenhydramine (Benadryl)] or, if severe, epinephrine. Transfusion may be resumed
Transfusion-related acute lung injury (TRALI)	Caused by antibodies to donor WBCs. Respiratory symptoms such as dyspnea, tachypnea, chest pain, and cough develop. Occurs 1–6 h after transfusion	Chest x-ray shows noncardiogenic pulmonary edema. Wheezing or rhonchi may be heard	Supportive care with oxygen or intubation if needed

Hypercoagulable States

Symptoms

Patients are generally asymptomatic until an event heralds diagnosis or thrombosis. Events may include deep venous thrombosis (DVT), pulmonary embolus (PE), superficial thrombophlebitis, or stroke.

Inherited disorders—factor V Leiden deficiency, protein C or S deficiency, antithrombin III deficiency, homocystinemia.

Acquired disorders—prolonged immobilization, tissue damage from surgery or fracture, disseminated intravascular coagulation (DIC), hyperlipidemia, multiple myeloma, lupus anticoagulant (antiphospoholipid syndrome), nephrotic syndrome (leading to loss of protein C/S), smoking, malignancy, oral contraceptive use, or pregnancy.

Diagnosis

Labs: CBC for platelet level, coagulation panel PT/aPTT, and calculated INR, protein C and S levels, thrombin level, antithrombin III level, bleeding time. Obtain genetic testing as needed and antinuclear antibody (ANA) for lupus. Consider a 50:50 mixing study to determine if anticoagulant is present. If present, test for lupus, which would indicate thrombotic tendency, not antithrombotic. Test for β-human chorionic gonadotropin (β-hCG).
Imaging: Obtain imaging of head (CT, MRI) if suspected CVA. Doppler flow ultrasound if DVT suspected. See Chapter 11 for other tests available.

Treatment

- Anticoagulation with heparin or low molecular weight heparin, enoxaparin (Lovenox), is indicated initially. This prevents further clot formation, but does not treat current clot. After 2–3 days, warfarin (Coumadin) may be started for oral anticoagulation. Keep the INR between 2 and 3. The duration of treatment varies depending on defect. Lifelong anticoagulation may be indicated, but courses may be as short as 3 months if the condition is found to be acquired and corrected.

- Thrombolytics are controversial and of limited proven benefit.
- Treat any condition that is possible such as lupus or renal failure.

Disseminated Intravascular Coagulation

A serious condition that occurs by systemic deposition of fibrin and consumption of coagulation factors. Causes vary but are classically due to gram-negative sepsis, amniotic fluid embolus, abruptio placenta, liver failure, and malignancy.

Diagnosis

Usually seen in the very ill; DIC may first be seen as bleeding at IV sites, ecchymosis, purpura, and distal limb discoloration. Bleeding may become brisk and occur from GI tract or surgery site.

Labs: When suspected, immediately obtain coagulation studies for PT/aPTT, which are both prolonged. Thrombin time is markedly prolonged. CBC shows decreased platelets. Fibrin split products are very high while fibrinogen is low. Above are the most important labs acutely, but the following may also be abnormal: D-dimer positive; increased bleeding time; schizocytosis; leukocytosis; increased LDH; decreased antithrombin III; decreased factors V, VIII, X, XIII; hematuria; and occult blood in stools.

Treatment

- Admission to the ICU.
- Treat the underlying cause. Consider high-dose, broad-spectrum antibiotics until infection is ruled out.
- Replace acutely lost blood with transfusion.
- Give fresh frozen plasma (FFP) for clotting factors. Cryoprecipitate is an alternative.
- Antithrombin III if FFP fails.
- Administration of platelets is not useful as they are destroyed due to systemic coagulation.
- Heparin may be considered if complications from clotting is suspected, *but never after head injury.*

Hemophilia

Hemophilia A and B are reflections of genetically deficient factors VIII and IX, respectively. Hemophilia A is five times more common than B.

Symptoms

Since this is an X-linked disorder, almost all affected are men. Degrees of severity exist and depend on the levels of the missing factor, <1% severe,

<5% moderate, and >5% mild. First episodes of bleeding often from either minor trauma or circumcision. Further bleeding occurs with minor cuts or scrapes and may be profuse, even life-threatening. Hemarthroses are a common complication and can be disfiguring because of calcium deposition and deformity.

Diagnosis

Labs: Coagulation studies show increased aPTT, but normal PT. CBC may show anemia and normal platelet count. Bleeding time is only sometimes prolonged. Factor VIII is low in hemophilia A; factor IX is low in hemophilia B. Female hemophilia A carrier state may be diagnosed by comparison of factor VIII level and von Willebrand's factor (VWF). Polymerase chain reaction (PCR) and genetic testing are also effective in detecting carriers.

Treatment

- Recombinant and immunoaffinity-purified forms of both factor VIII and IX are now available. These may be given at hemophilia centers, ERs, or refrigerated at home. Patients may now use home infusion if involved in minor trauma or hemarthrosis.
- Target factor activity following minor bleeding episode is >20%. Before surgery, target should be 100% with >50% maintained until healing is completed.
- Desmopressin (DDAVP) is also effective in acutely raising factor VIII levels, and may be used in mild hemophiliacs.
- Vaccinate for hepatitis at the time of diagnosis. Regular visits to hemophilia specialist are recommended.
- Genetic counseling as indicated.

Idiopathic Thrombocytopenic Purpura

Symptoms

Petechial hemorrhages, purpura, easy bruising, gingival bleeding, GI bleeding, recurrent and brisk nosebleeds, or spontaneous bleeding if platelet count <20,000. History may be positive for recent minor viral disease.

Diagnosis

Strictly a diagnosis of exclusion.
Physical exam: Petechiae, purpura, multiple ecchymoses, conjunctival hemorrhage, bleeding from minor trauma sites.
Labs: CBC shows normal WBCs and low platelets. Platelets may be significantly low to <20,000. Bleeding time often prolonged. PT/aPTT normal. Positive bound platelet-associated antibody (PA-IgG).
Imaging: CT head for possible intracranial bleeding if indicated.

Treatment

- Commonly self-limited to <2 months in younger patients. More common to progress to chronic form in older patients.

- Platelet transfusion only indicated for acute, profuse bleeding.

- Treat with corticosteroids (IV or oral) if platelet count <20,000 or <50,000 with symptoms. Intravenous immunoglobulin (IVIG) is used if steroids are not effective. Anti Rho(D) immune globulin (RhoGam) may also be tried instead of or including IVIG.

- Splenectomy is a last resort and generally reserved for chronic form that has failed other treatment.

Thrombotic Thrombocytopenic Purpura and Hemolytic Uremic Syndrome

Classic associations

Hemolytic uremic syndrome (HUS): Triad of hemolytic anemia, thrombocytopenia, and acute renal failure (ARF).

Thrombotic thrombocytopenic purpura (TTP): Pentad of HUS triad + fever and neurologic signs.

Symptoms

Much the same as other thrombocytopenic disorders with petechial hemorrhages, purpura, easy bruising, gingival bleeding, GI bleeding, recurrent and brisk nosebleeds, or other spontaneous bleeding if platelet count is decreased. Neurologic symptoms can include subtle changes such as confusion or severe headache. Focal, objective abnormalities are less frequent, but grand mal seizures and coma can occur. Age is often a clue to the disorder as HUS mainly occurs in children. Other past medical history may be disease-specific as follows:

HUS: Recent viral illness or infection with *Escherichia coli* 0157:H7 or *Shigella*.

TTP: Pregnancy, HIV positive, or oral contraceptive (OCP) use.

Diagnosis

Labs: CBC shows anemia and thrombocytopenia (often 35,000–100,000 range). LDH is elevated. Haptoglobin is decreased. Bilirubin is elevated. Peripheral smear may show schistocytes, burr cells, or helmet cells. Basic metabolic panel (BMP) often reveals renal failure (especially in HUS). Urinalysis may show blood, increased RBCs, or RBC casts.

Treatment

- Admission to the hospital or ICU is often needed.

- Supportive care with fluids and control of blood pressure is mandatory.

- Consider dialysis for significant renal failure.

- Mainstays of therapy include plasma exchange, FFP, or cryosupernatant.
- In refractory cases (or TTP) consider corticosteroids, vincristine, IVIG, rituximab (Rituxan), aspirin, and immunosuppresion with azathioprine or cyclophosphamide.
- DO NOT give platelet transfusion in TTP/HUS, they are contraindicated.

Answers

6.1 E. This patient has symptoms of multiple myeloma, which may be diagnosed by the investigation of three main areas: serum protein electrophoresis (SPEP) and/or urine protein electrophoresis (UPEP) for monoclonal spike, end-organ damage such as renal failure or lytic lesion on radiographic bone survey (*not* scintiography), or the presence of plasma cells on bone marrow biopsy.

6.2 E. Microcytic anemia is typically not seen in multiple myeloma unless another comorbid condition exists. Anemia, if present, tends to be normo or macrocytic. Other answers are typical for this disease.

6.3 A. This patient has symptoms and signs consistent with acute myelogenous leukemia. Diagnosis is supported by the demonstration of Auer rods on peripheral blood smear.

6.4 D. The most life-threatening complication of acute myelogenous leukemia (AML) is disseminated intravascular coagulation (DIC), which may be treated with fresh frozen plasma (FFP) or cryoprecipitate to replace clotting factors.

6.5 B. This patient has a long history of sickle cell disease, and multiple crises thus may likely have splenic dysfunction from autosplenectomy. This will cause increased vulnerability to encapsulated bacteria, commonly *Haemophilus, Pneumococcus, Meningococcus.*

Infections and Parasitic Diseases	139
Scabies	139
Candidiasis	140
Acne Vulgaris	141
Onychomycosis	142
Cellulitis/Erysipelas	143
Skin Abscess	145
Folliculitis	145
Impetigo	146
Viral Warts (Human Papillomavirus)	147
Skin Lesions	148
Squamous Cell Carcinoma	148
Basal Cell Carcinoma	149
Malignant Melanoma	150
Benign Skin Lesions	152
Psoriasis	155
Neurofibromatosis	157

Infections and Parasitic Diseases

Scabies

Symptoms

Itching and soreness between fingers and toes. Vesicles or papules may be seen.

Diagnosis

Physical exam: Look for burrow tracks between fingers or toes.
Labs: Scrap tracks and look under microscope. Classic picture is of microscopic parasite (see Figure 7.1).

Treatment

- Permethrin (Elimite, Acticin) or crotamiton (Eurax) topical cream applied from the neck to the soles of the feet. This is

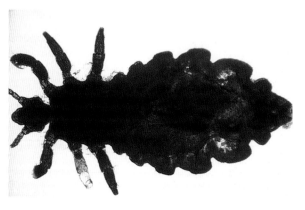

FIGURE 7.1 The female scabies mite.

Clinical Dermatology. Fifth edition. MacKie, RM. Copyright 2003. Oxford University Press.

left on, then washed off 12 h later. Reapplication in 1 week may be needed. Lindane (Kwell, Scabene) may also be used in this manner, but is somewhat more toxic and should not be used in the very young, pregnant, or old patients. Use precipitated sulfur in pregnant patients and ivermectin (Stromectol) in the immunocompromised.

- Diphenhydramine (Benadryl) for itching.

Q 7.1

Which treatment below is not indicated for cutaneous candidiasis?

A. Nystatin (Mycostatin).
B. Clotrimazole cream.
C. Econazole (Spectazole).
D. Ciclopirox (Loprox).
E. Griseofulvin.

Candidiasis

Symptoms

Erythematous, painful, itchy, well-demarcated patches, often in the intertriginous places. Lesions are often moist and malodorous and reveal classic "satellite lesions." History may reveal immunocompromised state (or risk factors) or diabetes.

Diagnosis

Usually a clinical diagnosis that can be made by exam.
Labs: Skin scrapings may be examined on potassium hydroxide slide. Branching pseudohyphae are pathopneumonic (see Figure 7.2).

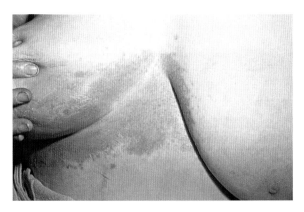

FIGURE 7.2 Inframammary candidiasis in a female diabetic patient.

Clinical Dermatology. Fifth edition. MacKie, RM. Copyright 2003. Oxford University Press.

Treatment

- Topical therapy often effective and include nystatin (Mycostatin), clotrimazole, econazole (Spectazole), ciclopirox (Loprox), sulconazole (Exelderm), or miconazole topicals. Ketoconazole (Nizoral) orally may be used if infection is refractory to topical treatments. If these are not effective or patient is immunocompromised, consider fluconazole (Diflucan) or itraconazole (Sporanox).

- Vaginal candidiasis is often treated with fluconazole (Diflucan) because of one-time convenient dosing.

Acne Vulgaris

Symptoms

Open or closed comedones, nodules, papules, pustules. Scarring may or may not be present.

Diagnosis

Characteristic appearance and history.

Physical exam: Lesions usually on face, forehead, neck, superior back, and anterior chest. Comedones and cystic lesions usually on erythematous base.

Treatment

- Should be stepwise. Anecdotal evidence exists that decreasing fat intake and basic daily hygiene show improvement. Wash face with nonoil-based soap at least twice per day.

- Start with benzoyl peroxide in the morning or at night. Increase to twice per day.

- Tretinoin (Retin-A) may be added, starting with the cream of lowest concentration and titrating up. Highly effective, but has several side effects such as sun sensitivity, reddening, severe drying, and interaction with benzoyl peroxide. These lessen with time, so counsel patient on compliance.

- Adapalene (Differin) cream or gel, tazarotene (Tazorac), or azelaic acid (Azelex) may be tried, but have similar side effects as Tretinoin.
- Antibiotic topicals such as erythromycin (Emgel, EryDerm), clindamycin (Cleocin-T), or metronidazole (Metrogel) may be effective.
- Systemic antibiotics such as tetracycline, minocycline, doxycycline, erythromycin, or TMP-SMX (Bactrim or Septra) are the next step. Avoid tetracyclines in young children/pregnant patients, and counsel that photosensitivity is the most common side effect.
- Consider systemic birth control pills for favorable side effect of reducing acne in women.
- Spironolactone may be effective because of antiandrogen properties, but watch for side effect of gynecomastia in men.
- As a last resort, referral may be considered to dermatology for isotretinoin (Accutane). Very effective, especially against severe, cystic form, but is very teratogenic. Patients must use at least two methods of birth control and be fully informed about the increased rates of cancer and psychiatric disturbances.
- All treatments take at least 4 weeks to show improvement and should not be expected to be immediate.

Q 7.2

A 51-year-old African American male comes to your clinic with complaints of yellow nails. He states nails on all his toes are thickened, yellow, and brittle. He has tried several over-the-counter medications, but nothing has helped. You consider placing him on an oral medication, what labs should be monitored during treatment?

A. BUN/creatinine.
B. Albumin, AST, ALT, PT/aPTT.
C. Na, K, Ca, Mg, Ph.
D. AST/ALT, platelet count.
E. Creatinine kinase (CK).
F. AST, ALT, and albumin alone.

Onychomycosis

Symptoms

Yellow, brittle, thickened nails, usually of the toes. Nonpainful, but may spread between nails and to opposite foot or hands.

Diagnosis

Labs: KOH preparation for branching hyphae is sensitive and specific. If negative, yeast culture is available, but takes 4–6 weeks and sensitivity is not much improved.

Biopsy also characteristic of yeast infection and may be the most sensitive technique, but often unnecessary.

Treatment

- Various topical regimens exist, but are widely regarded as ineffective against the vast majority of infections.
- Long-term oral therapies have been the classic treatments and include terbinafine (Lamisil), itraconazole (Sporanox), and fluconazole (Diflucan). Effectiveness varies with terbinafine (Lamisil) being the best, but also most expensive. Drawbacks include that treatment duration should be 12 weeks or longer. Obtain transaminases and CBC (for platelet count) at baseline and for routine monitoring while on terbinafine or transaminases, or on itraconazole. Intervals of monitoring are approximately 4–6 weeks. These medications are contraindicated with preexisting significant hepatic or renal disease. Have patient abstain from EtOH during therapy.
- Surgical excision of nail is an option if infection is restricted to only that nail, and this is acceptable to the patient.

Cellulitis/Erysipelas

Symptoms

Red, erythematous, painful, skin area without pustules or vesicles. Break in skin commonly identifiable, but not necessary for diagnosis. Often on extremities, but erysipelas more common on face.

Diagnosis

Physical exam: Macular/papular skin area with reasonably well-demarcated border. Area will be tender and warm, although should not significantly constrict the movement of underlying joint. Skin break may be obvious, but no fluctuance or expressible fluid should be present (consider accompanying abscess if these exist).
Labs: WBC may be increased. Culture any expressible fluid from skin breaks. Methicillin-resistant *Staphylococcus aureus* (MRSA) is now becoming common. Consider blood cultures as warranted.
Imaging: Unnecessary, unless exclusion of septic joint or osteomyelitis is considered. Ultrasound may reveal underlying fluid collection if present (see Figures 7.3 and 7.4).

Treatment

- Clean area and deroof any scab or skin break to evaluate for underlying abscess.
- Oral antiobiotics active against gram-positive bacteria are highly effective, and may be used on outpatient basis as first line. Use cephalexin (Keflex), TMP-SMX (Bactrim DS, Septra DS), dicloxacillin, erythromycin, or clindamycin.

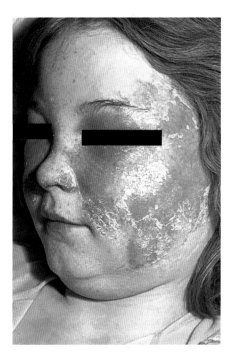

FIGURE 7.3 Erysipelas demonstrating well-defined borders and facial location.

Clinical Dermatology. Fifth edition. MacKie, RM. Copyright 2003. Oxford University Press.

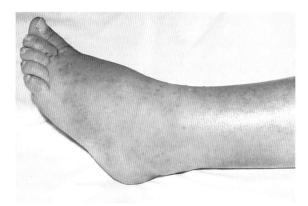

FIGURE 7.4 Cellulitis of lower extremity demonstrating swelling and erythema.

Clinical Dermatology. Fifth edition. MacKie, RM. Copyright 2003. Oxford University Press.

- Admission should be considered for toxic-appearing children, presence of sepsis, facial cellulitis, poor follow-up is likely, or suspicion of underlying bone infection.

- Inpatient management should include an IV regimen of penicillin G, nafcillin, clindamycin, cefozolin, or vancomycin for empiric therapy. If MRSA prevalence is high in the local area, consider more than one antibiotic such as IV clindamycin and PO TMP-SMX (Bactrim DS, Septra DS) as regimen. Vancomycin is also effective against MRSA, but requires good kidney function and has its own resistance patterns. New medications are evolving, including tigecycline (Tygacil) for IV use.

Skin Abscess

Symptoms

Formation of fluctuant mass, usually under skin break, or scab formation. Usually extremely tender to palpation and often surrounded by cellulitis or erysipelas. Deroofing of scab or opening of skin break may demonstrate pus or fluid drainage. Gentle pressure may be needed. History may reveal "skin popping" by drug user or prior skin break or superficial injury in the location over abscess.

Diagnosis

Usually a clinical diagnosis of the existence of abscess. If no obvious skin break is detected, needle aspiration may be used and can distinguish abscess from other cystic structures.

Labs: Culture all fluids from the abscess. Blood cultures are warranted as well, but are often negative.

Imaging: Ultrasound may be useful in demonstrating fluid-filled pocket under the skin.

If IV drug user, consider HIV or drug screen.

Treatment

- "The only way to treat an abscess is to cut an abscess." Incision and drainage are the standard of care, although antibiotics are warranted for accompanying skin infection (see cellulitis/erysipelas). Once drained, break up loculations with sterile instrument and pack with sterile packing (Iodoform Gauze). Change/repack q.d.-b.i.d. until healed. Packing ensures further fluid would not accumulate and healing will occur from the inside wall of abscess.

Folliculitis

Symptoms

Often occurring in groups, lesions may generally be <5 mm diameter, pruritic, erythematous, tender, and with central protrusion of hair shaft. Lesions may occur in bathing suit distribution such as in "hot-tub folliculitis."

Diagnosis

Culture of expressible fluid usually not necessary, but may reveal group A *Streptococcus*, *S. aureus*, or *Pseudomonas* (in hot-tub folliculitis).

Treatment

- Hot-tub folliculitis is usually self-limited, and systemic antibiotics do not shorten course.

- Topical mupirocin (Bactroban) may be used and is usually sufficient therapy.

- In more severe cases, give cephalexin (Keflex), erythromycin, or dicloxacillin.
- Recurrent folliculitis often indicates carrier state, which is most commonly in the anterior nares. Treat with mupirocin (Bactroban) topical t.i.d. for 5 days every month for 2 months to reduce outbreaks.

Impetigo

Symptoms

Classic "honey crusted" appearance of grouped lesions with mild surrounding erythema. Often lesions are tender, but generally nonpurulent. Distribution, especially in the young, is often around mouth, lower face, and on fingers/hands.

Diagnosis

Clinical diagnosis of typical appearance (see Figure 7.5).

Treatment

- Topical treatment with mupirocin (Bactroban) is often adequate for mild-to-moderate disease. Consider systemic antibiotics for the very young or severe cases. PO regimens include erythromycin, cephalexin (Keflex), and dicloxacillin.
- Cover or dress affected areas to keep children from scratching and auto-infecting other body parts.

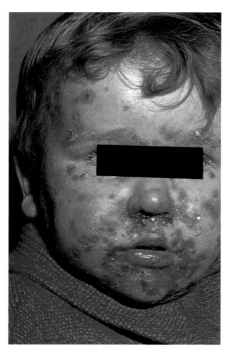

FIGURE 7.5 Classic Impetigo.

Clinical Dermatology. Fifth edition. MacKie, RM. Copyright 2003. Oxford University Press.

Viral Warts (Human Papillomavirus)

Symptoms

Nonerythematous skin colored or slightly hyperpigmented nodules. Often occur on hands, plantar surface of feet, genitals, or practically anywhere on the body. Caused by various serotypes of human papillomavirus (HPV).

Diagnosis

Physical exam: Verrrucous appearance. Plantar warts have characteristic "black dots" in the lesion itself, which consist of capillaries induced by the virus (see Figures 7.6 and 7.7).

Labs: Biopsy often not needed.

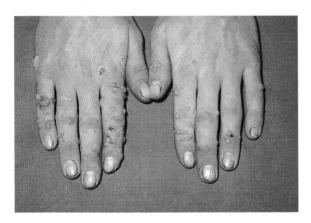

FIGURE 7.6 Multiple warts on hands.

Clinical Dermatology. Fifth edition. MacKie, RM. Copyright 2003. Oxford University Press

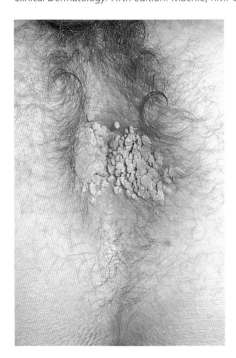

FIGURE 7.7 Extensive perivulvar warts.

Clinical Dermatology. Fifth edition. MacKie, RM. Copyright 2003. Oxford University Press.

Treatment

- Various treatments and topicals exist.
- In-office procedures include paring lesion down with a scalpel or razor, then applying electrocautery or cryotherapy. Have the patient return every week until lesion is cured. Some laser treatments also exist for stubborn plantar warts.
- Medications include salicylic acid 40% topical, trichloroacetic acid (Tri-Chlor), imiquimod (Aldara). In severe cases, podophyllin topical or Bleomycin injection may be used. Topicals take on the order of months, so do not expect quick results.

Skin Lesions

Squamous Cell Carcinoma

Symptoms

Small, usually isolated, lesions occur in sun-exposed areas and consist of exophytic nodules, which are commonly scaly, red, crusting, and occasionally bleed and become tender. Patient may have previously been treated or diagnosed with **actinic keratosis**.

Diagnosis

Characteristic appearance: Biopsy shows abnormal, cancerous cells all the way to the dermis (see Figure 7.8).

Treatment

- Prevention is the key.
- Otherwise, surgery is the best treatment for most lesions or those that occur in sensitive sites such as around the mouth, ear, or

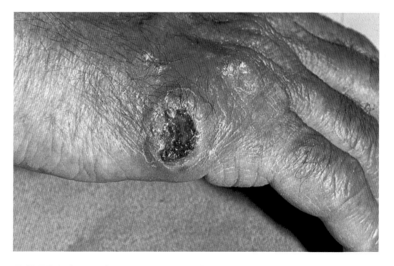

FIGURE 7.8 Invasive squamous carcinoma.

Clinical Dermatology. Fifth edition. MacKie, RM. Copyright 2003. Oxford University Press.

genitals. Surgical excision may be done in conjunction with biopsy of lesions with high initial malignancy suspicion, but care must be taken to include the whole lesion within the margins of the biopsy.

- Other techniques such as cryosurgery, electrodessication, topical 5-FU, and other topicals exist, but should only be used for low-risk lesions.

- Radiation therapy may be used for those lesions that involve cosmetically sensitive areas *and* are of low risk. Side effects, however, do exist, which may be intolerable to the patient.

- Moh's micrographic surgery is another option for skin cancer and involves specialty surgery referral. Indications include recurrent lesion, ill-defined borders, underlying tissue involvement, multiple clumped lesions, or lesion in prior radiation-exposed areas.

Basal Cell Carcinoma

Most frequent skin malignancy.

Symptoms

Often occurs in sun-exposed areas and on the face it appears like a small nodule or papule with translucent covering or ulceration, commonly with overlying telangiectasias. May have pearly white areas and bleed without healing.

Diagnosis

Characteristic appearance.

Biopsy is mandatory (see Figure 7.9).

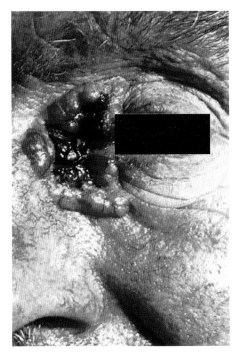

FIGURE 7.9 Basal cell carcinoma of left perinasal region.

Clinical Dermatology. Fifth edition. MacKie, RM. Copyright 2003. Oxford University Press.

Treatment

- Biopsy results, location, age, and cosmetic outcome must be taken into account when choosing treatment.

- Options include electrodessication, cryotherapy, local radiation, and surgical excision.

- Moh's micrographic surgery is an option, but involves specialty surgery referral.

Q 7.3

A 56-year-old male accountant returns to your office for followup after a previous biopsy revealed the presence of superficial spreading melanoma. He is fairly upset and desires to know more about the disease. According to the Breslow's and Clark's classification schemes for staging, what is the most important factor in prognosis?

A. Greatest diameter in millimeters.
B. Presence of other lesions in the same dermatome.
C. Depth of the lesion.
D. Vascular supply of the underlying skin region.
E. Immunologic state of the patient.

Malignant Melanoma

Symptoms

May be asymptomatic for years, hence the opportunity for lethal metastasis. Otherwise, lesions are usually discrete and occur in sun-exposed areas.

Diagnosis

Physical exam: Look for border irregularity, asymmetric shape, variegated color throughout lesion, elevation above skin surface, and large diameter (>6 mm).

Four main histologic types: Superficial spreading, nodular, acral-lentiginous, lentigo maligna.

Biopsy any suspicious lesion all the way to the subcutaneous fat, since grading/staging depends on depth.

Classification systems include the combination of two staging systems: **Breslow's,** which classifies based on depth of invasion in millimeters, and **Clark's,** which classifies based on anatomic skin level. The deeper in either system, the worse the prognosis.

Evaluate for metastatic spread to other systems with appropriate imaging. Melanoma spreads everywhere (see Figures 7.10–7.13).

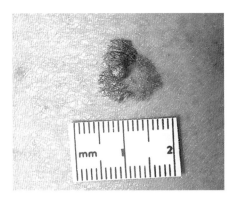

FIGURE 7.10 Superficial spreading melanoma.

Clinical Dermatology. Fifth edition. MacKie, RM. Copyright 2003. Oxford University Press.

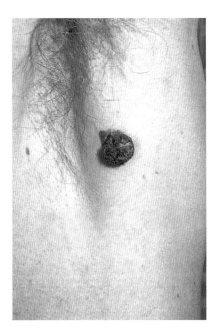

FIGURE 7.11 Nodular melanoma of left axilla.

Clinical Dermatology. Fifth edition. MacKie, RM. Copyright 2003. Oxford University Press.

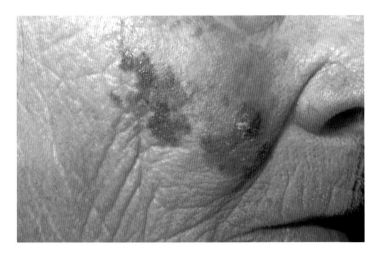

FIGURE 7.12 Lentigo maligna melanoma.

Clinical Dermatology. Fifth edition. MacKie, RM. Copyright 2003. Oxford University Press.

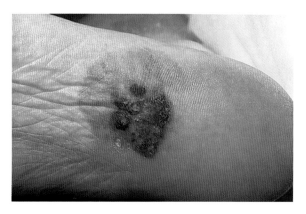

FIGURE 7.13 Acral melanoma.

Clinical Dermatology. Fifth edition. MacKie, RM. Copyright 2003. Oxford University Press.

Treatment

- Surgical excision is the treatment in all cases. Clear horizontal margin amount depends on the depth of lesion, and safe amounts are still somewhat in debate. Sentinel lymph node biopsy is sometimes done with or without regional lymph node dissection.

- For metastatic disease, radiation and chemotherapy are both effective.

- After treatment, surveillance measures include weekly patient skin checks, physician-conducted skin checks every 3–6 months, and yearly chest x-rays.

Q 7.4
Correctly pair the benign skin lesion with the skin malignancy it is associated with,

A. Seborrheic keratosis and basal cell carcinoma.
B. Compound nevus and melanoma.
C. Actinic keratosis and squamous cell carcinoma.
D. Acrochordons and squamous cell carcinoma.
E. Pyogenic granuloma and lentigo maligna melanoma.

Benign Skin Lesions

See Table 7.1.

TABLE 7.1 Common benign skin lesions

Lesion	Appearance/associations	Treatment	Appearance
Actinic keratosis	Associated with aging; appear very scaly, rough, nonpainful. Conversion to squamous cell cancer uncommon, but possible	Cryotherapy, electrodessication, laser therapy, dermabrasion, or trichloroacetic acid topical. Biopsy if not clinically obvious to exclude malignancy	See Figure 7.14
Seborrheic keratosis	"Stuck on" appearance of elevated nodule. Brown color and rough feel	Cryotherapy, electrodessication, shave biopsy, or topical trichloroacetic acid	See Figure 7.15
Hypertrophic scar formation (Keloid)	More common in dark-skinned individuals. Complication of late healing	Steroid injection, radiation therapy, dermabrasion, pressure dressings, or surgical removal and debulking	
Acrochordons (skin tags)	Small, often pedunculated, skin-colored lesions usually on opposing surfaces of skin such as under breasts, between legs, and axilla. Often also occur on lateral neck	Cryotherapy, shave biopsy, electrodessication	
Keratocanthoma	Usually rapid-onset, flesh-colored lesion with eventual central depression exhibiting plug of kertatinous material. Clinically similar to squamous cell cancer, but has no malignant potential	Excisional biopsy is most common, but 5-FU or steroid injection may also be effective with better cosmesis. Eventual involution often occurs	See Figure 7.16
Lipoma	Subcutaneous rubbery mass that feels unattached to overlying skin. Literally a benign fat cell tumor	Surgical removal. Recurrence is common, so repeat surgery may be needed	
Pyogenic granuloma	Usually, rapidly growing, often pedunculated mass, which is characteristically friable with frequent bleeding. May occur on extremities after minor skin trauma	Surgical excision, electrocaudery, or cryotherapy are the usual treatment	See Figure 7.17

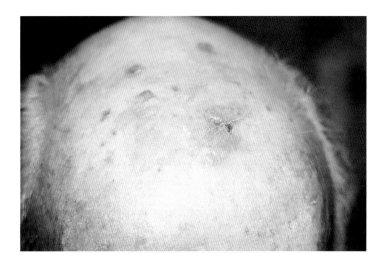

FIGURE 7.14 Actinic Keratoses on scalp.

Clinical Dermatology. Fifth edition. MacKie, RM. Copyright 2003. Oxford University Press.

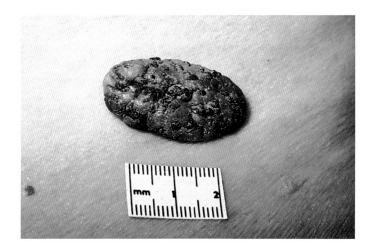

FIGURE 7.15 Classic Seborrheic Keratosis with "stuck on" appearance.

Clinical Dermatology. Fifth edition. MacKie, RM. Copyright 2003. Oxford University Press.

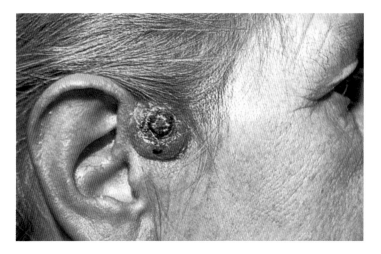

FIGURE 7.16 Keratocantoma of the right peri-aural skin.

Clinical Dermatology. Fifth edition. MacKie, RM. Copyright 2003. Oxford University Press.

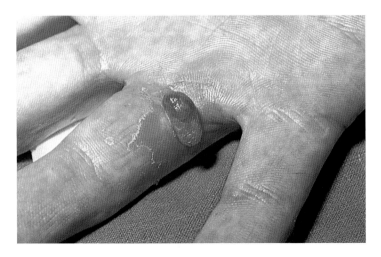

FIGURE 7.17 Pyogenic granuloma of finger.

Clinical Dermatology. Fifth edition. MacKie, RM. Copyright 2003. Oxford University Press.

Q 7.5

A 47-year-old Caucasian female comes to your clinic for the evaluation of worsening rash. Her symptoms include red, scaly, silvery, well-demarcated plaques mainly on the extensor aspects of extremities. She has noticed pitting of her nails during this time, which she cannot explain. She states her mother and sister both have similar rashes and they must have passed some sort of infection between them. You conduct a thorough medical history and records review, and discover she is on several oral medications including atenolol (Tenormin) for hypertension (HTN), oral contraceptive pills (OCPs), tretinoin (Retin-A) for acne, etanercept (Enbrel) for rheumatoid arthritis, and guaifenesin (Robitussin) for chest congestion. Which of these medications may be contributing to her condition?

A. Atenolol (Tenormin).
B. OCPs.
C. Tretinoin (Retin-A).
D. Etanercept (Enbrel).
E. Guaifenesin (Robitussin).

Psoriasis

Symptoms

Patients present with intermittent scaly, silvery, erythematous, well-demarcated, ovoid or circinate, patches, or plaques. Sometimes these are pruritic and may occur on the scalp, knee, nails, extensor surfaces of extremities, elbows, eyebrows, sacral area, buttocks, penis, axillae, umbilicus, or, more rarely, may be generalized. Family history may be positive for psoriasis or other immunologic abnormality. Flares may occur after direct skin injury (Koebner phenomenon), use of antimalarial agents, β-blockers, and lithium. Other medications may make the existing disease worse including angiotensin-converting enzyme inhibitors (ACEIs), nonsteroidal antiinflammatory drugs (NSAIDs), tetracycline, amiodarone, salicylates, and penicillins.

A variant includes psoriatic arthritis, which is a clinical entity that involves the joints and mimics rheumatoid arthritis.

Diagnosis

Physical exam: Scaly, silvery, flaking patch or papule as described earlier. Nails may show stippling, pitting, and onycholysis, which resembles onychomycosis.

Clinical diagnosis is usually adequate.

Biopsy is rarely indicated and exhibits immune involvement and characteristic appearance.

Labs: Fungal studies may/may not reveal overlying fungal infection; rheumatoid factor should be negative; leukocytosis and increased ESR may be present in acute flair; rarely anemia with vitamin B_{12}/folate or iron deficiency is present (see Figures 7.18 and 7.19).

Treatment

- Sun exposure and UVA/UVB phototherapy are commonly used with good results mainly in generalized disease. Add psoralen plus ultraviolet A (PUVA) for added efficacy.

- Topical moisturizers and occlusive dressings that are aimed at decreasing dryness are effective.

- Topicals such as corticosteroids, coal tar solutions, retinoids such as tazarotene (Tazorac) and calcipotriene (Dovonex), or topical immunomodulators such as tacrolimus (Protopic), anthralin, or pimecrolimus (Elidel) may be used for mild-to-moderate disease.

- For generalized or severe disease, methotrexate (classic), cyclosporine, or newer systemic immune modulating therapies such

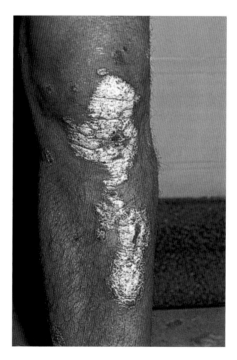

FIGURE 7.18 Typical appearance of psoriasis vulgaris occurring on the leg.

Clinical Dermatology. Fifth edition. MacKie, RM. Copyright 2003. Oxford University Press.

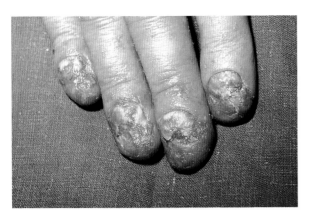

FIGURE 7.19 Severe destructive psoriasis of the finger nails. Note pitting, onycholysis, and destruction of nails.

Clinical Dermatology. Fifth edition. MacKie, RM. Copyright 2003. Oxford University Press.

as alefacept (Amevive), efalizumab (Raptiva), or etanercept (Enbrel).

- Refer to dermatology as needed.

Neurofibromatosis

Type I: von Recklinghausen disease.
Type II: Bilateral acoustic neurofibromatosis.

Symptoms/Diagnosis

Symptoms vary depending on type. Family history is often positive for autosomal dominant inheritance in either type.

Type I:
- **Café-au-lait macules** ($\geq$6 if prepubertal, $\geq$15 if adult) measuring 5 mm or more
- Two or more neurofibromas
- Axillary or inguinal freckling
- Two or more Lisch nodules of the eye (hamartomas of the iris)
- Optic glioma
- Characteristic osseous lesions (long bone cortical thinning, mild scoliosis)
- First-degree relative with neurofibromatosis type 1 (NF1).

Also may be associated with learning disabilities or attention deficit hyperactivity disorder (ADHD).

Imaging: Obtain screening plain films of spine, long bones, skull. Obtain MRI of brain including optic nerves and spine.

Examine retina with slit lamp.

Type II:
- Bilateral acoustic/vestibular schwannomas.
- Family history of NF2.

- Family history of neurofibroma, meningioma, glioma, or unilateral schwannoma.

Imaging: MRI of the brain.

Consider brainstem auditory evoked response (BAER) with audiologic evaluation.

Treatment

- Type I

    - General outpatient follow-up with symptomatic control as needed.

    - Referral to neurosurgeon for complications of CNS tumor or glioma.

    - Consider psychological referral for learning disability if present.

    - Referral to neurosurgery/orthopedic surgery for scoliosis as needed.

- Type II

    - Annual exams including neurologic, ophthalmologic, and audiologic.

    - Hearing aids as needed.

    - Speech therapy as needed.

    - Neurosurgery evaluation for any CNS tumors.

- Families with either type will benefit from genetic counseling.

Answers

7.1 E. Griseofulvin is generally ineffective and not recommended in the treatment of candidiasis. This is likely due to candidiasis being caused by a yeast, and griseofulvin being more effective against dermatophytes.

7.2 D. This patient likely has onychomycosis. Treatment regimen is most effective if systemic, and may include terbinafine (Lamisil), itraconazole (Sporanox), or fluconazole (Diflucan). Terbinafine and itraconazole require baseline and periodic monitoring of transaminases/platelet level or transaminases alone, respectively.

7.3 C. Breslow's staging system relies on depth of the lesion in millimeters and Clark's relies on anatomic skin layer involvement, both of which are measures of skin depth. Both these systems correlate greater depth with poorer prognosis.

7.4 C. There is an association between malignant transformation of actinic keratosis and squamous cell carcinomas.

7.5 A. This patient likely has psoriasis. β-blocking agents have been implicated in the worsening of psoriasis, and is likely contributing to this patient's condition. A trial of alternate hypertension (HTN) medication will likely produce improvement.

8   Musculoskeletal System

Systemic Lupus Erythematosus	160
Rheumatoid Arthritis	162
Internal Derangement of the Knee	164
Afflictions of the Shoulder	165
Bursitis	167
Tendonitis	167
Infectious Tenosynovitis of the Hand	168
Ganglion Cyst	169
Rhabdomyolysis	169
Myositis	170
Collagen Vascular Diseases	170
Osteoporosis	172
Developmental Musculoskeletal Deformities	173
Spondylosis	174
Ankylosing Spondylitis	174
Intervertebral Disc Herniation	175
Spinal Stenosis	176
Malignant Metastases	177
Skull Fracture	177
Fractures	178
Infective Arthritis	179
Temporomandibular Joint Syndrome	180
Ankle Sprain	181
Osteoarthritis	182

Systemic Lupus Erythematosus

Symptoms

A multiorgan, systemic disease that occurs more often in African American women, manifesting as the symptoms shown in Table 8.1.

Diagnosis

Diagnosis is based on a combination of signs/symptoms and laboratory testing. Table 8.2 shows the criteria from the American College of Rheumatology. Systemic lupus erythematosus (SLE) diagnosis needs 4 of the 11 criteria during any period of observation.

TABLE 8.1 Common symptoms of SLE

System	Symptoms
Constitutional	Fatigue, fever, weight loss
Skin	Malar (butterfly) rash, photosensitive rash, alopecia, mucous membrane lesions, Raynaud's phenomenon, purpura, urticaria
Musculoskeletal	Arthritis (multiple joints), arthralgia, myositis
Renal	Hematuria, proteinuria, cellular casts
Hematologic	Anemia, thrombocytopenia, leukopenia
Lymph	Lymphadenopathy, splenomegaly
Neurological	Seizures, transverse myelitis, cranial neuropathies, peripheral neuropathies
Psychiatric	Psychosis, depression, anxiety
Gastrointestinal	Nausea, vomiting, abdominal pain, peritonitis
Cardiac	Pericarditis, endocarditis, myocarditis, pericardial effusion

TABLE 8.2 Criteria for the diagnosis of SLE

Criteria	Description
Malar rash	Rash on face in "butterfly" pattern, sparing the nasolabial folds
Discoid rash	Erythematous, raised patches with scaling and follicular plugging. Scarring possibly present
Photosensitivity	Skin rash made worse by sun exposure
Oral ulcers	Painless oral or pharyngeal ulcers
Arthritis	Nonerosive, swollen, tender joints. Two or more in peripheral areas
Serositis	Pleuritic chest pain, pleural rub, or pleural effusion. Pericarditis, pericardial effusion, ECG changes, or cardiac rub
Renal disorder	Protienuria >500 mg per 24 h or >3+ on dipstick. Cellular casts in urine
Neurologic disorder	Seizures or psychosis in the absence of other reasons for either
Hematologic disorder	Hemolytic anemia, reticulocytosis, or leukopenia, lymphopenia, or thrombocytopenia on two or more occasions
Immunologic disorder	Anti-dsDNA, anti-SM, antiphospholipid antibody as measured by anticardiolipin antibody IgG and IgM. Presence of lupus anticoagulant. False-positive testing for syphilis (VDRL)
Antinuclear antibody (ANA)	ANA titer positive

Anti-SM, anti-Smith; dsDNA, double-stranded deoxyribonucleic acid.
SLE diagnosis needs 4 of the 11 criteria during any period of observation.

Source: Summarized from Hochberg, MC. Updating the American College of Rheumatology Revised Criteria for the Classification of Systemic Lupus Erythematosus (letter). *Arthritis Rheum* (1997) 40:1725.

Treatment

- Sunscreen and UV light avoidance for those who are photosensitive.

- Skin manifestations respond well to topical (intermediate-to-high strength) glucocorticoids.

- Mild disease, arthralgias, mild fevers, and other symptoms may respond well to nonsteroidal antiinflammatory drugs (NSAIDs). Short-course glucocorticoids are commonly used clinically, although no specific evidence has shown benefit.

- Antimalarials, classically hydroxychloroquine (Plaquenil), are the next step for mild-to-moderate disease. In practice, several antimalarial regimens have shown good response.

- Systemic corticosteroids are indicated for more serious, multiorgan disease. Prompt initiation may prevent irreversible damage to the kidneys and liver. Hospitalization and high-dose IV corticosteroids may be indicated.

- Other immunomodulating medications may be added if disease is thought to be severe or progressive. These include cyclophosphamide (Cytoxan), methotrexate (Trexall), chlorambucil (Leukeran), cyclosporine (Gengraf), or nitrogen mustard. Use of these medications should be attempted only with the guidance of a rheumatologist.

- Intravenous immunoglobulin (IVIG) may be helpful in those with severe thrombocytopenia.

- If steroids are used, minimize dose and length of therapy to avoid steroid-associated side effects.

- Remember to vaccinate and refer for routine ophthalmologic exams.

Q 8.2

A 59-year-old Latino female comes to your outpatient office practice with complaints of neck pain and paresthesias of her arms and fingers. She states that the neck pain radiates to the occiput and is made worse by forward flexion. Paresthesias have progressed over a period of months and are described as nonpainful feelings of pins and needles in the forearms and hands. Her past medical history is significant for rheumatoid arthritis, hypertension, lumbar vertebral osteoarthritis and several bone spurs, and hyperlipidemia. Based on this history, what is the most likely diagnosis of her symptoms?

A. Atlantoaxial subluxation.
B. Bone spur formation in the cervical region.
C. Occult cervical fracture.
D. Degenerative disease causing nerve compression of the cervical region.
E. Anxiety.

Rheumatoid Arthritis

Symptoms

Pain, morning stiffness, deformity, heat, and resistance to motion occur in multiple joints including shoulders, wrists, knees, elbows, ankles, feet, and subtalar joints. Deformity, especially of hands, is often noticed in later stages. Systemic symptoms may be present as well and include fatigue, depression, malaise, anorexia, rheumatoid nodules, and entrapment neuropathies.

Comorbid conditions include **atlantoaxial joint subluxation**, carpal tunnel syndrome, Baker's cyst rupture, episcleritis, Sjögren's syndrome, pulmonary fibrosis, hepatosplenomegaly, Hashimoto's thyroiditis, pleuritis, lung nodules, pericarditis, and myocarditis.

Diagnosis

Physical exam: Inflamed, stiff joints, especially in the hands. In later stages, classic hand deformities show metacarpophalangeal (MCP) and proximal interphalangeal (PIP) involvement producing **"Swan-neck"** finger deformity, "Boutonnière's deformity," ulnar deviation of the fingers, and **sparing of the distal interphalangeal (DIP) joints** (see Figure 8.1).

Diagnosis is made by the combination of history, physical exam, x-ray, and laboratory results.

Table 8.3 shows the criteria from the American College of Rheumatology.

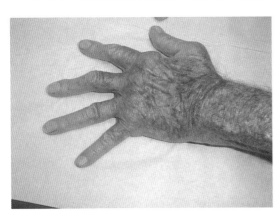

FIGURE 8.1 Rheumatoid arthritis of the hand showing ulnar deviation and Swan-neck deformity of the fingers. Note relative sparring of the distal interphalangeal (DIP) joints.

Courtesy: Charlie Goldberg, MD. University of California, San Diego School of Medicine, San Diego VA Medical Center.

TABLE 8.3 Criteria for RA diagnosis

Criteria	Description
Morning stiffness	Lasting >1 h
Arthritis in three or more joints	Soft tissue swelling or effusion in the wrist, PIP, MCP, elbow, knee, ankle, or MTP
Hand joint involvement	Involvement of the wrist, MCP, or PIP joints
Symmetric arthritis	Both right and left joints involved
Rheumatoid nodules	Subcutaneous nodules in the areas surrounding affected joints
Serum rheumatoid factor (RF) positive	Positive RF
Radiological changes	Typical erosions or loss of density in affected joints

Diagnosis should include four or more criteria which are required to be present for ≥6 weeks.

MCP, metacarpophalangeal; MTP, metatarsophalangeal; PIP, proximal interphalangeal.

Source: Summarized from Saraux A, Berthelot M, Chales G, Le Henaff C, Thorei JB, Hoang S, et al. Ability of the American College of Rheumatology 1987 Criteria to Predict Rheumatoid Arthritis in Patients with Early Arthritis and Classification of these Patients Two Years Later. *Arthritis Rheum* (2001)44:2485–91.

Labs: CBC for mild anemia, ESR/CRP usually elevated, antinuclear antibody (ANA) positive in 20%–30% patients, rheumatoid factor (RF) is as shown in Table 8.3, comprehensive metabolic panel (CMP) for electrolytes, renal, and liver involvement.

Joint aspiration and fluid analysis.

Imaging: Obtain plain radiographs of chest, cervical spine, and affected joints as needed.

Treatment

- NSAIDs should be used for first-line therapy, but should not be used alone.

- Glucocorticoids are very effective in rheumatoid arthritis (RA) treatment but have long-term side effects. Thus, they may be useful in shorter courses for acute flares or as "bridging" therapy when disease-modifying antirheumatic drugs (DMARDs) are started. Intraarticular injections may also be used for acute flares of joint symptoms.

- DMARDs are the mainstay of therapy and include methotrexate (Trexall), hydroxychloroquine (Plaquenil), sulfasalazine (Azulfidine), leflunomide (Arava), infliximab (Remicade), and etanercept (Enbrel). Sulfasalazine or hydroxychloroquine often are started first, but in more severe cases, methotrexate or combination therapy may be the first-line treatment.

- Monitoring is common for each DMARD and often done with periodic CBCs and surveillance for infection.

- Nonmedicinal treatments such as rest, acupuncture, and hot baths, have shown some benefit but research is still lacking.

Internal Derangement of the Knee

See Table 8.4.

Imaging: MRI is the best modality for all the above, since it allows the visualization of ligaments. Plain x-rays may assess fracture.

Treatment

- NSAIDs acutely and subacutely. Further pain control may be necessary at the time of injury. Rest, ice, and elevation may help with initial swelling.

- Definitive treatment is surgery and repair. Posterior cruciate ligament (PCL) injuries are often deferred without surgery.

- Physical therapy and rehabilitation are often useful.

- Brace may symptomatically help in the interim but has not been shown to improve outcomes.

TABLE 8.4 Common knee injuries

Derangement	Injury	Physical exam
Anterior cruciate ligament (ACL) tear	Twisting or rotary motion of the knee. Often in planting since this is a sequential motion, the description should "then" be turning motions	*Lachman test*—Best overall test. Flex knee to 30°, stabilize the femur, and apply anterior/posterior force to proximal tibia. Positive test is "soft" or "boggy" endpoint. *Anterior drawer sign*—In 90° flexion, lower leg is stabilized and anterior force applied to tibia, anterior laxity with "boggy" endpoint indicates positive
Posterior cruciate ligament (PCL) tear	Fall while foot is plantar-flexed with knee in flexion or as a dashboard injury in motor vehicle accident	*Post-drawer sign*—In 90° flexion, stabilize the lower leg and apply posterior force to anterior tibia, posterior laxity with "boggy" endpoint indicates positive
Medial collateral ligament (MCL)	Stress or blow to knee on the lateral side. Often occurs in football-tackling injuries	*Valgus stress test*—Place knee in 30° flexion and apply valgus stress to lower leg; medial laxity or pain indicates positive
Lateral collateral ligament (LCL)	Skiing, football, or soccer injuries	*Varus stress test*—Place knee in 30° flexion and apply varus stress to lower leg; lateral laxity or pain indicates positive
Meniscal tear	Running, basketball, or unknown injury	*Apley compression test*—In prone position with knee in 90° flexion, place downward force on heel to load knee; pain or click on rotation of foot indicates positive. *McMurray test*—While supine, begin with 90° flexion and simultaneously apply varus and valgus stress while extending and flexing knee. Pain or clicking indicates positive

Afflictions of the Shoulder

See Table 8.5.

Imaging: Shoulder x-ray (three views) is indicated if acute injury is suspected. Rotator cuff tear or pathology is sometimes visible by the narrowing of joint space. Shoulder arthrography has historically been useful but is now being replaced by MRI/MR arthrography. Ultrasound may demonstrate large tears but is limited with tears <1 cm. If suspicious of tear, obtain MRI.

Treatment

- Pain control with NSAIDs.

- **Rotator cuff and impingement:** Injection of painful area with mix of local anesthetic and steroid is often useful. This reduces inflammation and provides immediate relief. Be certain not to inject tendons. Rest from inciting event. Refer for physical therapy. Consider surgery after conservative treatment failure.

- **Anterior dislocation:** May be treated with gentle traction on the arm or "hanging weight." Humoral head often relocates after a

TABLE 8.5 Common shoulder injuries

Derangement	Injury	Physical exam
Rotator cuff tear	Fall on outstretched arm, fall on shoulder, excessive pulling (lawn mower engine starting), etc. SITS muscles of rotator cuff: **S**upraspinatus, **I**nfraspinatus, **T**eres minor, **S**ubscapularis	Test range of motion, strength of motion, and isolate muscles as needed. Specific tests are as follows: *Drop arm test*—fully abduct the shoulder and have patient actively, slowly lower extended arm to side. Pain on attempt or "dropping" of the arm indicates supraspinatus weakness/tear *Isometric supraspinatus test*—with elbow flexed 90°, abduct the shoulder 45° and have the patient attempt abduction against isometric resistance; pain indicates positive *Isometric infraspinatus test*—with shoulder hanging to side and elbow flexed 90°, have the patient externally rotate against isometric resistance; pain indicates positive
Impingement	Rotator cuff tendon inflammation	*Hawkin's test*—stabilize the shoulder with one hand, 90° flex the shoulder and 90° flex the elbow. Pain on internal rotation indicates impingement *Passive painful arc maneuver*—with arm at side, in full internal rotation, and elbow flexed at 90°, stabilize the shoulder with one hand and passively flex the shoulder. Pain or shrugging indicates impingement *Empty can test*—with shoulder flexed at 90° with extended elbow and hand in pronation; pain with attempting full flexion against resistance indicates impingement
Biceps tendonitis	Repetitive motion or weightbearing on flexed arm. May occur with the occupation of repetitive lifting	*Speed's test*—with extended elbow and shoulder flexed to 30°, have patient flex shoulder against resistance. Pain indicates positive *Yergason's test*—With shoulder hanging at side and elbow flexed to 90° and forearm in full pronation, grasp patient's hand (as if to shake) and have patient supinate against resistance; pain indicates positive
Dislocation	Anterior dislocation occurs with blow to lateral or posterior shoulder, often repetitive. Posterior dislocation is associated with seizures, electrocutions, and motor vehicle accidents	Look for deformity and prominent humoral head. Often acutely painful *Apprehension test*—with abduction of the shoulder to 90° and flexion of elbow 90°; fear of dislocation or pain on external rotation and anterior pressure to shoulder indicates positive

few minutes. A short duration in a sling is usually adequate for full recovery. If recurrent, consider referral to orthopedist for possible surgery to tighten ligaments.

- Surgery is indicated for posterior shoulder dislocation and repair of rotator cuff tears.

- Physical therapy and rehabilitation are often useful.

Bursitis

Symptoms

Pain, tenderness, and mildly limited range of motion of the affected joint. Bursa may have effusion present, which may become infected. History is often positive for overuse or repeated direct trauma when not otherwise seen, such as in the "weekend warrior."

Diagnosis

Physical exam: Tender area to direct palpation over bursal area. Pain is generally superficial and easily evoked. If infection is present, erythema, effusion, swelling, and fluctuance are evident. Common sites are olecranon, prepatellar, subdeltoid, trochanteric, and radiohumeral.

Labs: Generally unnecessary, but CBC shows leukocytosis with infection.

Treatment

- NSAIDs are helpful for pain.
- Rest, ice, compression, and elevation (RICE) may be helpful acutely.
- Treat infection if present with broad-spectrum oral antibiotics; cover for skin bacteria.
- Injection with steroid/lidocaine mix may help pain and speed healing.

Tendonitis

Symptoms

Pain and tenderness of tendon commonly at the origin of muscle or insertion of tendon. Often after exertion and made worse by flexion of nearby joints. History is often positive for overuse in sporting event or vigorous repetition.

Diagnosis

Physical exam: Tenderness on isolated contraction of the affected muscle and tendon. Weakness elicited by same maneuver, but tendon integrity should be preserved.

Imaging: If in doubt, MRI is the best visualization modality. Often not needed. Plain x-ray may show calcific deposits in repeated or chronic tendonitis.

Treatment

- Limit affected muscle use and exertion. This may be done with sling or counseling.
- NSAIDs are often helpful for pain.
- Advance to physical therapy after patient is pain free.
- For epicondylitis, forearm bands may be helpful in long-term recovery but work by limiting range of motion.

- Injection of steroid/lidocaine mix to the surrounding tendon sheath provides acute relief.

- Complete healing generally takes 4–6 weeks.

Q 8.3

A 21-year-old Caucasian female comes to the ER for evaluation of a cat bite she received from her new kitten 4 days ago. Her vital signs are now normal and she is afebrile. Exam reveals a swollen, very tender right finger with erythema extending down the tendon sheath into the wrist. The finger seems to be in a semiflexed position and exhibits pain on passive extension. What is the next step in management?

A. Incision and drainage of any superficial abscesses possible and oral antibiotics.
B. IV antibiotics and admission for observation.
C. Bone scan of hand.
D. Capture and quarantine of the animal for observation with the consideration of rabies prophylaxis for the patient.
E. Surgical consultation.

Infectious Tenosynovitis of the Hand

Symptoms

Pain, limited range of motion, swelling, and red streaking from infected finger. History commonly shows skin break or minor trauma to finger or hand along tendon sheath. Cat bites are common source.

Diagnosis

Physical exam:
Kanavel's signs

1. Symmetric swelling along tendon sheath.

2. Tenderness and erythema along tendon sheath.

3. Semiflexed posture of the involved finger.

4. Severe pain on passive extension.

Labs: CBC shows leukocytosis. Obtain cultures before antibiotics. Cultures often positive for *Staphylococcus* and *Streptococcus* spp.
Imaging: Plain x-rays of hand depending on mode of injury.

Treatment

- Surgical incision and drainage of tendon sheath should be done as soon as possible.

- IV antibiotics initiated after surgery may include IV penicillin or cephalosporin.

- Place hand in Murphy's splint during recovery (hand kept above level of the heart).

- NSAIDs or opiate pain control as needed.
- Refer to orthopedics or plastic surgeon.

Ganglion Cyst

Symptoms

Painful or nonpainful rubbery mass over joints, commonly of wrist or hand.

Diagnosis

Physical exam: Rubbery, discrete subcutaneous mass over the joint or tendon sheath.

Treatment

- Reassurance that the mass is benign and common.
- Aspiration with 18-gauge needle is effective acutely, but counsel the patient that it will likely recur.
- Surgical excision is the only definitive method of removal and must be done in the OR. Recurrence is, however, common. Recovery is usually fast without complication.

Rhabdomyolysis

Symptoms

Severe muscle aches, tenderness, and dark urine. History is often prominent for comorbid inciting event such as crush injury, compartment syndrome, heat stroke/injury, shock, and rarely, use of statin drugs. Classic scenario is of alcoholics who fall and remain in the same position for long periods of time, effectively sustaining a crush injury. If severe, these symptoms may be accompanied by mental status change or evidence of other organ damage.

Diagnosis

Physical exam: Tender muscles. Muscular injury may be obvious. Evaluate for compartment syndrome even if it is not the inciting event.

Labs: CBC may show hemoconcentration, creatine kinase (CK) is significantly elevated, urine positive for myoglobin (may be followed), and CMP may show electrolyte abnormalities of Na, K, Ph, Ca. Abnormalities in Ph and Ca may be followed, lactate dehydrogenase (LDH) is elevated (may be followed), aspartate aminotransferase and alanine aminotransferase (AST and ALT) are often >3 times normal (may be followed), and PT/aPTT/INR may show liver injury or early disseminated intravascular coagulation (DIC); arterial blood gas (ABG) shows metabolic acidosis.

Treatment

- Most important initial step is to start IV fluids. Generous bolus at first, then at least two times maintenance. Follow urine myoglobin, which should turn positive indicating when to normalize the rate of fluid administration.

- Monitor for pulmonary edema or adult respiratory distress syndrome (ARDS) in severe cases. Give furosemide (Lasix) as needed.

- Treat seizures with benzodiazepines as needed.

- Manage concurrent organ damage and its effects.

- DIC may be an indication of eminent crash; be vigilant.

- Alkalinization of the urine with sodium bicarbonate is controversial but helps clear myoglobin more effectively; consider in severe cases.

Myositis

See Table 8.6.

Collagen Vascular Diseases

See Table 8.7.

TABLE 8.6 Disorders of myositis

Disease	Associations	Diagnosis	Treatment
Polymyositis/ dermatomyositis	Proximal muscle **weakness and pain**; difficulty raising arms, ascending stairs, brushing teeth. Characteristic skin rash may accompany	Based on history, physical exam, and labs showing **increased CK**, lactate dehydrogenase (LDH), AST/ALT, creatinine, ESR, aldolase. EMG and muscle biopsy clinch the diagnosis	**Prednisone** is the classic choice and may require long-term use. Refractory cases may benefit from methotrexate, azathioprine, cyclophosphamide, chlorambucil, or cyclosporine. Use lowest effective dose for shortest interval
Polymalgia rheumatica	Proximal muscle **pain without weakness**; soreness in pelvic or pectoral girdle. AM stiffness or after inactivity. **Temporal arteritis** may be comorbid	ESR and CRP often very elevated. Normocytic anemia. CK normal. EMG normal. Arterial biopsy for temporal arteritis	Prednisone is very effective and dramatic response can be diagnostic. Long-term maintenance is usually required, use lowest effective dose

TABLE 8.7 Common collagen vascular diseases

	Associations	Diagnosis	Treatment
Marfan syndrome	Tall, gangly limbs, long/thin fingers, pectus deformity, high-arched palate, **scoliosis**. Associated with heart abnormalities such as aortic dissection, aortic regurgitation/insufficiency, mitral regurgitation/prolapse. Eye manifestations include subluxation of lens, myopia, or retinal detachment	Plain x-rays of spine for scoliosis during childhood. Annual echocardiograms for premorbid aortic root dilatation	Multidisciplinary surveillance for aortic or vascular dilatation, ophthalmologic disorders, and spinal malformations. Treat individual abnormalities with surgery. β-Blockers and calcium-channel blockers along with the avoidance of strenuous exercise may be advised. Consider exogenous estrogen to induce premature puberty in girls to avoid excess height
Ehlers–Danlos syndrome	Several different types with variable genetic genotypes/phenotypes. Hyperflexibility of joints (often hands), hyperextensible skin, poor wound healing, easy bruising, and, rarely, subcutaneous spheroids. Vascular involvement may be present, but less common	Most often clinical, unless genetic analysis is done. Pedigree with affected relatives should be analyzed. Many different inheritances and mutations may produce variations on disease	Reassurance that for mild disease there will likely never be disability. For more severe disease, treat individual conditions

Q 8.4

According to current recommendations, when should screening for osteoporosis take place?

A. Beginning at age 50 if average risk.
B. Beginning at age 55 if average risk.
C. Beginning at age 60 if average risk.
D. Beginning at age 65 if average risk.
E. No age is specified but should be based on risk factor assessment.

Q 8.5

According to the World Health Organization (WHO) guidelines, what level of bone mineral density (BMD) constitutes osteoporosis?

A. BMD not more than 1 standard deviation below peak adult bone mass (PABM). T-score >-1.
B. BMD between 1 and 2.5 standard deviations below PABM. T-score between -1 and -2.5.
C. BMD value more than 2.5 standard deviations below PABM. T-score ≤-2.5.
D. Osteoporosis with T-score ≤-2.5 plus one or more fragility fracture.
E. Age >65 years with any fracture of a long bone or vertebra.

Osteoporosis

Symptoms

Often an asymptomatic disease until there is complication of fracture. Fractures may commonly be seen in hip or vertebrae. Spine may develop many "microfractures" developing into severe kyphoscoliosis, which may progress to respiratory compromise in late stages. Risk factors include personal history of fragility fracture, low body weight, current smoking, use of oral corticosteroid therapy for more than 3 months, estrogen deficiency at an early age (<45 years), poor health/frailty, northern areas, low calcium intake (lifelong), low physical activity, and alcohol in amounts >2 drinks per day.

Diagnosis

See Table 8.8.

DEXA scanning and elucidation of the *T*-score is commonly used for the classification of bone mineral density (BMD).

Plain bone or spine x-rays should be sought on any suspected fracture.

Recommendations on screening show little variations among expert groups. The United States Preventive Services Task Force (USPSTF) and the National Osteoporosis Foundation (NOF) recommend universal screening of all women over the age of 65, and screening of postmenopausal women under age 65 with one or more risk factors (not including being female, White, and postmenopausal). The NOF further recommends screening of postmenopausal women that present with fragility fractures. Recommendations have not been made for repeat or interval testing.

Treatment

- Oral calcium/vitamin D intake throughout life, but is highly recommended especially after menopause. Calcium dose is generally 1200 mg/day with vitamin D 400–800 IU/day.

- Recommend regular strength training exercise.

TABLE 8.8 World Health Organization (WHO) criteria for diagnosis of osteoporosis

Normal	BMD not more than 1 standard deviation below PABM. *T*-score >−1
Osteopenia	BMD between 1 and 2.5 standard deviations below PABM. *T*-score between −1 and −2.5
Osteoporosis	BMD value more than 2.5 standard deviations below PABM. *T*-score ≤ −2.5
Severe osteoporosis	Osteoporosis with *T*-score ≤−2.5 plus one or more fragility fractures

BMD, bone mineral density; PABM, peak adult bone mass.

- Bisphosphonates such as alendronate (Fosamax), risedronate (Actonel), pamidronate (Aredia) are effective at both prevention and treatment. These drugs should be taken while upright (sitting/standing) for at least 30 min and on an empty stomach to avoid common GI side effects.

- Calcitonin (Miacalcin) has shown good effectiveness with little side effects.

- Raloxifene (Evista) is a selective estrogen receptor modulator (SERM) that is approved for postmenopausal osteoporosis, although common side effects include hot flashes and possible deep vein thrombosis (DVT).

- Progesterone and estrogen hormone replacement therapy (HRT) have shown positive effects on BMD in postmenopausal women but has recently been shown to cause disproportionate cardiovascular and breast cancer risks by the Women's Health Initiative study. However, it is still commonly used for short-term relief of menopausal symptoms and if all other options for osteoporosis have been exhausted.

Developmental Musculoskeletal Deformities

See Table 8.9.

TABLE 8.9 Developmental hip deformities

	Diagnosis	Treatment
Hip dysplasia	Often at birth with positive Barlow/Ortolani test. Unequal number of thigh folds and uneven height of knees. For neonates obtain **hip ultrasound**, for older infants plain x-rays in anteroposterior (AP) and frog lateral leg positions. CT, MRI may be beneficial	Positioning in "frog leg" position with hip flexed and abducted. Double or triple diapers effective in neonates, older infants may require **Pavlik harness**. In infants >6 months, closed reduction and hip spica cast are indicated. Duration usually 1–3 months
Legg–Calvé–Perthes disease (avascular necrosis of femoral head)	Presents as "painless limp" around 7 years. Plain x-rays in AP and frog lateral positions are usually adequate to diagnose. MRI may catch early disease, but not adequate to follow course	Abduction brace for most. Surgical correction for severe cases
Slipped capital femoral epiphysis (SCFE)	Classically, overweight male adolescent. Pain in thigh or knee (referred) with external rotation of hip. Plain x-rays in AP and frog lateral positions show abnormality	Surgery including internal fixation and pinning, osteotomy, and hip spica cast immobilization

Spondylosis

Degeneration of the intervertebral disc spaces (osteoarthritis) leading to increased weightbearing on alternate intervertebral joints and osteophyte formation.

Symptoms

Localized back pain commonly in lumbar and cervical regions. If advanced, may produce radicular pain including sciatica or in dermatomal distribution. Progression may lead to neurogenic claudication and signs of spinal stenosis.

Diagnosis

Physical exam: Tenderness at the level of defect, increased pain on back extension. Pain is exacerbated by ipsilateral bending to the side with the affected joints.
Labs: CBC and ESR are usually normal.
Imaging: Plain spinal x-rays reveal intervertebral disc degeneration and osteophyte formation. MRI and CT are not indicated unless spinal stenosis is suspected.

Treatment

- NSAIDs and tylenol are the mainstays of treatment.
- Physical therapy such as core muscle strengthening, transcutaneous electro-nerve stimulation (TENS), and ultrasound therapy have shown benefit in the short term.
- Surgery (spinal fusion) is indicated for significant neurologic symptoms although long-term benefit is controversial.
- Decompression laminectomy may be used if stenosis is suspected.

Ankylosing Spondylitis

Symptoms

Insidious-onset lower back pain and stiffness are the hallmarks of the disease. Morning stiffness is present that is relieved by activity. Pleuritic chest pain and constricted chest expansion may be reported. Constitutional symptoms such as fever, weight loss, and fatigue may be present and correlate with back pain flares. Rarely, anterior uveitis and cardiovascular abnormalities are present in history.

Diagnosis

Physical exam: Tenderness on palpation of sacroiliac (SI) joint, limited range of motion of SI joint, and relative loss of lumbar lordosis. Decreased chest expansion is often present. Heart exam should be focused on the presence of murmur indicating aortic valve sclerosis.

Labs: Antigen testing for HLA-B27 (common); ESR/CRP is often elevated. CBC may show a mild normocytic anemia.

Imaging: Plain x-rays (including oblique view) of lumbar spine may show "bamboo" spine with squaring of vertebrae. Early disease seen by sclerosis of SI joint while late disease is seen by ankylosis and osteopenia. Peripheral joints showing symptoms should be imaged as well. MRI may be used if plain radiography is inconclusive. Increased signal in the area of the SI joint indicating surrounding edema may be present.

ECG is recommended but may be inadequate if valvular disease is present. Consider echocardiography if murmur exists.

DEXA scan is indicated for possible osteoporosis.

Treatment

- Physical therapy with focus on strengthening back extensors is effective.

- NSAIDs are the mainstay of therapy with indomethacin (Indocin) most common. Good response supports diagnosis.

- Interarticular corticosteroid injection provides temporary relief.

- Other antirheumatic drugs such as etanercept (Enbrel), sulfasalazine (Azulfidine), and methotrexate (Trexall, Rheumatrex) have showed excellent benefit in recent studies.

Intervertebral Disc Herniation

Symptoms

Localized back pain and radiating neurological pain. While the vast majority is mild to moderate, severe herniation accompanied by nerve impingement may result in sensory or motor symptoms. History may reveal heavy lifting or traumatic event. "Red flag" symptoms include bowel/bladder incontinence, fever, weight loss, bilateral sensory or motor dysfunction, or saddle anesthesia.

Diagnosis

Physical exam: Tenderness at herniation site. Flexion or extension at the site may produce radicular symptoms. Straight leg raise or crossed straight leg raise reproduces radicular symptoms (not back pain). Sensory or motor dysfunction may be seen in spinal nerve root distribution.

Imaging: Plain x-rays are rarely indicated in acute work-up unless red flag symptoms present. After 4–8 weeks of continued symptoms despite therapy, anteroposterior (AP) and lateral views may be obtained. MRI is the best technique for evaluation and may show disc herniation or nerve compression. Recent studies have shown significant proportion of individuals with disc herniation in the asymptomatic population raising the question of causation of symptoms.

EMG may reveal nerve root compression and slowed conduction after acute phase.

Treatment

- NSAIDs and physical therapy are the mainstays of therapy. Corticosteroid injection may also reduce local inflammation and treat acutely.
- Surgery (laminotomy, microdiscectomy, spinal fusion, or laminectomy) is needed in only a small proportion of individuals with progressive, acute neurologic dysfunction, chronic progressive pain, or refractory chronic symptoms.
- **Cauda equina syndrome** is an emergent condition that is characterized by a patchy loss of sensory and motor function of the lower extremities. Classic signs are saddle anesthesia, loss of bowel/bladder function, and leg weakness. It requires prompt neurosurgical consultation and constitutes an emergency.

Spinal Stenosis

Symptoms

Nonspecific lower back pain is usually the inciting complaint, followed by lower extremity complaints such as fatigue, pain, numbness, or weakness. Often occurring on walking or running, these symptoms are loosely referred to as "neurogenic claudication."

Diagnosis

Physical exam: Symptoms are classically reproduced by back extension and relieved by flexion. Neurologic exam may be normal if patient is seated during the exam; thus a repeat exam should be done after the patient has walked.

Imaging: Plain x-rays are not adequate for diagnosis but may show disc space narrowing and general degeneration of the joints. Spondylolisthesis (anterior slippage of one vertebra upon another) may be evident if present. MRI is the much preferred modality of imaging, and most clearly demonstrates narrowing of the spinal canal. CT with injection myelography is also useful, but is invasive.

EMG may demonstrate nerve root compression, but is often not needed.

Treatment

- Conservative therapy with NSAIDs, weight loss, and back strengthening may be tried initially.
- Injection therapy including epidural and/or soft tissue injection with a mix of local anesthetic and corticosteroid have provided some relief, although is rarely long lasting.
- Decompressive surgery, commonly with laminectomy, is the definitive treatment that has shown good outcomes. Recent meta-analysis, however, has not proved long-term benefits as compared with nonsurgical treatments.

Malignant Metastases

Symptoms

Bone pain, commonly in spine, may be the presenting symptom (may be associated with fracture). Pain may be in other areas including the hip, femur, ribs, sternum, or humerus. Rarely in smaller bones. History may show prior treatment for cancer or risk factors for cancer. Common primary sites include **prostate, breast, and lung**.

Diagnosis

Physical exam: Tenderness to palpation over bone in affected area. Swelling, erythema, warmth, or deformity may accompany a pathologic fracture.
Labs: CBC to evaluate for signs of infection. Serum and ionized calcium increased. Alkaline phosphatase increased.
Imaging: Plain x-ray useful in evaluating for fracture, but nuclear medicine bone scan (skeletal survey) is most important. Bone scan will show lytic lesions.

Biopsy the lesion as well as the suspected sight to evaluate the grade of carcinoma.

Treatment

- Treat according to the best treatment guidelines for primary sight. This often includes local radiation therapy and chemotherapy. By the time bone metastases are seen, advanced stage is usually present. Therapy is often palliative.

- Give pain control with narcotics as needed. Do not limit regimen for fear of dependence.

Skull Fracture

Symptoms

Pain and bruising are cardinal symptoms. May be accompanied by change in vision, double vision, alteration of consciousness, clear otorrhea or rhinorrhea, or movable fracture regions of face. History often reveals traumatic closed head injury such as in motor vehicle accidents.

Diagnosis

Physical exam: Bruising "battle's sign"—postauricular ecchymosis, "Raccoon eyes"—periorbital ecchymosis, and facial bone crepitus.
Imaging: Plain x-rays of head and cervical spine. Multiple views may be needed to visualize fractures. CT may also reveal fractures and is inevitably done for the evaluation of intercranial bleeding. MRI will also show fractures, but is less commonly done acutely (see Figure 8.2).

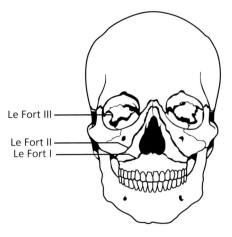

FIGURE 8.2 Le Fort classification of facial fractures.

Oxford Handbook of Emergency Medicine. Third edition. Wyatt J.P. et al. Copyright 2006. Oxford University Press.

Treatment

- Surgical correction with neurosurgeon, ENT, or plastic surgeon.
- Wires and stabilization bars may be placed temporarily for stabilization.
- Give adequate pain control.

Fractures

See Table 8.10 and Figure 8.3.

TABLE 8.10 Common fractures

Fracture	Description	Common context	Management
Boxer's fracture	Fracture of fifth metacarpal neck	Closed fist punch of hard surface or object	Closed reduction and ulnar gutter splint. If good opposition of ends not accomplished, consider open reduction internal fixation (ORIF)
Colle's fracture	Fracture of distal radius. Often dorsally displaced and dorsally angulated	Fall on outstretched hand	Closed reduction with eventual long arm cast
Greenstick fracture	Incomplete fracture of children's immature bones	Fall or direct trauma often to forearm	If angulation is insignificant, casting not needed. Otherwise, long arm cast
Salter–Harris fractures	Pediatric fracture with break affecting the physis. Five types exist	Multiple	Closed reduction in types I and II, higher types require ORIF

(continued)

TABLE 8.10 Common fractures

Fracture	Description	Common context	Management
Clavicle fracture	Majority occur in middle one-third, next most common in distal one-third, and rarely in medial one-third	Multiple. Common football injury	Ipsilateral sling often adequate. Figure-of-eight cast or surgery only needed if significant misalignment seen
Rib fracture	Often hairline or complete. Evaluate for pneumothorax	Blunt trauma to ribcage such as in car accident. If in pediatric patient, posterior/lateral location, consider child abuse	Pain control is commonly all that is needed. Treat complications
Vertebral body fracture	Compression fracture involving the body of vertebrae. May be in "burst" or "wedge" pattern	Osteoporosis in the elderly is common. Car accident in the young	Pain control and bedrest acutely. Evaluate the need for steroids secondary to spinal compression. Closed management common if uncomplicated. Vertebroplasty/kyphoplasty if not
Hip fracture	Several types exist, but most involve femoral neck and danger to vascular supply	"Step off" mechanism common in the elderly. Seated "dashboard" injuries in car accident in young	ORIF because of delicate blood supply
Tibia/fibula fracture	Often occur together and involve proximal and distal ends	Rotation of foreleg common mechanism. Common skiing fracture	Closed management unless complicated or open

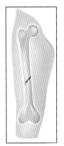 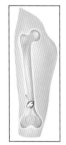 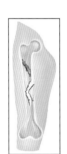 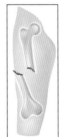

Oblique   Comminuted   Spiral   Compound

FIGURE 8.3 Common fracture patterns.

Infective Arthritis

Symptoms

Pain, fever, tenderness, limited range of motion, erythema, and effusion are common in septic joint. Causes are many, but history may reveal *Neisseria gonorrhoeae* infection, trauma, immunodeficiency state, recent joint surgery, penetrating wound (such as cat bite), or recent significant bacteremia.

Diagnosis

Physical exam: Often mono- or pauci-articular. Swelling, erythema, effusion, and limited range of motion are common. Fever, myalgias, and obvious inoculation site may be seen.

Labs: Aspiration of joint fluid and Gram stain is mandatory. Fluid analysis often reveals increased WBCs and bacteria. Protein and glucose are not reliable for diagnosis. Culture the aspirate and obtain sensitivities. Evaluate fluid for crystal presence indicating gout or pseudogout. If sexually active, young patient, test for *gonorrhea*.

Treatment

- Drainage of purulent joint fluid is most important. This may be done by aspiration, but most common in the OR by orthopedic surgery.
- Treatment should be according to suspected organism on Gram stain, regimen often includes vancomycin. Add ceftriaxone (Rocephin) if *gonorrhea* is a possibility.
- Narrow regimen according to sensitivities and culture results. Course of antibiotics often 4–6 weeks and may be longer depending on the host.
- Surgically remove any infected artificial joints.

Temporomandibular Joint Syndrome

Symptoms

More common in women of third or fourth decade, symptoms include jaw pain, clicking, tenderness on mastication, headache, earache, or neck pain. History may reveal comorbid conditions such as anxiety, fibromyalgia, rheumatoid arthritis, osteoarthritis (OA), gout, or other arthropathy.

Diagnosis

Physical exam: Tenderness to palpation of temporomandibular joint (TMJ) and muscles of mastication. Audible clicking on mastication. Assess jaw range of motion.

Imaging: Plain x-rays of TMJ are rarely useful. MRI may show disc and position, but clinical correlation of displaced disc and symptoms are poor. Therefore, disc position not necessarily significant. Single-contrast videoarthrography rarely needed but shows joint dynamics in detail.

Treatment

- NSAIDs may be effective but generally not enough if used alone.
- Tricyclic antidepressants taken at night are often helpful, with amitriptyline (Elavil) being most efficacious. Oral muscle relaxants such as cyclobenzaprine (Flexeril) may be helpful.
- Steroid injection of TMJ is efficacious acutely. Use mix of methylprednisolone and lidocaine for best effect.

- Botulinum toxin (Botox) injection has recently shown benefit.
- Long-term treatment of comorbid psychiatric disorders will likely improve this syndrome.
- Surgical referral indicated for refractory cases or those with significant displacement or damage to disc.

Q 8.6

A 15-year-old African American male comes to your office with complaints of twisting his ankle during sports practice and now feeling like he cannot walk on it. He describes the mechanism of injury to be inversion while traveling forward. On exam, there is ecchymosis of the anterior lateral aspect of the ankle with marked concurrent swelling. The area is generally very tender, with instability demonstrated by provocative testing and inability to bear weight. The patient refuses adequate evaluation of drawer signs. You obtain an x-ray of the ankle, which showed no fracture. What is the next step in management?

A. RICE therapy and NSAIDs.
B. RICE therapy, NSAIDs, and stabilization brace.
C. Obtain MRI of ankle and consider referral to orthopedic surgery.
D. Obtain CT of ankle.
E. RICE therapy, NSAIDs, and physical therapy consultation.

Ankle Sprain

Symptoms

Pain and feeling of looseness of the joint are the most common symptoms. Often acutely swollen with mild erythema. Subacutely may become ecchymotic. History commonly reveals injury with inversion or other event. Prior ankle sprain is the main risk factor for new injury.

Diagnosis

Physical exam: Tender to palpation over the injured ligament. May show swelling, ecchymosis, erythema, and limited range of motion. Provocative testing includes inversion, eversion, plantar/dorsiflexion, and abduction and adduction. Ankle anterior and posterior drawer signs should be tested.

Imaging: Often unnecessary unless fracture suspected. Stress x-rays and arthrography may be helpful for extent of tear, but rarely used since advent of MRI. MRI is useful in grade 2–3 sprains to evaluate extent of tear (if in question).

Ligaments involved in ankle sprain:

1. Anterior talofibular ligament.
2. Calcaneofibular ligament.
3. Posterior talofibular ligament.

TABLE 8.11 Grades of ankle sprain

Grade	Tear	Treatment
Grade 1	Mild sprain or stretching of ligaments	RICE, NSAIDs for pain. Stabilization wrapping followed by return to function
Grade 2	Partial tear	RICE, pain control, and stabilization brace. Consider imaging and physical therapy
Grade 3	Complete tear (rupture)	Obtain MRI to confirm, casting or brace is indicated. Refer to orthopedic surgery

NSAIDs, nonsteroidal antiinflammatory drugs; RICE, rest, ice, compression, elevation.

Treatment

See Table 8.11.

- Adequate pain control is essential.
- Physical therapy referral is helpful in rehabilitation.

Osteoarthritis

Symptoms

Classically, pain that worsens during the day. Arthritis is noninflammatory but often limits the range of motion and is characterized by a dull ache in or around the joints. In advanced disease, erosion may produce inflammatory picture including swelling and erythema of joints. Risk factors include obesity, advanced age, female sex, previous joint injury, and family history.

Diagnosis

Physical exam: Tenderness on passive range of motion may be seen. Crepitus is a sign of advanced disease. **Heberden's nodes** (bony enlargement) may be seen on DIP joints of hands if involved.

Labs: No specific lab tests exist for OA although exclusion of other arthropathies may be indicated with screening labs. ESR is not reliable for diagnosis.

Imaging: Plain x-rays of joint in question often show narrowing of joint space and osteophyte formation. Erosion, formation of subchondral cysts, and sclerotic walls may develop later. MRI may show greater detail of these changes but is commonly not needed due to the reliability of plain x-rays.

Aspiration of joint often not needed and shows noninflammatory process with normal WBCs. Crystal disorders and inflammatory arthritis may be excluded (see Figure 8.4).

Treatment

- Weight reduction, heat to affected joint, and occupational modification or assistance is the first step in treatment.
- NSAIDs and tylenol are the pharmacologic mainstays of treatment. In the elderly, monitor for GI bleeding or renal failure.

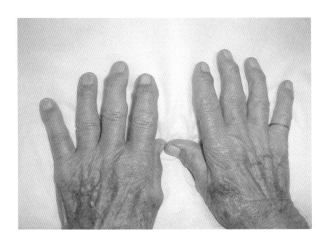

FIGURE 8.4 Heberden's nodes seen on distal interphalangeal (DIP) joints of patient with osteoarthritis (OA).

Courtesy: Charlie Goldberg, MD. University of California, San Diego School of Medicine, San Diego VA Medical Center.

- Cyclooxygenase (COX)-2 inhibitors (NSAIDs) have been an acceptable alternative to regular NSAIDs in the past, although recent concerns have been raised on safety regarding cardiovascular risks. Benefits include less GI symptoms and risk of bleeding. Monitor closely if these are used.

- Topical capsaicin cream is often helpful.

- Opioid analgesics are rarely indicated for OA.

- Intraarticular corticosteroid injections often improve symptoms although repeated injection commonly needed. Limit to three to four injections per year, never exceeding 12 injections per any one joint.

- Intraarticular injection of hyaluronic acid has been shown to provide some relief, but further investigation is needed to define the benefit.

- Surgery, including total joint arthroplasty, is acceptable and effective when the disease has proven to be refractory to medical therapy. Symptom reduction and joint mobility are often significantly improved.

Answers

8.1 E. Answers A–D are each separate criteria used to diagnose systemic lupus erythematosus (SLE). Syphilis screening testing is often false positive, and is a separate criterion for the diagnosis of SLE if present.

8.2 A. Atlantoaxial subluxation is a well-known complication occurring in rheumatoid arthritis patients, and may present with several signs and symptoms including neck pain radiating cephalad and peripheral paresthesias.

8.3 E. This patient is exhibiting all four Kanavel's signs of infectious tenosynovitis of the hand including symmetric swelling along tendon sheath, tenderness and erythema along tendon sheath, semiflexed posture of the involved finger, and severe pain on passive extension. This infection is more common with bites from an animal with long needle-like teeth, such as a cat, with the ability to puncture deep into tissue. Treatment should include prompt evaluation for operative incision and drainage.

8.4 D. The United States Preventive Services Task Force (USPSTF) and the National Osteoporosis Foundation (NOF) recommend universal screening of all women over the age of 65 and screening of postmenopausal women under age 65 with one or more risk factors (not including being female, White, and postmenopausal). The NOF further recommends screening of postmenopausal women that present with fragility fractures.

8.5 C. According to World Health Organization (WHO) guidelines, osteoporosis is present when bone mineral density (BMD) falls below 2.5 standard deviations from peak adult bone mass (PABM). Often seen as DEXA bone scan T-score of <-2.5. Answer D would constitute severe osteoporosis.

8.6 C. This patient exhibits signs of likely grade 2 or 3 anterior talofibular ligament injury. Instability of ankle on provocative testing and inability to bear weight should raise questions of complete tear of the ligament (grade 3). Thus, evaluation with MRI with possible referral to orthopedic surgery is indicated.

Infectious Diseases

Intestinal Infections	186
Streptococcal Sore Throat	187
Streptococcal Infections	188
Staphylococcal Infections	188
Escherichia coli Infections	189
Haemophilus influenzae Infection	189
Pseudomonas Infection	189
HIV Infection and AIDS	190
Pneumocystis Pneumonia	192
Kaposi's Sarcoma	193
Varicella	195
Herpes Simplex	196
Measles	198
Childhood Exanthems	200
Syphilis	202
Sexually Transmitted Diseases	203
Tinea (Dermatophytosis)	203
Candidiasis	204
Mycoses	205
Hepatitis	205
Mumps	207
Hand, Foot, and Mouth Disease	208
Infectious Mononucleosis	209
Molluscum Contagiosum	211
Cat Scratch Disease	211
Cytomegalic Inclusion Disease	212
Adenovirus	212
Rhinovirus	213
Toxoplasmosis	213

West Nile Virus	214
Rocky Mountain Spotted Fever	215
Malaria	216
Lyme Disease	218
TORCHES Infections During Pregnancy	218
Osteomyelitis	219
Incubation Periods and Infectivity	221

Intestinal Infections

See Table 9.1.

TABLE 9.1 Common intestinal infections

Etiology	Associations	Treatment
Viral (adenovirus, rotavirus, Norwalk-like virus, etc.)	Low-grade fever, nausea/vomiting, nonbloody diarrhea, abdominal cramps; look for history of sick contacts	Hydration is key; either orally or IV. Bismuth subsalicylate
Campylobacter infections	Subtypes denote common location, i.e., pylori, jejuni, coli, etc.; cause nausea/vomiting, diarrhea, abdominal cramps; may rarely see **Guillain–Barré** syndrome after illness	Rehydration Ciprofloxacin, azithromycin, erythromycin.
Clostridium difficile	Severe diarrhea, fever, abdominal cramps. History often positive for hospital stay, recent antibiotic use. Send a stool sample for *C. difficile* toxin if suspected	Isolate the patient Rehydration Metronidazole is first line Vancomycin is second
Food poisoning/gastroenteritis (*Shigella, Salmonella, Escherichia coli* species (0157:H7, enterotoxigenic, etc.), *V. parahaemolyticus, C. perfringens, Y. enterocolitica, S. aureus, B. cereus*	Obtain history relating to suspected meal time, <24 h likely toxin, >24 h likely invasive bacteria. Symptoms commonly fever, abdominal cramps, diarrhea (bloody or not), nausea/vomiting. History may reveal illness in individuals who shared the suspected meal	Rehydration Treatment is controversial. Do not treat *E. coli* 0157:H7 with antibiotics Loperamide (Imodium) controversial as it may make disease worse if toxigenic. If antibiotics used, ciprofloxacin, TMP/SMX, not necessary here other broad spectrum.
Giardia lamblia	Bloating, flatulence, nausea/vomiting, loose/greasy/foul-smelling stools, weight loss; history of time spent outdoors; check stool for ova/parasites	Rehydration Tinidazole (Tindamax) Metronidazole (Flagyl) Nitazoxanide (Alinia)

Streptococcal Sore Throat

Symptoms

Sore throat, decreased oral intake, malaise, fever, tender anterior cervical lymph nodes, halitosis. History often reveals sick contacts or day care exposure.

Diagnosis

Physical exam: Fever, anterior cervical lymphadenopathy, exudative tonsillitis, and posterior pharyngeal erythema.

Clinical Tool

See Table 9.2.

- Rapid streptococcal test from tonsilar swab has good sensitivity and specificity with modern tests.
- Throat culture is the gold standard, but takes 2–3 days for result.
- Monospot for mononucleosis is often warranted.

Treatment

- Penicillin is the standard. Oral Pen V if compliant, IM penicillin benzathine G if not.
- Macrolides such as erythromycin or azithromycin are second line or considered in Pen-allergic patients.
- If given amoxicillin and a rash develops, the patient likely has mononucleosis and not strep throat.
- Nonsteroidal antiinflammatory drugs (NSAIDs) have been shown to be most effective for the pain, sore throat, and myalgias; otherwise, lozenges, throat sprays, rest may help symptoms.

TABLE 9.2 Clinical tool for determination of streptococcal throat infections

Risk factor	Points
Anterior cervical lymphadenopathy	1
Fever	1
Tonsillar exudate	1
Absence of cough	1
Age <15 years	1
Age 15–45 years	0
Age >45 years	−1

Scoring: −1 or 0 points: streptococcal infection ruled out (2%); 1–3 points: order rapid test and treat accordingly; 4–5 points: probable streptococcal infection (52%), consider empiric antibiotics.

Streptococcal Infections

See Table 9.3.

TABLE 9.3 Common streptococcal infections

Disease	Prototypic antibiotic/treatment
Cellulitis	Pen G
Necrotizing fasciitis	Pen G + clindamycin
Impetigo	Antibacterial ointment (Mupirocin)
Wound infection after trauma	TMP/SMX DS or clindamycin
Streptococcal toxic shock syndrome	Pen G + clindamycin
Pneumonia	Azithromycin
Scarlet fever	Penicillin
Intrapartum group B Streptococcus (GBS) prophylaxis	Penicillin or ampicillin
Meningitis	Ceftriaxone or ampicillin or Pen G. These ± vancomycin
Otitis media	Amoxicillin
Sinusitis	Amoxicillin or amoxicillin/clavulanate (Augmentin)

Staphylococcal Infections

See Table 9.4.

TABLE 9.4 Common Staphylococcal infections

Disease	Prototypic antibiotic/treatment
Endocarditis	(Nafcillin + gentamicin) or vancomycin
Osteomyelitis	Vancomycin
Mastitis	Continued nursing + dicloxicillin or TMP/SMX DS
Toxic shock syndrome	Remove tampons (common source), nafcillin, IVIG, ± vancomycin
Cellulitis	Dicloxicillin
Scalded skin syndrome	Nafcillin
Hordeolum (stye)	Hot packs ± nafcillin/oxacillin (if internal)
Conjunctivitis	Ophthalmic drops of gatifloxacin, levofloxacin, or moxifloxacin

Escherichia coli Infections

See Table 9.5.

TABLE 9.5 Common *E. coli* infections

Disease	Prototypic antibiotic/treatment
Urinary tract infection	TMP/SMX DS (Bactrim, Septra) or ciprofloxacin
Gastroenteritis 0157:H7	No treatment
Gastroenteritis—Traveler's diarrhea	Azithromycin or ciprofloxacin, loperamide (Imodium), bismuth subsalicylate

Haemophilus influenzae Infection

See Table 9.6.

TABLE 9.6 Common *H. influenzae* infections

Disease	Prototypic antibiotic/treatment
Epiglottitis	Ceftriaxone (Rocephin)
Otitis media	Amoxicillin
Pneumonia	Azithromycin

Pseudomonas Infection

See Table 9.7.

TABLE 9.7 Common *Pseudomonas* infections

Disease	Prototypic antibiotic/treatment
Otitis externa (swimmer's ear)	Ofloxacin ear drops
Contact lens wearer's conjunctivitis	Gentamicin eye drops + piperacillin eye drops to infected eye around the clock
Cystic fibrosis-pneumonia	Tobramycin + piperacillin
Cystic fibrosis-pneumonia suppression	Inhaled tobramycin (1 month on, 1 month off)
Sepsis related to burns	Vancomycin + amikacin + piperacillin, debridement

Q 9.1

A 37-year-old Asian male comes to the homeless clinic complaining of recent cough, fever, decreased appetite, and chest congestion. He states he has been having unprotected intercourse with other men and has previously been diagnosed with HIV although has not been taking any medication. He is febrile and mildly tachycardic with an O_2 saturation of 94%. His exam reveals right basilar rhonchi and increased egophony of the right lung base. On laboratory testing, his CD4 count is found to be 180 mm^3. What is the most likely finding on chest x-ray?

A. Right lower lobe opacity indicative of lobar infiltrate.
B. Right-sided lymphadenopathy with granuloma formation.
C. Right-sided upper lung round mass indicative of fungal infection.
D. Right-sided diffuse, lacy infiltrate.
E. Right-sided diffuse perihilar infiltrate and interstitial shadowing.

Q 9.2

What is the next step in the management of this patient?

A. Start highly active antiretroviral therapy (HAART) alone.
B. Start HAART and IV trimethoprim/sulfamethoxazole (TMP/SMX) therapy.
C. Start IV TMP/SMX therapy alone.
D. Start INH, pyridoxine, and HAART.
E. Start INH and pyridoxine.

HIV Infection and AIDS

Symptoms

After early transmission patients are most commonly asymptomatic for a period of weeks. When antibodies form, an acute viral-like illness with generalized malaise, low-grade fever, and myalgias may be reported. After seroconversion, an asymptomatic period with generalized lymphadenopathy may last for a variable amount of time, after which, "class B" conditions may appear, such as oral/vaginal candidiasis, herpes zoster, oral hairy leukoplakia, peripheral neuropathy, cervical dysplasia, fever/diarrhea >1 month, and idiopathic thrombocytopenic purpura. After the progression of disease to include diagnosis of AIDS (see below), almost any symptom/sign may be seen and are usually indicative of one of the AIDS-defining illnesses.

Diagnosis

Do a complete physical exam and document any abnormal findings.
According to the Centers for Disease Control and Prevention recommendations, AIDS is present in those patients with CD4 counts <200 mm^3 or

one or more AIDS-defining illnesses (commonly *Pneumocystis* pneumonia, Kaposi's sarcoma, candidiasis of the esophagus, trachea, bronchi, or lung, toxoplasmosis of the brain, etc.).

Labs: Enzyme-linked immunosorbent assay (ELISA) antibody testing for screening. If reactive, confirm with second ELISA. If still reactive, obtain Western blot analysis. ELISA seroconversion typically takes 4–10 weeks for positive result.

CD4 count is the key to therapy and prognosis. Obtain accompanying viral load.

Obtain screening labs such as CBC, Chem-20, hepatitis panel, cytomegalovirus (CMV) antibodies, toxoplasmosis antibodies, RPR/VDRL, purified protein derivative (PPD), etc.

Imaging: Chest x-ray (CXR) for pneumonia, CT head for toxoplasmosis (ring-enhancing lesion). Other imaging as clinically necessary.

Treatment

- Treat HIV directly with highly active antiretroviral therapy (HAART). Regimens consist of three drug combinations. Drugs include zidovudine, lamivudine, efavirenz, fosamprenavir, ritonavir, nelfinavir, abacavir, nevirapine, as well as others.

When to Start HAART

See Table 9.8.

Prophylaxis in HIV

See Table 9.9.

- Follow disease with serial visits and CD4/viral load counts every 3–6 months.
- All pregnant women should be screened for HIV status and placed on zidovudine (AZT) if positive.
- Consider referral to infectious disease specialist.

TABLE 9.8 Thresholds for starting HAART therapy

CD4 count	HIV symptoms present?	Start highly active antiretroviral therapy (HAART)?
Any	Yes	Yes
<200 mm³	Yes/no	Yes
>200, <350 mm³	No	Offer
>350 mm³ (viral load >100,000 cop/ml)	No	Consider
>350 mm³ (viral load <100,000 cop/ml)	No	No

TABLE 9.9 Prophylaxis in HIV/AIDS patients

Indication	Disease	Prophylaxis
HIV+	Influenza	Annual vaccination
HIV+	Pneumococcal pneumonia	Vaccination
HIV+	Hepatitis B virus	Vaccination
HIV+	Hepatitis A virus	Vaccination
HIV+ with no history of exposure/vaccination	Chickenpox or varicella zoster	Vaccination
CD4 <200 mm³	*Pneumocystis carinii* pneumonia	trimethoprim/sulfamethoxazole (TMP/SMX) daily or dapsone or aerosolized pentamidine.
CD4 <100 mm³ and Toxoplasmosis IgG positive	*Toxoplasmosis gondii*	TMP/SMX DS daily
CD4 <50 mm³	Mycobacterium avium complex (MAC)	Azithromycin weekly
HIV+ and PPD ≥5 mm diameter or contact with person with active TB	Tuberculosis	INH + pyridoxine for 9 months

---

Q 9.3

A 23-year-old Caucasian female is beginning prenatal care at your clinic and her HIV screen has returned positive. What is the next step in the management of this patient?

A. Obtain CD4 count and viral load studies.
B. Confirm the result with Western blot analysis.
C. Confirm the result with repeat ELISA antibody testing.
D. Obtain screening TB testing, toxoplasma antibodies, CD4 count, viral load, CBC, Varicella antibodies, hepatitis screen testing, and complete vaccination history.
E. Confirm the result with repeat ELISA testing in 8–10 weeks.

Pneumocystis Pneumonia

Symptoms

Insidious onset of dyspnea on exertion, weakness, fatigue, malaise, fever/chills, scantly productive cough. This is a common AIDS-defining illness and often occurs with CD4 count <200 mm³. Consider other reasons for immunocompromised state including humeral cancers and chemotherapy.

Diagnosis

Physical exam: Diffuse rhonchi and possible rales if effusion present. Tachypnea may be present.

Labs: Obtain arterial blood gas (ABG) if hypoxemia suspected, lactate dehydrogenase (LDH) levels often increased. Diagnosis often by saline-induced sputum sample and staining although bronchoalveolar lavage may be necessary; *Pneumocystis carinii* cysts will be seen. Check for HIV if not previously diagnosed (see earlier), obtain CD4 count.

Imaging: CXR reveals diffuse perihilar infiltrates and interstitial shadowing. Rarely a consolidation is seen. Effusion, abscesses, cavitations, or pneumothorax may also be seen depending on the degree of disease (see Figure 9.1).

Treatment

- Prevention is the standard and should include trimethoprim/sulfamethoxazole (TMP/SMX) (Bactrim, Septra), dapsone, or aerosolized pentamidine (Pentam) if CD4 <200 mm^3.

- Give oxygen.

- Give steroids if the patient is acutely ill. Prednisone is a good choice and is proven to decrease mortality.

- TMP/SMX or dapsone/TMP are first-line antibiotics. Treatment course is 21 days.

- D/C prophylaxis if CD4 rises >200 mm^3 for >3 months.

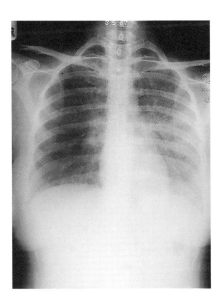

FIGURE 9.1 Chest x-ray showing *Pneumocystis carinii* pneumonia.

Problem-orientated Clinical Microbiology and Infection. Second edition. Humphreys H, Irving WL. Copyright 2004. Oxford University Press.

Kaposi's Sarcoma

Disease caused by human herpesvirus 8 (HHV8) and is most often found in the immunocompromised (AIDS), endemic (African) form, or elderly men.

Symptoms

Often presents with reddened, vascular skin lesion. On head, neck, trunk in HIV patients, or feet and lower extremities in older men. Tumors may be tender or pruritic and can also occur on mucous membranes, in lymph nodes, or viscera.

Diagnosis

Physical exam: Multicentric red-blue violaceous tumors on the skin. Tumors may be pruritic and tender and in HIV patients tend to appear on the face, arms, and trunk. Lesions may be in mucous membranes, viscera, or lymph nodes as well.

Labs: HIV testing as described earlier, biopsy is gold standard from the lesion. HHV8 antibody testing is usually positive, and Southern blot analysis or polymerase chain reaction (PCR) may be done on biopsy to confirm.

Imaging: Obtain CXR and CT for disseminated disease (see Figure 9.2).

Treatment

- Treat HIV infection as indicated.

- Local disease may be amenable to surgery, radiotherapy, CO_2 laser, cryotherapy, or intralesional chemotherapy. Generalized disease may be treated with chemotherapy. Antiviral medications are still unproven, but show promise.

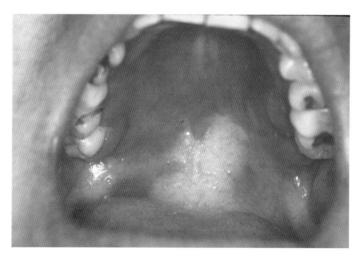

FIGURE 9.2 Kaposi's sarcoma.

Problem-orientated Clinical Microbiology and Infection. Second edition. Humphreys H, Irving WL. Copyright 2004. Oxford University Press.

Varicella

Symptoms

Primary infection usually in children. Symptoms include vesicular, erythematous, pruritic, lesions starting on the trunk and moving toward extremities (centripetally). Low-grade fever, malaise is common. Vesicles finally rupture and crust over (indicating the end of contagious stage).

Reactivation varicella (called zoster or shingles) usually presents with similar lesions, but are confined to a single dermatome. Commonly preceded by localized pain of the dermatome affected. After acute illness, shingles may leave residual pain called "postherpetic neuralgia."

Diagnosis

Physical exam: Lesions are vesicular papules with erythematous base. Rupture of vesicle with crusted top is usual. Appearance of "dew drop on a rose petal" (see Figures 9.3 and 9.4).

Most often clinical diagnosis although multinucleated giant cells may be present on Tzanck smear of scrapings (rarely done).

Treatment

- *Chicken pox*: For children <12 years, supportive care and treatment of symptoms is adequate. (Do not give aspirin to avoid risk of Reye syndrome).

- Postexposure prophylaxis should be initiated in high-risk patients (such as pregnancy, immunocompromised, or >15 years without

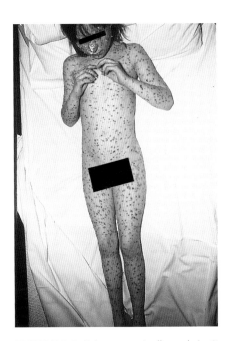

FIGURE 9.3 Primary varicella rash in 8-year-old female.

Problem-orientated Clinical Microbiology and Infection. Second edition. Humphreys H, Irving WL. Copyright 2004. Oxford University Press.

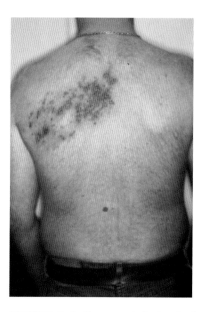

FIGURE 9.4 Characteristic Varicella zoster distribution demonstrating thoracic nerve root involvement.

Problem-orientated Clinical Microbiology and Infection. Second edition. Humphreys H, Irving WL. Copyright 2004. Oxford University Press.

history of disease) with varicella zoster immunoglobulin (VZIG) within 96 h of exposure.

- Treat adolescents, immunocompromised, or pregnant patients with **acyclovir (Zovirax)** or **valacyclovir (Valtrex)** to shorten the course.

- Live attenuated vaccine is now being recommended for children and adolescents to avoid primary disease. However, do not vaccinate pregnant women with this live vaccine.

- *Varicella zoster (shingles).* Should be treated with antiviral medications such as acyclovir (Zovirax) or valacyclovir (Valtrex) within 72 h of eruption. Give oral steroids to control symptoms. Topical capsaicin or topical lidocaine (Lidoderm) may be effective for acute pain relief.

- Postherpetic neuralgia may be treated with NSAIDs, tricyclic antidepressants (TCAs) such as amitriptyline (Elavil), and gabapentin (Neurontin).

Herpes Simplex

Herpes simplex virus (HSV)-1 usually perilabial.

HSV-2 usually genital.

These may often be switched.

Symptoms

Fever blisters are commonly preceded by 3–5 days of characteristic pain or tingling in the affected area, then nonvesicular blister forms and often crusts

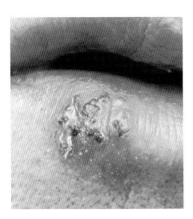

FIGURE 9.5 Herpes simplex virus-1 (HSV-1) lesion on lip.

Problem-orientated Clinical Microbiology and Infection. Second edition. Humphreys H, Irving WL. Copyright 2004. Oxford University Press.

over (see Figure 9.5). History often reveals triggers such as stress, excessive light exposure, trauma, menstruation, or fever.

Diagnosis

TZANCK smear reveals multinucleated giant cells.

Pap smear may reveal suspicious giant cells.

Viral culture, EIA, or PCR (more sensitive) may be done on fluid from the lesion.

Serology: Direct fluorescent antibody (DFA), ELISA, and radioimmunoassay (RIA), and compliment fixation testing may be done on scrapings of the lesion but these tests don't distinguish HSV types. However, primary HSV confers a ≥4-fold increase in titer over the convalescent baseline. Recurrent infection has no increase over the convalescent baseline; thus, the titer increase may be able to distinguish primary from recurrent lesions.

Type-specific serologic antibody testing (immunoblot, western blot, and glycoprotein-G blocking RIA) is available and can show the presence of IgM and IgG antibodies to HSV I and II. However, the clinical utility is limited because HSV I and II may occur either on the oral area or in the genitals. Because of this, the results should be interpreted with consideration that only 85%–90% of genital herpes lesions are of type II.

Indications for obtaining type-specific serology:

- Evaluation and surveillance of asymptomatic long-term sexual partners of infected individuals, especially if pregnant
- Recurrent, undiagnosed genital lesions
- Differentiation of primary versus recurrent disease
- Screening of high risk groups (semen donors, candidates for immunosuppresion, high risk HIV persons, frequent STD clinic patients)

Treatment

- Symptomatic care and pain reduction usually adequate for oral labial lesions. Use capsaicin topical (Zostrix) or NSAIDs as needed for pain.

- If severe, consider treatment within 72 h of onset with antivirals. Use acyclovir (Zovirax) or valacyclovir (Valtrex) or famciclovir (Famvir).
- Suppressive therapy for patients with genital disease reduces the number of outbreaks and may give psychological benefit.
- Pregnant patients with the history of genital disease should be placed on suppressive therapy with valacyclovir (Valtrex) at the end of pregnancy. Perform C-section if active lesions are present on genital tract while in labor.

Measles

Symptoms

Classic triad of symptoms, including **cough, coryza, and conjunctivitis,** appear first. These are commonly accompanied by fever, malaise, photophobia, and **Koplik's spots** on oral mucosa. Rash appears generally on head and spreads down. Onset of rash ~2 weeks after exposure and patient remains contagious until ~4 days after the onset of rash.

Diagnosis

Physical exam: Increased temperature common and resolves 2–3 days after rash onset. Red, morbilliform, blanching rash begins as discrete lesions on head or neck that then coalesce. Pharyngitis and lymphadenopathy may be present (see Figures 9.6 and 9.7).

Labs: Serologic testing for immunoglobulin G (IgG) and IgM is the most widely used technique for diagnosis and involves diagnosing specific

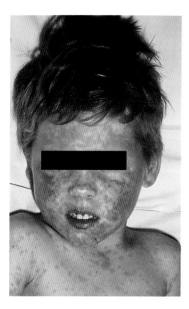

FIGURE 9.6 Primary measles infection.

Problem-orientated Clinical Microbiology and Infection. Second edition. Humphreys H, Irving WL. Copyright 2004. Oxford University Press.

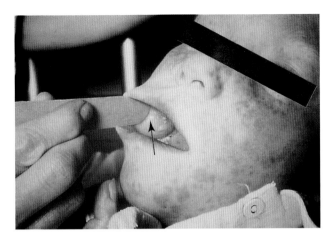

FIGURE 9.7 Koplik's spots on oral buccal mucosa.

Problem-orientated Clinical Microbiology and Infection. Second edition. Humphreys H, Irving WL. Copyright 2004. Oxford University Press.

peaks in these antibodies. Viral culture of lesion requires special facilities, but it may also be used. CBC may show leukopenia, lymphopenia, or thrombocytopenia.

Imaging: Obtain CXR for possible lung involvement.

Associated condition that develops years later is **subacute sclerosing panencephalitis (SSPE)**.

Treatment

- Supportive care with antipyretics, antitussives, and NSAIDs.

- High-risk individuals (pregnancy, HIV, immunosuppressed, etc.) may benefit from postexposure prophylaxis including measles immunoglobulin or live-attenuated measles vaccine. However, do not give measles, mumps, rubella (MMR) or live virus vaccine to pregnant women.

- Give vitamin A in endemically vitamin A–deficient areas.

- Report to local health department.

Q 9.4

A 6-year-old Asian American male is admitted to the general pediatric ward of your hospital with the diagnosis of Kawasaki's disease. He has been receiving high-dose aspirin and IVIG and has steadily improved. What life-threatening complication is this therapy aimed at?

A. Coronary artery aneurysm.
B. Long-term lymphoma development.
C. Pericardial effusion and tamponade.
D. Peripheral extremity skin desquamation.
E. Cardiac valvular embolism and ischemic stroke.

Childhood Exanthems

See Table 9.10.
See Figures 9.8 and 9.9.

TABLE 9.10 Common childhood exanthems

Disease	Associations	Rash	Diagnosis	Treatment
Rubella	Commonly vaccinated for in MMR. Intrapartum infection causes "**congenital rubella syndrome**" in child and includes cataracts, PDA, VSD, hearing loss, etc.	Descending "**blueberry muffin**" rash of infant	Serum IgM and IgG testing. Viral culture may also be used	Postnatal infection: Symptomatic treatment only Congenital rubella: Supportive treatment and contact isolation Vaccinate to prevent. Do not vaccinate pregnant women with MMR
Roseola	Abrupt moderate–high fever. After fever, rash appears	Appearance of maculopapular, nonpruritic, blanchable rash on the trunk, arms, and neck. Short course of hours to days	Serum antibody testing or serum PCR for HHV-6/HHV-7 may also be indicative	Symptomatic care with antipyretics, etc. Self-limited illness
Erythema infectiosum (Fifth disease)	Associated with only mild fever, pruritus, mild arthralgias. Complications include transient **aplastic crisis**, significant joint involvement, and chronic anemia. Hydrops fetalis may occur if acquired during pregnancy	"Slapped cheek" appearance of facial rash. Rash develops into reticulated lacy pattern on trunk and extremities. Once rash appears on face, patient is no longer infectious	IgM antibody indicates acute infection. Less common, but more reliable is testing viral DNA in fetal blood	Symptomatic as needed IVIG in refractory cases or those with significant complications
Kawasaki's disease (mucocutaneous lymph node syndrome)	Fever ≥5 days, bilateral conjunctivitis, cervical lymphadenopathy, characteristic "strawberry" tongue, hand/foot swelling, and desquamation. **Coronary artery aneurysms** of main concern	Polymorphous rash, which may appear as scarlatiniform, morbilliform, or erythema multiforme. Rash may desquamate in groin area	Clinical diagnosis Labs may show leukocytosis, thrombocytosis, anemia, elevated CRP, ESR. Obtain ECG and echocardiogram to evaluate possible aneurysms	High-dose aspirin Consider IVIG to decrease incidence of cardiac abnormalities Follow-up echocardiograms

CRP, C-reactive protein; ESR, erythrocyte sedimentation rate; HHV, human herpesvirus; IVIG, intravenous immunoglobulin; MMR, measles, mumps, rubella; PCR, polymerase chain reaction; PDA, patent ductus arteriosus; VSD, ventral septal defect.

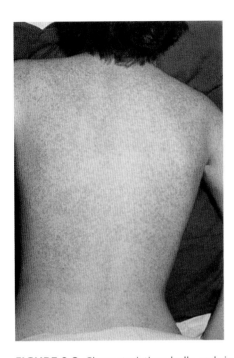

FIGURE 9.8 Characteristic rubella rash in adult female.

Problem-orientated Clinical Microbiology and Infection. Second edition. Humphreys H, Irving WL.
Copyright 2004. Oxford University Press.

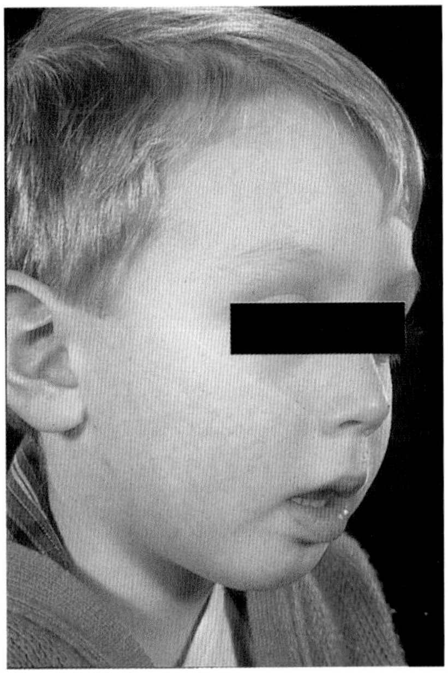

FIGURE 9.9 "Slapped cheek" appearance of erythema infectiosum.

Problem-orientated Clinical Microbiology and Infection. Second edition. Humphreys H, Irving WL.
Copyright 2004. Oxford University Press.

Syphilis

Symptoms

Primary: Painless chancre (or ulcer) on the genitals. Lasts 2–6 weeks and then heals with scarring.

Secondary: Often overlaps with chancre stage, nontender, rash appears usually on **hands and soles of the feet**. Rash is contagious if break in skin present. Accompanied by patchy alopecia, condyloma lata (gray–white lesions on mucous membranes), generalized lymphadenopathy, anorexia, and headache.

Tertiary: Involves other organ systems such as central nervous system (CNS) (neurosyphilis), cardiac system, bones, and skin.

Diagnosis

Primary: Darkfield microscopy of fluid from chancre may demonstrate spirochete. Screening nontreponemal tests are VDRL or RPR. Positive result should be confirmed with treponemal testing: Fluorescent treponemal antibody absorption (FTA-ABS) or microhemagglutination treponemal pallidum (MHA-TP). Follow disease with VDRL or RPR titers, since FTA-ABS/MHA-TP turn positive for life after disease.

Secondary: Positive serologic testing and clinical signs of rash, condyloma lata, characteristic symptoms, generalized lymphadenopathy, or hepatomegaly.

Latent: Asymptomatic stage often between secondary and tertiary.

Tertiary: Involvement of extragenital organ systems. CNS involves neurosyphilis, which may be seen as **tabes dorsalis**, characteristic gait, paresis, paralysis, visual, or hearing disturbance. Cardiac involves the presence of murmur, aneurysms, or valvular abnormalities. Bones may show Charcot joints, osteomyelitis. Skin shows gummas (destructive granulomatous pockets) and possible secondary infections. Serologies may be negative in this stage. Consider lumbar puncture if tertiary stage is suspected. VDRL may be performed on cerebrospinal fluid (CSF) along with treponemal tests.

Congenital: Can lead to meningitis, **saber shins**, **Hutchinson teeth**, and **interstitial keratitis** (see Figure 9.10).

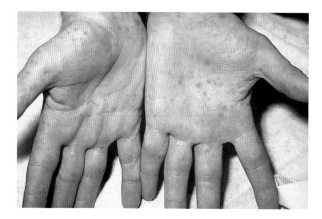

FIGURE 9.10 Typical rash of secondary syphilis on hands.

Clinical Dermatology. Fifth edition. MacKie RM. Copyright 2003. Oxford University Press.

Treatment

- Classic and still very effective is **penicillin G** IM. Alternatives include doxycycline or azithromycin.
- Primary and secondary syphilis should get 2.4 million units IM ×1.
- Tertiary or latent syphilis >1 year should receive Pen G 2.4 million units q. week ×3 weeks.
- Neurosyphilis is very difficult to treat and should get 3–4 million units q. 4 h ×10–14 days.
- Watch for **Jarisch–Herxheimer reaction** of acute febrile illness sometimes seen at the beginning of treatment due to destruction of spirochetes.
- Congenital syphilis should be treated with aqueous crystalline Pen G for 14 days.
- Follow with quantitative VDRL/RPR.

Sexually Transmitted Diseases

See Table 9.11.

Tinea (Dermatophytosis)

Symptoms

Fungal infection almost anywhere on the body. This includes *Tinea capitis*, *T. corporis*, *T. versicolor*, *T. cruris*, *T. pedis*, *T. barbae*. These have varied presentations, but often involve color change, reddening of skin, flaking, alopecia, and pruritus. History often positive for contacts with similar symptoms.

Diagnosis

Clinical diagnosis often made based on appearance.

Skin scraping and exam with potassium hydroxide (KOH). Branching hyphae should be seen if positive.

Treatment

- Topical preparations of azole medications generally effective except against *T. capitis* or nail infections. These include miconazole (Monistat), clotrimazole (Lotrimin), and econazole (Spectazole).
- Oral azoles indicated for *T. capitis*, nail infections, or refractive cases. These include griseofulvin, fluconazole (Diflucan), terbinafine (Lamisil), ketoconazole (Nizoral), or itraconazole (Sporanox).
- Liver function and enzyme testing should be evaluated before starting oral medications.
- Expect long course of 4–6 weeks before cure.

TABLE 9.11 Common STD's

Disease	Associations	Diagnosis	Treatment
Gonorrhea	Urethritis/epididymitis in men, urethritis, cervicitis, or PID in women. Disseminated form possible as well as pauci-articular septic arthritis	Gram stain of purulent fluid for gram-negative diploccoci. DNA probes and PCR also widely used and sensitive. Culture possible, but special medium needed	Ceftriaxone IM or ciprofloxacin PO. Always treat for Chlamydia as well. "Gut and Butt" regimen
Chlamydia	Urethritis/epididymitis in men, urethritis, cervicitis, or PID in women. Other forms of Chlamydia produce pneumonia, trachoma, and psittacosis. Also associated with **lymphogranuloma venereum**	DNA probes and PCR widely used. Culture and direct antigen testing also used	Doxycycline or azithromycin. Always treat for gonorrhea as well. "Gut and Butt" regimen
Chancroid	Associated with **painful** chancre. Uncommon in the United States	Culture and Gram stain for organism. PCR testing also available	Ceftriaxone IM or azithromycin
Trichomoniasis	Frothy, green cervical discharge and fishy odor in women, often asymptomatic in men	Wet prep slide with visualization of organism most common. "Whiff test" positive. PCR, culture, ELISA, DNA probes are also available	Metronidazole (Flagyl)
Genital warts (Condyloma acuminate)	Associated with HPV types 6 and 11, only rarely with higher-risk types	Clinical diagnosis usual. Acetowhite color change positive. PCR may be done on biopsy, but rarely needed	Excision, cryotherapy, CO_2 laser, or electrodesiccation are all common and effective. Imiquimod (Aldara), podophyllin, podofilox (Condylox), and trichloroacetic acid are topical options

In all sexually transmitted diseases (STDs), treat partner as well as patient.
ELISA, enzyme-linked immunosorbent assay; HPV, human papillomavirus; PCR, polymerase chain reaction; PID, pelvic inflammatory disease.

Candidiasis

Symptoms

Erythematous, painful, itchy, well-demarcated patches often in the intertriginous places. Lesions are often moist and malodorous and often reveal classic "satellite lesions." History may reveal immunocompromised state (or risk factors) or diabetes. Do not forget to ask about these.

Diagnosis

Usually a clinical diagnosis that can be made by exam.
Labs: Skin scrapings may be examined on KOH slide. Branching pseudohyphae are pathopneumonic (see Figure 9.11).

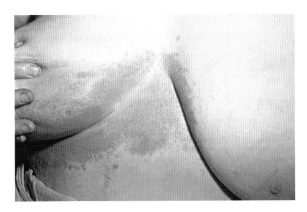

FIGURE 9.11 Inframammary candidiasis in a female diabetic patient.

Clinical Dermatology. Fifth edition. MacKie RM. Copyright 2003. Oxford University Press.

Treatment

Topical therapy often effective and includes Nystatin (Mycostatin) cream powder; this also comes in combination with a topical steroid (or may be mixed) to add itch relief. Clotrimazole cream (Lotrimin, Mycelex) or miconazole (Micatin) are second line.

Mycoses

See Table 9.12.

Hepatitis

See Table 9.13.

TABLE 9.12 Common mycoses infections

Disease	Associations	Treatment
Histoplasmosis	**Midwestern United States**. History may show contact with birds or their droppings. Vast majority are asymptomatic. May be reactivated in immunocompromised	Ketoconazole (Nizoral) if mild Amphotericin-B if disseminated or severe
Coccidioidomycosis	**Southwest United States**. Contracted by contact with dust, soil, or cave exploration. Many cases asymptomatic	Amphotericin-B, ketoconazole (Nizoral), itraconazole (Sporanox), fluconazole (Diflucan) depending on severity
Blastomycosis	**Mississippi and Ohio river valleys**. Soil-dwelling organism. Pulmonary, skin, genital, and re-activation forms	Itraconazole (Sporanox), ketoconazole (Nizoral), or amphotericin-B for severe disease

TABLE 9.13 Characteristics of hepatitis by type

Hepatitis type	Transmission route	Symptoms/ associations	Diagnosis	Treatment
Hep A	Oral-fecal. Occurs in outbreaks of contaminated food and during travel to Latin American or Third World countries	Acute, flu-like illness with abdominal pain and nausea. Often asymptomatic especially in the young. Never chronic!	Anti-HAV IgM positive for acute or recent infection. Anti-HAV IgG indicates prior infection. Antibody is protective	IVIG useful for prevention after exposure. Otherwise, supportive care for acute infection. Vaccinate those at risk
Hep B	Blood or body fluid contact as through sex, drug use (needles), or perinatally	Acute illness has fever, malaise, jaundice, anorexia, etc. Often acutely asymptomatic. May progress to chronic form and cirrhosis or liver cancer. Associated with polyarteritis nodosa	See below	Vaccinate. No indication to treat acute disease. Chronic form treated with Lamivudine or interferon-α. Do not expect cure, but suppression of viral load
Hep C	Blood or body fluid contact as through sex, drug use (needles), or perinatally	Acute illness has fever, malaise, jaundice, anorexia, etc. Fifty percent progress to chronic form. Associated with *Lichen planus*	Anti-HCV antibody shows prior infection. HCV quantitative RNA testing determines virus in blood. If positive, obtain genotype to match with prognosis	Acute: Interferon-α to prevent progression Chronic: Pegylated interferon-α 2b + ribavirin

HAV, hepatitis A virus; HCV, hepatitis C virus; IVIG, intravenous immunoglobulin.

TABLE 9.14 Hep B markers

Marker	Interpretation
HbsAg	Acute or chronic disease
Anti-HBsAg	Antibody conferring immunity
HbeAg	Indicates infectivity
Anti-HBeAg	Antibody indicating low infectivity
IgM anti-HbcAg	Antibody indicating new infection
IgG anti-HbcAg	Antibody indicating old infection

Hepatitis B Markers

See Table 9.14 and Figure 9.12.

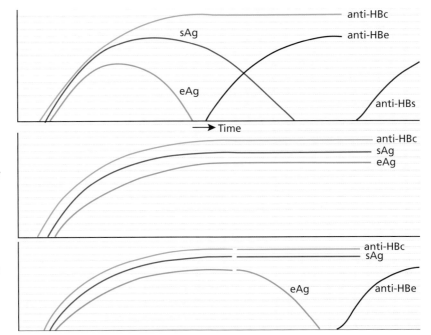

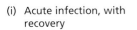

(i) Acute infection, with recovery

(ii) Acute infection followed by chronic carriage, highly infectious, at risk of liver damage

(iii) Acute infection, chronic carriage, but spontaneous (or interferon-induced) seroconversion from eAg to anti-HBe

FIGURE 9.12 Acute hep B infection with recovery.

Problem-orientated Clinical Microbiology and Infection. Second edition. Humphreys H, Irving WL. Copyright 2004. Oxford University Press.

Mumps

Symptoms

Acute febrile illness with the swelling of parotid glands prominent. Sore throat, pain in parotids with eating sour food, mild fever, and malaise are usual. May be accompanied by swelling of testes.

Diagnosis

Physical exam: Swelling of parotid gland and cervical lymph nodes. Elevated temperature common, but moderate. Orchitis may be seen. Meningismal signs including neck tenderness and nuchal rigidity are rare.

Labs: Viral isolation may be done from throat swab, urine, blood, or CSF. If mental status changes and meningismal signs, obtain spinal fluid for testing (see Figures 9.13 and 9.14).

Treatment

- Vaccinate to prevent.
- Usually supportive for acute illness.
- Isolate and keep children home from school until 9 days after the onset of symptoms (contagious period).
- Subfertility uncommon and infertility rare.

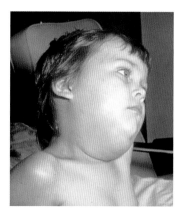

FIGURE 9.13 Parotitis of mumps.

Problem-orientated Clinical Microbiology and Infection. Second edition. Humphreys H, Irving WL. Copyright 2004. Oxford University Press.

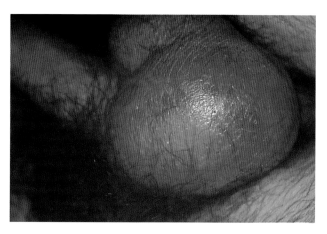

FIGURE 9.14 Orchitis of mumps.

Problem-orientated Clinical Microbiology and Infection. Second edition. Humphreys H, Irving WL. Copyright 2004. Oxford University Press.

Hand, Foot, and Mouth Disease

Symptoms

Acute illness usually of childhood involving vesicular lesions of the mouth, palms of hands, and soles of feet. Usually accompanied by low-grade fever, malaise, and fussiness. History often reveals sick contacts.

Diagnosis

Physical exam: Mouth lesions or ulcers, small, vesicular lesions on palms and soles of feet. See Figures 9.15 and 9.16.
Labs: Virus may be isolated from lesions, but is usually not done. Causative organism is of the coxsackievirus family.

Treatment

- Supportive with NSAIDs and Tylenol.

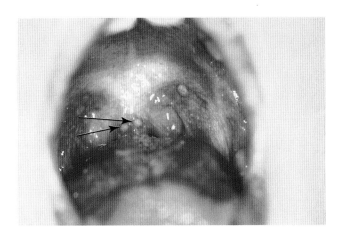

FIGURE 9.15 Typical oral lesions.

Problem-orientated Clinical Microbiology and Infection. Second edition. Humphreys H, Irving WL. Copyright 2004. Oxford University Press.

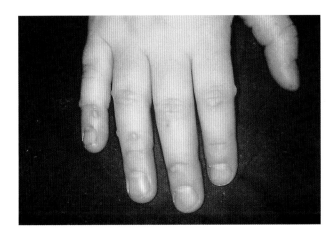

FIGURE 9.16 Typical hand vesicles.

Problem-orientated Clinical Microbiology and Infection. Second edition. Humphreys H, Irving WL. Copyright 2004. Oxford University Press.

Infectious Mononucleosis

Symptoms

Marked fatigue, sore throat, noticeable swollen lymph nodes, anorexia, low-grade fever, and malaise. History often positive for group living such as military recruits, college students, or campers.

Diagnosis

Physical exam: Pharyngitis with erythema and possibly tonsillar exudates. Marked tonsillar swelling: "kissing tonsils." Palpable cervical lymphadenopathy. Palpable spleen may be present indicating enlargement. Look for characteristic rash that may have developed after prior misdiagnosis and treatment of strep throat with amoxicillin.

Labs: Monospot test of IgM heterophile antibodies against Epstein–Barr virus useful in telling acute infection. Usually negative after 6 months. CBC may show lymphocytosis/leukocytosis with atypical lymphocytes, thrombocytopenia.

Imaging: Splenic ultrasound for suspected splenomegaly or to follow course. CT abdomen not needed unless recent injury makes rupture likely (see Figures 9.17 and 9.18).

Treatment

- Supportive care.
- Avoid contact sports or situations of high-risk abdominal injury to avoid possible splenic injury for 3 weeks after the onset of disease. If patient has had clinical documentation of enlarged

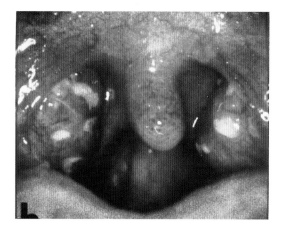

FIGURE 9.17 Tonsillar swelling in acute mononucleosis.

Problem-orientated Clinical Microbiology and Infection. Second edition. Humphreys H, Irving WL. Copyright 2004. Oxford University Press.

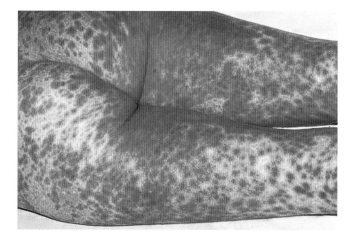

FIGURE 9.18 Morbilliform eruption caused by administration of ampicillin to a patient with infectious mononucleosis.

Clinical Dermatology. Fifth edition. MacKie RM. Copyright 2003. Oxford University Press.

spleen, follow-up ultrasound for the resolution of splenomegaly indicated.

- Oral steroids (prednisone) are used by some and may decrease lymphadenopathy and tonsillar size although this is unproven.

Molluscum Contagiosum

Symptoms

Discrete, flesh-colored lesions with umbilicated top. Often occur in children on inner thighs. Spread very easily from person to person by direct contact or sex. May be reactivated in HIV or immunocompromised patients.

Diagnosis

Physical exam: May be aided by cryotherapy revealing umbilicated top to lesion. Magnification also used. May have white core (see Figure 9.19).

Treatment

- Cryotherapy, electrodessication, or excision are all effective.
- Topical treatments include imiquimod (Aldara), podofilox, trichloroacetic acid, tretinoin, salicylic acid, or podophyllin applied in office. None have been researched but many are clinically used.

Cat Scratch Disease

Symptoms

Inoculation site usually presents as macule that progresses to papule or pustule. The most prominent feature that develops weeks after infection is **lymphadenopathy**, usually of head, neck, or upper extremities. Malaise and

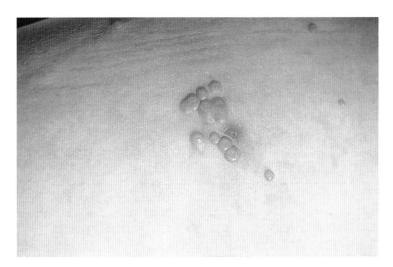

FIGURE 9.19 Molluscum contagiosum showing pearly lesions and central umbilication.

Clinical Dermatology. Fifth edition. MacKie RM. Copyright 2003. Oxford University Press.

fever may be present. History often prominent for contact with cats/kittens with bite or scratch. Eye or encephalitic forms do exist.

Diagnosis

Physical exam: Significant lymphadenopathy and increased temperature.
Labs: Blood culture useful, but the organism, *Bartonella henselae*, is difficult to grow. Histopathology of inoculation site shows characteristic dermis changes. Serologies exist but are often not clinically useful. Skin testing is no longer considered useful due to a variety of reasons.

Treatment

- Multiple antibiotics effective, including azithromycin, erythromycin, doxycycline, TMP/SMX, rifampin, or ciprofloxacin.
- Supportive care with NSAIDs or Tylenol as needed.

Cytomegalic Inclusion Disease

Symptoms

Often asymptomatic, presentation varies widely. Often acute, overlooked viral illness in normal adults with symptoms of fever, malaise, nausea, vomiting, arthralgias, fatigue, chest congestion, or diarrhea. More prominently affects immunocompromised patients (AIDS, transplant recipients) with retinitis, pneumonitis, encephalitis, and other conditions. One of the TORCH [toxoplasmosis, other (hepatitis B, coxsackie, varicella), rubella, cytomegalovirus, and herpes simplex virus, HIV, syphilis]. infections and may lead to fetal stillborn, CNS involvement, deafness, or other birth defects.

Diagnosis

Labs: Fibroblastic cell culture for virus, but may take weeks. Immunofluorescent techniques do exist. CBC may reveal leukopenia or thrombocytopenia with lymphocytosis.
Imaging: Consider skull plain films or CT head for intracerebral calcifications in congenital disease.

Treatment

- Usually symptomatic treatment for normal adults.
- For high-risk groups, consider antiviral medications such as ganciclovir, foscarnet, or cidofovir. Valacyclovir may be used for prophylaxis in bone marrow transplant patients.

Adenovirus

Symptoms

Acute viral illness with cold-like symptoms is usual. Low-grade fever, malaise, nausea, vomiting, chest congestion may be present. May cause upper respiratory tract infection (URI), lower respiratory tract, conjunctival, and

GI symptoms. Often more serious in neonates or immunocompromised patients.

Diagnosis

Physical exam: Pharyngitis, anterior cervical shotty lymphadenopathy, rhinorrhea, nasal blockage, and mild fever.
Labs: Viral culture from pharyngeal swab or stool possible.

Treatment

- Symptomatic with NSAIDs or Tylenol for fever.
- Hydration is important.

Rhinovirus

Symptoms

Common cold symptoms that include rhinitis, runny nose, sore throat, nasal congestion, facial pain, ear pain, or other minor URI symptoms.

Diagnosis

Vast majority may safely be clinically diagnosed as common cold or viral rhinitis.
Screen for other etiologies such as bacterial sinusitis as necessary.

Treatment

- Symptomatic care is the standard.
- Needless to say, antibiotics are ineffective.
- Decongestants, antihistamines, mucolytics all may be used. NSAIDs, OTC analgesics, lozenges, or throat spray are all widely used for sore throat pain.

Toxoplasmosis

Symptoms

Several different forms. Congenital form is worse when acquired during first trimester of pregnancy. Includes symptoms ranging from asymptomatic to jaundice, microcephaly, mental retardation, seizures, visual defects (**chorioretinitis**), or death in the first month of life. Ocular form is seen as chorioretinitis and eyesight difficulties. If acquired while mother was pregnant, often shows much later in life. Acute form in immunocompromised patients may have CNS symptoms such as **focal neurologic deficits**, seizures, mental status changes, visual changes, encephalitis, or meningeal symptoms. Acute infection in normal host may show symptoms of mild viral illness. Look for history of exposure to cat feces (litter boxes) or ingestion of undercooked pork.

Diagnosis

Physical exam: Increased temperature, focal neurologic signs, change in mental status, signs of increased intracranial pressure (increased BP, papilledema). Generalized lymphadenopathy. Retinal exam may show yellow, white, fluffy cotton patches.

Labs: Demonstration of the organism (a protozoan) in blood, body fluids, or placenta is diagnostic. ELISA and PCR testing are also useful in finding acute infection. Serologies that detect IgM and IgG are also available and may be useful to detect infection in pregnant patients.

Imaging: CT scan of head with contrast may show intracranial **ring-enhancing lesion**. **Intracranial calcifications** also may be seen. MRI also useful. Ultrasound of fetus may show suspicion, which can be tested for by amniocentesis (See Figure 9.20).

Treatment

- Prevention of congenital form by instructing pregnant women to avoid litter boxes, cats, eating raw meat.

- Otherwise, give sulfadiazine (Microsulfon), pyrimethamine (Daraprim), or leucovorin (folinic acid). Regimens include months of treatment and in immunocompromised (AIDS) may require maintenance regimen after treatment. Use TMP/SMX for prophylaxis in AIDS patients with CD4 counts <100 and positive IgG titer. Pregnant women may start one of these drugs after 16th week.

- Supportive care and admission to hospital should be considered.

West Nile Virus

Symptoms

Transmitted by mosquitoes, this acute flu-like illness may present with fever, flaccid paralysis, headache, neck pain, vomiting, myalgias, muscle weakness, maculopapular rash, diarrhea, or altered mental status. Presentation may resemble Guillain–Barré syndrome. Timing is usually late spring.

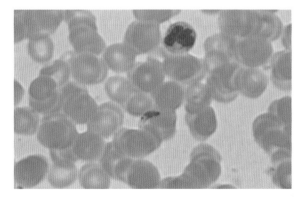

FIGURE 9.20 Tachyzoite of *Toxoplasma gondii*.

With permission Nivaldo Medeiros, MD.

Diagnosis

Physical exam: Encephalitis form may be severe and involve high fever, altered mental status, meningeal signs, and other conditions.

Labs: Lumbar puncture may be characteristic of viral meningitis (pleocytosis with lymphocytic predominance, increased protein). ELISA may be done on CSF. Test the serum for West Nile antibodies.

Treatment

- Supportive as needed.
- If infection is severe or the patient is elderly, consider hospitalization.

Q 9.5

A 21-year-old Caucasian female presents to your office complaining of 4-day history of fever, myalgias, arthralgias, and headache after a recent camping trip as camp counselor to her little sister's girl scout troop. She has not thrown up during this illness, but does endorse nausea. Her vital signs are BP 120/84, HR 88, temperature 39.0°C (102.2°F), RR 18. Her exam is normal except for a maculopapular rash on the wrists and ankles. The rash is blanchable, nonpruritic, and nonpainful. She denies noticing the rash before. What is the best course of treatment for this patient?

A. Metronidazole (Flagyl) orally.
B. Adequate PO fluid intake and supportive care.
C. Ciprofloxacin orally and supportive care.
D. Doxycycline orally.
E. Rabies immunoglobulin IM.

Rocky Mountain Spotted Fever

Symptoms

Classic triad is **headache, fever, characteristic rash**. However, other symptoms include nausea/vomiting, abdominal pain, myalgias, lymphadenopathy, and CNS symptoms. History often reveals tick bite or time in the outdoors.

Diagnosis

Physical exam: Mild fever, photophobia; rash may be macular, maculopapular, or petechial in appearance. Rash is centripetal (starts on extremities and moves toward trunk).

Labs: CBC for hematocrit and platelets, which may be low. WBC count is not helpful because of common variation. Chem-7 may show electrolyte abnormalities especially in advanced cases. Antibody testing possible, but usually not helpful early because of typical late antibody response. Skin biopsy possible, but rarely used. Cultures are not available outside large research centers.

Treatment

- Antibiotics include doxycycline (as with most rickettsial diseases), tetracycline, or chloramphenicol in kids.
- Supportive care as needed with tylenol and NSAIDs.

Q 9.6

A 22-year-old male army soldier who has returned from a recent deployment to East Africa comes to the ER with complaints of ongoing fevers/chills, myalgias, malaise, headache, and mild nausea. He states his fevers began ~1 week before returning from Africa and seem to come and go. His trip was otherwise uneventful, and he states he has not taken any medicine throughout the recent past. His vital signs are now BP 134/90, temperature 39.6°C (103.2°F), RR 18, HR 102. Exam is unremarkable except for generalized myalgias and mild hepatomegaly. Laboratory investigation with thick/thin blood smears demonstrates malarial schizonts. What potentially fatal reaction may occur from therapy?

A. Hemolysis if glucose-6-phosphatase deficient.
B. Jarisch–Herxheimer reaction if parasite load is high enough.
C. Stevens–Johnson syndrome if allergic to chloroquine.
D. Flash pulmonary edema if glucose-6-phosphatase deficient.
E. Inadequate effect on parasite if given chloroquine to chloroquine-resistant organism.

Malaria

Types include *Plasmodium falciparum, P. vivax, P. malariae, P. ovale*. Most severe and lethal is *P. falciparum*. Types vary by endemic area although cross-over is common.

Symptoms

Episodic fever, chills, malaise, fatigue, headache, and nausea. Seizures and CNS involvement may be present in severe forms and are extremely serious. The protozoan disease is transmitted by the female anopheles mosquito, thus history of exposure to these pests is common. Look for travel to endemic areas (commonly Africa or tropical regions). If patient is from endemic area and has had malaria before, disease is often much milder.

Diagnosis

Physical exam: Cycles of temperature elevation every 36–72 h depending on type. Hepatomegaly or splenomegaly may be felt.

Labs: Malarial thin and thick blood smears examined for the presence of schizonts or gametocytes. Take at least three samples 6–12 h apart, best if obtained during fever spike. PCR and indirect fluorescent antibody (IFA) testing may yield type. Rapid malarial antigen tests have recently become available in the US and show promise of a more rapid test for *plasmodium* parasites, however, they are still not as sensitive or specific as thin/thick blood smears. Otherwise, CBC will likely show anemia, leukopenia or leukocytosis, and possibly thrombocytopenia. Hepatic function panel may show elevated liver transaminases. Chem-7 can be used to evaluate and follow renal function (see Figures 9.21 and 9.22).

Treatment

- Avoid mosquitoes by using DEET-based repellent and barrier precautions.

- Avoid the disease by taking chemoprophylaxis correctly. Mefloquine (Lariam), Malarone (atovaquone/proguanil), or doxycycline all must be started days to weeks before traveling and be continued weeks after return.

- Treatment of active disease consists of killing active protozoa and liver stage parasites. Chloroquine (in sensitive areas), primaquine, quinidine, quinine, doxycycline, tetracycline, mefloquine,

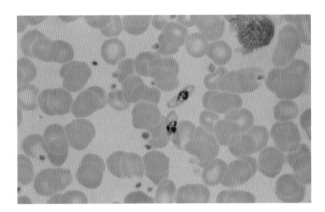

FIGURE 9.21 Two macrogametocytes of *Plasmodium falciparum.*

With permission Nivaldo Medeiros, MD.

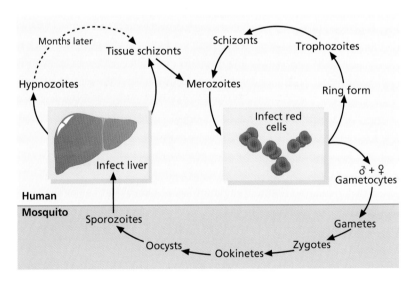

FIGURE 9.22 Lifecycle of malaria parasite.

Problem-orientated Clinical Microbiology and Infection. Second edition. Humphreys H, Irving WL. Copyright 2004. Oxford University Press.

pyrimethamine/sulfadoxine (Fansidar), Malarone (atovaquone/proguanil), or combinations of these are often very effective. Side effects are common and include GI upset, nausea/vomiting, headache, vivid dreams, lost memory, or insomnia.

- Make sure patient does not have glucose-6-phosphatase deficiency (G6PD) before starting therapy (to avoid hemolysis).

- Admit to hospital for monitoring in nonendemic patients. Transfer to ICU if seizures occur.

Lyme Disease

Tick-borne organism: *Borrelia burgdorferi*.

Symptoms

Stage 1: Localized disease often with characteristic target-like rash (**erythema chronicum migrans**). Also includes acute flu-like illness.

Stage 2: Early disseminated disease may involve symptoms of any organ system; CNS and cardiac system are most common. Look for meningitis symptoms, focal deficits, and heart block, and pericarditis.

Stage 3: Involves arthritis and chronic neurological syndromes.
History often indicates tick bite, although to transmit Lyme tick must be on for 12–24 h.

Diagnosis

Physical exam: Increased temperature common. Target like macular rash.
Labs: ELISA serum tests for IgM or IgG to *B. burgdorferi*. Follow positive result with Western blot. REMEMBER this test may be negative in first stage, thus cannot acutely be used for the evaluation of a tick-bite victim. CSF culture may be done and is diagnostic although may take some time (see Figure 9.23).

Treatment

- All three stages can be treated with doxycycline, or amoxicillin in children, for 3–4 weeks. Consider corticosteroids in stage 2. Cefuroxime, ceftriaxone (Rocephin), or cefotaxime (Claforan) may also be used IV or IM in stages 2 or 3.

- Consider ICU admission and/or cardiac monitoring in stage 2.

- Consider prophylactic dose of doxycycline in all tick-bite patients.

TORCHES Infections During Pregnancy

See Table 9.15.

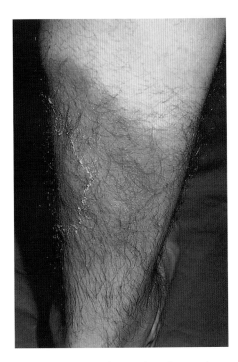

FIGURE 9.23 Erythema chronicum migrans on leg of patient with Lyme disease.

Clinical Dermatology. Fifth edition. MacKie RM. Copyright 2003. Oxford University Press.

TABLE 9.15 TORCHS infections of pregnancy

Disease	Sequelae
Toxoplasmosis	Retinitis, intracranial calcifications, mental retardation, jaundice, stillbirth
Other (hepatitis B, coxsackie, varicella)	Specific for disease. Varicella may cause limb hypoplasia
Rubella	Deafness, cataracts, microphthalmia, cardiovascular defects such as ventral septal defect (VSD) and patent ductus defects
Cytomegalovirus (CMV)	Deafness, micropthalmia, cerebral calcifications, mental retardation
Herpes	Skin lesions, encephalitis, conjunctivitis
HIV	Transmission to infant
Syphilis	Rhinitis, saber shins, Hutchinson teeth, interstitial keratitis, and skin lesions

Osteomyelitis

Symptoms

Symptoms are often localized and may include pain, overlying skin break-down, swelling, erythema, or drainage. Constitutional symptoms such as fever, malaise, arthralgias, or headache may be present. History may reveal source of bacteremia, comorbid vascular insufficiency, or recent operation or prosthetic device.

Diagnosis

Physical exam: Local inflammation, erythema, swelling, tenderness, ulceration, and drainage often are present in acute form. Chronic form may be asymptomatic.

Labs: Definitive diagnosis is made by aspiration or bone biopsy and culture. Blood cultures often positive. CBC shows leukocytosis in acute infection. Erythrocyte sedimentation rate (ESR) or C-reactive protein (CRP) often elevated.

Imaging: No single modality may be used for diagnosis or to rule out infection. Radiographs show characteristic appearance although often negative until weeks into infection. Nuclear medicine bone scan often helpful but nonspecific. CT scan may be used; MRI is the best overall modality (see Figure 9.24).

Treatment

- Empiric therapy guided by organism identification and sensitivities are best.

- Empiric regimens include nafcillin [if non methicillin-resistant *Staphylococcus aureus* (MRSA)], vancomycin (if MRSA), ciprofloxacin, or levofloxacin. Start these, or combinations of these, after bone is cultured. Duration often 4–6 weeks or longer in chronic form.

- Surgical debridement and removal of necrotic tissue or hardware is essential.

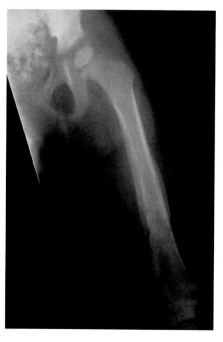

FIGURE 9.24 X-ray of femoral osteomyelitis in child.

Problem-orientated Clinical Microbiology and Infection. Second edition. Humphreys H, Irving WL. Copyright 2004. Oxford University Press.

- Revascularization surgery is beneficial in those patients who are candidates.
- Place patient on bed rest and place cast if necessary.
- Amputation is the last resort.

Incubation Periods and Infectivity

See Figure 9.25.

Incubation period usually <1 week

Staphylococcal enteritis	1–6 h
Salmonella enteritis	6–48 h (usually 12–24 h)
Bacillary dysentery (*Shigella*)	1–7 days (usually 1–3 days)
Botulism	12–96 h (usually 18–36 h)
Cholera	12 h–6 days (usually 1–3 days)
Gas gangrene	6 h–4 days
Diphtheria	2–5 days
Gonorrhoea	1–12 days (usually 3–5 days)
Legionnaires' disease	2–10 days (usually 7 days)
Meningococcaemia	1–7 days (usually 3 days)
Scarlet fever	1–4 days
Yellow fever	3–6 days

Incubation period usually 1–3 weeks

Brucellosis	7–21 days
Chickenpox	7–23 days (usually ≈14 days)
Lassa fever	3–16 days
Leptospirosis	2–21 days (usually 7–12 days)
Malaria (falciparum)	7–14 days (occasionally longer)
Malaria (vivax, malariae, ovale)	12–40 days (occasionally >1 year)
Measles	10–18 days (rash usually 14–18 days)
Mumps	14–18 days
Pertussis (whooping cough)	5–14 days (usually 7–10 days)
Poliomyelitis	3–21 days (usually 7–10 days)
Rubella	14–21 days
Tetanus	1 day–3 months (usually 4–14 days)
Typhoid	8–21 days
Typhus	4–21 days

Incubation period usually >3 weeks

Amoebiasis	2 weeks–many months
Hepatitis A	3–5 weeks (usually 4 weeks)
Hepatitis B, hepatitis C	6 weeks–6 months
HIV	3 weeks–3 months (anti-HIV appears)
Infectious mononucleosis	4–6 weeks
Rabies	4 days–2 years (usually 3–12 weeks)
Syphilis	10 days–10 weeks (usually 3 weeks)

FIGURE 9.25 Continued

Duration of infectivity of infectious diseases

Chickenpox	5 days before rash until last vesicle crusts
Hepatitis A	2 weeks before until 1 week after jaundice starts
Measles	From initial symptoms to 5 days after rash appears
Mumps	3 days before to 1 week after salivary swelling
Pertussis	3 days before to 3 weeks after start of symptoms (3 days if on erythromycin)
Rubella	1 week before to 5 days after onset of rash
Scarlet fever	10–21 days from onset of rash (1 day if on penicillin)

FIGURE 9.25 Incubation periods of selected infectious diseases.

Answers

9.1 E. This patient is showing several features of infection with *Pneumocystis carinii* infection including fever, cough, decreased appetite, and chest congestion. He has a decreased CD4 count to <200 mm^3 as well, which indicates he is at particular danger of developing the disease from this opportunistic organism. Chest x-ray of *P. carinii* infection characteristically has a perihilar infiltrate and interstitial shadowing. Although the other answers may be possible, would not indicate the likely *P. carinii* infection in this patient.

9.2 B. Since this patient has a CD4 count of <200 mm^3 and is showing symptoms of infection, highly active antiretroviral therapy (HAART) is indicated. Also, the patient likely has pneumonia from *P. carinii* infection, which is best treated with trimethoprim/sulfamethoxazole (TMP/SMX) IV for 21 days.

9.3 C. This patient has had one positive ELISA screen, which indicates confirmation with a repeat blood sample from the patient. This should be done immediately to avoid undue stress as in answer E. Western blot analysis may be used for confirmation, but standard practice is only to complete this after a second sample for ELISA has been taken.

9.4 A. Coronary artery aneurysm is the life-threatening complication of Kawasaki's disease and must be evaluated for with initial and repeat echocardiography in affected patients.

9.5 D. This patient exhibits symptoms of rocky mountain spotted fever including headache, fever, and rash. Her history of recent camping trip indicates possible exposure to tick bite.

9.6 A. Hemolysis is a potentially fatal reaction that occurs in patients with glucose-6-phosphatase deficiency (G6PD) after being given chloroquine-related treatment. Since malaria itself has some degree of hemolysis by the mechanism of disease, vigilant monitoring of therapy must take place in individuals of unknown G6PD status. Answer E details a potentially fatal result of disease, not therapy.

10   Emergency and Trauma

Eye Injuries	224
Foreign Body in the Eye	224
Chemical Burns of the Eye	224
Blunt Trauma to the Eye	225
Wounds/Bites	226
Foreign Bodies	227
Food Poisoning	227
Poisonings	228
Toxic Effects of Substances of Common Use/Abuse	229
Treatment of Nonmedicinal Substance Ingestion	230
Adverse Effects of Medicinal and Biologic Substances	231
Rape/Crisis Adjustment	232
Cranial Injuries	233
Internal Injuries, Abdomen, and Pelvis	234
Frostbite	235
Hypothermia	236
Heat Stroke	239
Complications of Surgery	240
Hemorrhage Complicating Surgery	240
Postoperative Infection	241
Other Complications of Surgical Procedures	241
Burns	241
Concussion	245

Eye Injuries

Foreign Body in the Eye

Symptoms

Extreme pain from corneal abrasion to mild sensation of scratchy or foreign body–like sensation. Tearing, hyperemia, and photophobia are common. Obvious bleeding and rarely ruptured globe are obvious. History often reveals metal work, welding, wood shop work, or other activities with high risk for particulate projectiles to be lodged into the eye.

Diagnosis

Fluorescein eye drops with Wood's lamp is very useful in detecting foreign body or abrasion. Slit lamp is also mandatory if abrasion or foreign body is found. Evert the eyelid to evaluate for hidden foreign bodies under the lid. **Imaging:** Consider a CT of the orbits. DO NOT DO AN MRI unless absolutely sure that no metal is in the eye!

Treatment

- Copious ocular irrigation for 15 min is the standard of care, but usually recommended just after initial injury. May be completed later if the patient is not sure of when the injury occurred.

- With slit lamp or magnification, use a cotton swab or small tissue forceps to extract any bodies that are immediately visible. If the foreign body very small, may attempt to use a large bore needle to remove them, but this technique should be reserved only for the very experienced!

- Topical anesthetic [e.g., proparacaine 0.5% ophthalmic (Alcaine)] is certainly warranted. Give erythromycin, tobramycin, or bacitracin-polymyxin B eye drops for antibacterial coverage. Give systemic opioids for pain relief. Avoid contact lens use and consider a 24–72 h eyepatch. Follow up with ophthalmologist in 1–2 days.

Chemical Burns of the Eye

Symptoms

Excruciating pain usually following obvious splash, spray, or other exposure to noxious chemicals. Profuse tearing, hyperemia, photophobia, swelling, and pain are almost always present. Obtain history for alkali or acid burn. Do not forget that chemical fumes can cause burns as well.

Diagnosis

For diagnosis, immediately flush eye for 15–30 min without delay or pause. Careful slit lamp or magnified exam after topical anesthesia with agents such as proparacaine 0.5% ophthalmic (Alcaine).

Treatment

- Initially, flush with copious amounts of water or NS for 15–30 min. Do not delay flushing for diagnosis.
- Give topical anesthetic for complete eye exam with magnification or slit lamp.
- Consider cycloplegic drugs (e.g., atropine 1% ophthalmic) to reduce iritis and iris spasm, which may be very painful.
- Give topical antibiotics.
- Treat with generous oral pain medicines.
- Follow up with ophthalmologist in 24 h.

Blunt Trauma to the Eye

Symptoms

Pain, swelling, hyperemia, photophobia, tearing, and contusion will be obvious. History of event should reveal exact mechanism.

Diagnosis

Physical exam: Do a superficial exam of the bony orbits to evaluate for fracture. Examine for extraocular movements. Positive exam or lack of eye movement suggests possible orbital fracture as well as possible globe injury.

Never forcibly open the eyelids since this may aggravate a globe injury.

Generously anesthetize with systemic agents such as meperidine (Demerol) and do a complete eye exam. Stop exam if significant anterior chamber hemorrhage (hyphema), or globe rupture found.

Imaging: Consider CT of the head to evaluate for fracture.

Evaluate and treat for foreign bodies as above.

Treatment

- Initially, control pain with meperidine (Demerol) or morphine. IM/IV more effective than PO route, because of the short time to onset.
- Dilate pupil with short-acting mydriatic such as cyclopentolate 1% ophthalmic (Cyclogyl) and phenylephrine 2.5% ophthalmic (Neo-Synephrine ophthalmic).
- Topical antibiotic drops should be started according to the regimen for foreign bodies.
- Referral to ophthalmologist in <24 h is often needed. Consider stat consult and transport if significant injury.
- Treatment of anterior chamber hemorrhage (hyphema) includes the measurement of intraocular pressure and administration of a carbonic anhydrase inhibitor (acetazolamide) if needed.
- Use of aminocaproic acid (Amicar) may reduce recurrent bleeding.

- Avoid nonsteroidal antiinflammatory drugs (NSAIDs) in anesthetic regimens as this may cause further bleeding.

- Eyepatch/shield until evaluation by ophthalmology or 72 h in mild injury.

Wounds/Bites

Symptoms

Obvious bleeding or laceration. Signs of superficial infection such as erythema, swelling, red streaking up an extremity, pain, and decreased range of motion.

Diagnosis

Physical exam: Evaluate for drainage tract or fluctuance, which may indicate abscess.

If bite is in the hand, consider tenosynovitis (see Chapter 8).

Wound culture/sensitivities of any expressible fluid from infected-looking wound.

Consider blood cultures.

Imaging: Plain x-rays on any wound that is suspected of having foreign body.

Consider bone scan and plain x-rays to evaluate for underlying osteomyelitis if wound is infected.

Treatment

- **Generously irrigate**. This alone may help most against future infection.

- Take into account the time course from injury to when the patient presents. Determine the level of cleanliness of the wound. Follow recommendations for tetanus and rabies prophylaxis in Chapter 1 of this book.

- If wound is infected, consider debridement of the surrounding tissue.

- Tetanus and rabies prophylaxis as indicated.

- Antibiotics: Give Augmentin (amoxicillin/clavulanate), trimethoprim-sulfamethoxazole (TMP-SMX) DS, or clindamycin (Cleocin). Erythromycin or clarithromycin (Biaxin) are second line.

- Referral is indicated for deep hand infections or tenosynovitis for immediate operative debridement.

- Suture or staple wounds loosely to close. In high-tension areas, consider mattress suturing for strength; in deep wounds consider multiple layer closure. Consider referral to plastic surgery if large laceration on face. Never close a dirty or infected wound!

TABLE 10.1 Common sites of foreign bodies

Location	Associations/treatment
Ear	Straighten the external ear canal by pulling the tragus or pinna. Irrigation is the first step. Extract using alligator forceps, ear probes, or glue on end of Q-Tip if possible.
Nose	Have the patient try to hold one nostril and blow object out. Consider sedation for young, combative patients. Topical vasoconstrictor/anesthetic such as tetracaine/cocaine may help to dislodge object. Extract using forceps when possible.
Trachea	Decreased/absent breath sounds on one side of chest or wheezing on exam. Cough may or may not be present. Order a chest x-ray (CXR) to visualize. Attempt to dislodge with abdominal thrusts. Bronchoscopy with extraction is the gold standard.
Pharynx/larynx	Protect the airway! If occluded, attempt abdominal thrusts on children and adults or back blows/abdominal thrusts on infants. Look for cyanosis, inability to make noise, decreased consciousness. Consider cricothyroidotomy if significant time passes without breathing
Esophagus or GI tract	Determine if the object is blunt or able to pass through the gut. Order CXR, acute abdominal series. Endoscopy if object may be extracted from above. Consider surgery if the object has passed the stomach, causing active bleeding; has embedded in the wall of gut; is not passing over time; or is obstructing. Consider watchful waiting by serial x-rays if the object is small, blunt, and rapidly passing down the gut

Foreign Bodies

See Table 10.1.

Food Poisoning

Symptoms

Nausea, vomiting, diarrhea (bloody or not), fever, malaise, avoidance of PO intake, and abdominal cramps are common. History usually reveals eating questionable food or sharing meal with other sick contacts. Look for recent meals of left-over rice (*Bacillus cereus*), undercooked poultry (*Salmonella*), undercooked hamburger (*E. coli* 0157:H7), or raw oysters (*Shigella*).

Diagnosis

Labs: Stool Hemoccult testing may show positive results if diarrhea is bloody, although false-negative results are also possible. CBC for leukocytosis or lymphocytosis. Chem-7 for electrolyte levels.

Stool studies such as ova/parasites, leukocytes, reducing substances, and culture.

Blood cultures if admitted to the hospital.

Treatment

- Often empiric based on history. Bismuth subsalicylate (Pepto) may be tried first and may provide some antiinflammatory action.
- Antibiotics are controversial and not proven effective. Consider only in case of prolonged illness state, if known or highly suspected susceptible organism is present, or if other treatments have failed.
- Ciprofloxacin (Cipro) has broad-spectrum coverage. TMP-SMX (Bactrim, Septra) is also active against many likely organisms.
- Do not give loperamide (Imodium) or antiemetics too soon as it may worsen the course if etiology is a toxin-producing organism such as *Shigella*, *Clostridium perfringens*, or *B. cereus*. Give in later course of illness if dehydration suspected.
- Hydration is the standard treatment. Orally if tolerated or IV if needed.

Poisonings

Symptoms

Almost any presentation is possible, but often symptoms include loss of or decreased consciousness, lethargy, coma, altered breathing, blurry vision, and others. Classic acronym is "Hot as a stove, Red as a beet, Dry as a bone, Mad as a hatter," indicating anticholinergic overdose.

Diagnosis

Labs: Drug screen is one of the first steps. Chem-7 and CBC.
   ECG for arrhythmias and placement of cardiac monitoring.

Treatment

- Above all: Remember your ABCs! Intubate if necessary.
- If the agent is identified and an antidote exists, give it (see Table 10.3). Otherwise, follow these guidelines:
  - Activated charcoal is the first line and absorbs most substances excluding heavy metals.
  - Bowel irrigation with polyethylene glycol may be considered, but is rarely used because of long time-course and unsure absorption of toxin. May be useful in heavy metals or drug "mules."
  - Emesis is rarely if ever the right answer on the test. Contraindicated in caustic or inflammatory agents or if patient is seizing or with impaired gag reflex. Short time course required from ingestion to be effective.
  - Gastric lavage if short time course from ingestion and patient is awake with intact gag reflex or intubated. May be used in suicide attempts with pill ingestion, but make sure pills will fit in the lavage tube.

- Alkalization of blood/urine is used generally for aspirin, phenobarbital and tricyclic antidepressants. Improves elimination.

- Hemodialysis is definitive treatment. Used after significant amount of time passed from ingestion or significant toxic effect occurring. Use with theophylline, methanol, lithium, barbiturates, or ethylene glycol.

Toxic Effects of Substances of Common Use/Abuse

See Table 10.2.

TABLE 10.2 Characteristics of commonly used recreational drugs

Class	Examples	Effects
Hallucinogens	LSD (lysergic acid diethylamide) "magic mushrooms," PCP (Phencyclidine), Peyote	Psychosis, audio/visual hallucinations, delusions, paranoia, arrhythmias
Depressants	EtOH, marijuana, "moonshine," benzodiazepines, barbiturates	Depressed mood, altered consciousness, relaxed feeling, paranoia, amotivational syndrome
Stimulants	Amphetamines, "ice," cocaine, crank, PCP	Stimulation and elevation of mood, erratic/dangerous behavior, psychosis, aggression, delusions (of grandeur), paranoia, tachycardia, mydriasis (dilation), hypertension
Opioids	Heroin, narcotics, Rx pain medications	Pain control, high feeling, euphoria, respiratory depression, miosis (constriction), constipation, chronic sensitization
Inhalants (huffing)	Glues, fuel vapors, paint vapors (especially metallic colors)	Euphoria, dizziness, slurred speech, ataxia, respiratory depression, arrhythmias

Q 10.1

You are working in the ER of a major metropolitan trauma center when several patients start to come in with symptoms including recurrent vomiting, tearing of eyes, and uncontrolled salivation. More and more patients start arriving by ambulance with similar symptoms. After seeing several patients, you determine they were all in the same bus station and all report a malodorous hazy mist inside the building preceding the onset of symptoms. The worst patients also have shown uncontrolled urination, defecation, dyspnea, air hunger, and bradycardia. By history and physical exam, you suspect acute organophosphate poisoning, which is later confirmed by lab studies. What is the next step in the management of these patients?

A. Neostigmine (Prostigmin).
B. Pralidoxime (2-PAM).
C. Edrophonium (Tensilon).
D. Amyl nitrite.
E. Copious IV fluids and supplemental oxygen.

Treatment of Nonmedicinal Substance Ingestion

See Table 10.3.

TABLE 10.3 Treatment of selected substance ingestion

Substance	Treatment
Heavy metals including lead, mercury	EDTA or dimercaprol
Iron	Deferoxime
Acetone	Removal from source, GL, O_2, and fluids
Carbon monoxide	100% O_2
Cyanide	Emesis or lavage; amyl nitrite→sodium nitrite→sodium thiosulfate
Ethylene glycol (automobile antifreeze), methanol	E_tOH drip (or PO), fomizole
Ethanol	Emesis or GL; IV glucose, fluids, consider dialysis
Benzene	Respiratory support, benzodiazepine for seizures, transfusion if anemia severe (may cause long-term effects)
Organophosphates (herbicides/insecticides)	2-PAM (pralidoxime) or atropine
Rat poison	Vitamin K

EDTA, ethylenediaminetetraacetic acid; GL, gastric lavage.

Q 10.2

A 20-year-old male college student comes to the ER the day after an end-of-semester kegger complaining of severe GI upset, profuse diarrhea, and fever. He states the party was hosted at a campground on a nearby lake. He reports drinking heavily, but claims he "normally can hold his liquor" quite well. Stool studies include ova and parasite analysis, which shows the organism *Giardia lamblia*. What treatment below is contraindicated in this patient?

A. Metronidazole (Flagyl).
B. Trimethoprim-sulfamethoxazole (TMP/SMX) DS (Bactrim DS).
C. Ciprofloxacin (Cipro).
D. Nitazoxanide (Alinia).
E. IV fluids and supportive care.

Adverse Effects of Medicinal and Biologic Substances

See Table 10.4.

TABLE 10.4 Effects of various biologically active agents

Substance	Effect	Substance	Effect
Acetaminophen	Liver damage	HMG CoA reductase inhibitors (statins)	Muscle aches, rhabdomyolysis, liver toxicity
α_1-Blockers	Orthostatic hypotension (first dose)	Isotretinoin (Accutane)	Suicidal tendencies, pregnancy-teratogen
Aminoglycoside	Oto/renal toxicity	INH (Isoniazid)	Peripheral neuropathy, lupus, vitamin B_6 deficiency
Amiodarone	Pulmonary fibrosis, thyroid problems	Lithium	Hypothyroidism, diabetes insipidus
Aspirin	GI bleed	Loop diuretics	Hypokalemia, hypocalcemia
β-Blockers	Asthma exacerbation, depression, alopecia	MAO-inhibitors	Reaction with wine, aged cheese, many drug/drug interactions
Bupropion	Seizures	Metronidazole	Photosensitivity, abd cramping, flushing/ nausea with EtOH
ACE inhibitors	Cough, pregnancy-renal agenesis	Metformin (Glucophage)	Lactic acidosis
Calcium channel blockers	Heart block	Methotrexate	Myelosupression, pulmonary fibrosis
Chloramphenicol	Aplastic anemia, gray baby	Niacin	Flushing
Clindamycin	Psudomembranous colitis (*Clostridium difficile*)	Oxytocin	SIADH
Carbamazepine (Tegretol)	SIADH, aplastic anemia, agranulocytosis	Phenytoin (Dilantin)	Pregnancy-teratogen
Colchicine	GI upset, diabetes insipidus	Progesterone	Spotting, weight gain, depression
Cimetidine	Inhibits hepatic enzymes, gynecomastia, Increased warfarin effect	Sildenafil (Viagra)	Blue vision, contraindication with nitrates
Cyclosporine	Nephrotoxicity	SSRIs	GI upset, delayed ejaculation, insomnia
Allopurinol	Gout flare, GI upset, rash, Stevens–Johnson syndrome (rare)	Tetracycline	Pregnancy—teeth staining

(continued)

TABLE 10.4 Effects of various biologically active agents

Substance	Effect	Substance	Effect
Digoxin	GI upset, bradycardia	Thiazide diuretics	Hypercalcemia, gout exacerbation
Finasteride	Pregnancy—male genital malformation	Trazodone	Priapism
Fluoroquinolones	Pregnancy—cartilage damage in fetus	Rifampin	Orange tears/urine/sweat
Heparin	Heparin-induced thrombocytopenia	Phenergan	Dystonic reaction
Ketoconazole	Gynecomastia	Warfarin	Warfarin skin necrosis, birth defects
Meperidine (Demerol)	Seizures, coma, toxic metabolite build-up	Vancomycin	"Red Man" syndrome
Disulfiram (Antabuse)	Severe nausea/vomiting, flushing on EtOH use	Valproic acid (Depakene)	Hepatotoxicity, pancreatitis, teratogen
Estrogen/progesterone contraceptives	Hypercoagulability	Opioids	Respiratory depression, CNS depression, addiction, constipation

ACE, angiotensin-converting enzyme; CNS, central nervous system; EtOH, ethyl alcohol; MAO, monoamine oxidase; SIADH, syndrome of inappropriate antidiuretic hormone secretion; SSRIs, selective serotonin reuptake inhibitors.

Rape/Crisis Adjustment

Diagnosis

History must include last menstrual period, time of last consensual coitus, contraceptive status.

Rape kits should be sought and include necessary bags, probes, and culture media to successfully handle samples from the victim and the victim's clothing.

Document patient's mental state and the recount of the event in her own words as accurately as possible. Do not assume anything and do not *ad lib*.

Collect patient's clothing.

Speculum exam with nonlubricated; water-moistened speculum.

Collect samples from vagina, rectum, mouth, under the fingernails, and locations of obvious trauma. Analyze samples by wet mount for the presence of sperm.

Pregnancy test immediately and in 2 weeks.

Obtain gonorrhea and *Chlamydia* testing, rapid plasma reagin (RPR) or VDRL for syphilis immediately and at 6 weeks after the event.

HIV blood testing immediately, and at 90 days and 120 days after the event.

Hepatitis panel immediately, and at 6 weeks and 6 months after the event.

Wood's lamp can be used to evaluate for seminal fluid.

EtOH and drug screen.

Depending on the state and circumstances, a chain of custody of evidence may be needed. As a general rule, give the evidence to the local authorities after placing each sample in separate, sealed, labeled containers.

Treatment

- Obtain history in very nonthreatening, nonconfrontational manner.

- Consult trauma/sexual assault counselor.

- Offer emergency contraception.

- Prophylaxis for *Gonorrhea/Chlamydia* and *syphilis* with ceftriaxone (Rocephin) IM ×1, azithromycin PO ×1, and penicillin G IM ×1.

- Treat bacterial vaginosis, if found, with metronidazole (Flagyl).

- Consider hep B immunoglobulin (HBIG) if exposure is known to be of high hep B risk.

- HIV prophylaxis is controversial and generally not recommended unless exposure is known to be of high risk.

- Treat physical pain/nausea/sleep disturbance as needed.

- Ensure extensive support network of patient.

- Ensure patient's physical safety if discharged from hospital.

- Close follow-up is absolutely necessary.

Cranial Injuries

Symptoms

Often obvious, but may have occurred hours/days ago and constitute a closed head injury. Loss of consciousness (LOC) and decreased consciousness is common as well as seizures, focal disturbances, ataxia, apraxia, decreased concentration, vomiting, headache, and amnesia of the event. Trauma to the spinal cord may cause paraplegia or quadriplegia that correlates with a certain spinal level.

Diagnosis

Physical exam: Note any bruising or skull bone crepitus indicative of fracture. Do not manipulate the temporal bones too much to avoid laceration of the middle meningeal artery if present. Raccoon eyes and Battle's sign may indicate basilar skull fracture. Ear exam for hemotympanum. Note CSF rhinorrhea or otorrhea. Examine the optic disks for "blurring" indicating increased intracranial pressure (ICP). Exam should include checking entire spinal column for step-offs or deformities. Inline stabilization should be used during exam.

Record Glasgow coma score.

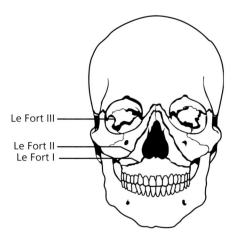

Le Fort III

Le Fort II
Le Fort I

FIGURE 10.1 Le Fort classification of facial fractures.

Oxford Handbook of Emergency Medicine. Third edition. Wyatt JP. Illingworth RN, Grahm CA. Copyright 2006. Oxford University Press.

Imaging: Plain skull x-ray may show fracture. To evaluate cervical injury: Obtain a cross-table cervical spine x-ray. Make sure you see T1, which constitutes an adequate study. If inadequate, CT the neck to clear it.

Obtain a head CT for bleeds although the slow ones may not immediately be seen. Look for signs of increased ICP or midline shift of ventricles. Consider repeating hours later (see Figure 10.1).

Treatment

- Remember your ABCs at first.
- Scalp lacerations often bleed profusely, but these are not your first priority.
- Decrease ICP with hyperventilation, consider mannitol or Lasix, but these medications may be tricky in shock. Rely on neurosurgery to help.
- IV steroids to reduce CNS (and spinal cord) edema. This alone may improve outcome.
- Consult neurosurgeon.
- See Chapter 1 on related topics.

Internal Injuries, Abdomen, and Pelvis

Symptoms

Pain in the abdomen or pelvis is usually present, but the patient may have impaired sensation or consciousness. Look for hypotension, decreasing blood pressure, decreased/decreasing consciousness, expanding abdomen, peritoneal signs, and dependent bruising.

TABLE 10.5 Diagnostic modalities for evaluation of internal injuries

	Diagnostic peritoneal lavage (DPL)	Ultrasound FAST exam	CT scan
Advantages	Early diagnosis and 98% sensitive	Early diagnosis; noninvasive and repeatable; 86%–97% accurate	Most specific for injury; 92%–98% accurate
Disadvantages	Invasive; misses injury to diaphragm or retroperitoneum	Operator-dependent; bowel gas and subcutaneous air distortion, misses diaphragm, bowel, and some pancreatic injuries	Cost and time; misses diaphragm, bowel tract, and some pancreatic injuries

Source: Adapted from *Advanced Trauma Life Support for Doctors*, sixth edition. American College of Surgeons Committee on Trauma. Student Course Manual. Chapter 5; Table 1, p. 166.

Diagnosis

Physical exam: "There should be a finger or tube placed in every orifice" to check for bleeding or fluid drainage. Evaluate for pelvis fracture by manual manipulation, but limit this maneuver to only once.

Imaging: Pelvic fractures should have a plain AP x-ray. Remember, it is hard to break a pretzel in one place—the same is true of the pelvis—always look for the second fracture site if one is found.

Penetrating abdominal injuries including gunshots and penetrating knife wounds should go directly to laparotomy.

See Table 10.5 for other diagnostic modalities.

Treatment

- If internal disruption of the organs is confirmed by the above testing, celiotomy is indicated. If tests above are negative but hypotension continues and bleeding into the peritoneum or retroperitoneum is suspected, celiotomy is indicated. In short, have a low threshold for taking to the OR.

- Before pelvis fracture fixed, stabilize it by pelvic braces or a simple tightly drawn sheet. Consider angiography to evaluate for circulation/deep venous thrombosis (DVT) around pelvis.

Frostbite

Symptoms

Usually distal extremities or appendages exposed to cold. When frostbite occurs, appendage becomes hard; white, without signs of circulation; and anesthetic. Pain is not a symptom but may indicate "frostnip."

Diagnosis

Generally a clinical diagnosis, but as rewarming starts various methods to evaluate microcirculation damage exist: thermography, angiography, digital plethysmography, and radioisotope vascular and bone scanning. These are generally helpful for the surgeon to make decisions about what and where to cut.

Blistering often starts 4–6 h after rewarming. Proximal bloody blisters are a negative prognostic indicator and indicate deep tissue damage. Distal serum-filled blisters are better and may indicate only superficial damage.

Treatment

- Make sure the patient is in no danger of refreezing the appendage as this may cause much more damage. If still in the high-risk environment, do not thaw the appendage!
- Slow (over the course of 20–30 min) rewarming with the use of warm (40°C, 104°F) water should be done. Expect tissue to turn pink and blotchy. It is advisable to monitor heart function for arrhythmias during this procedure if possible. Do not rub or massage the tissue.
- Give opioid analgesics during rewarming, since it can be very painful.
- After rewarming, the appendage should be kept warm and dry. Blisters should remain intact for 7–10 days.
- Give tetanus prophylaxis as indicated.
- No antibiotics are warranted unless infection is noted.
- No nicotine or other vasoconstrictors.
- Referral to surgery is usually indicated at some stage.

Hypothermia

Symptoms

Wide variations of clinical presentations exist. Commonly, mental status change (ataxia, amnesia, apathy, and dysarthria), LOC, psychiatric disturbance (delusions), and shivering. History is often suggestive of cold exposure, lack of clothing, drugs/EtOH exposure, infection, hypothyroidism, recent anesthesia, or immobility.

Diagnosis

Physical exam: By definition, temperature ≤35°C (95°F). Best temperature taken is rectal. Low BP may also be present.

Labs: CBC, metabolic panel, hepatic function tests, TSH, glucose, illicit drug screen, EtOH level, ABG, and blood cultures.

ECG: Characteristic J (Osborne) waves indicating delayed repolarization are classic. Arrhythmias such as AFib and bradycardias are also common. The lethal arrhythmia is usually ventricular fibrillation.

Imaging: None specific for hypothermia, but consider chest x-ray (CXR) for pulmonary infection, and other infections (see Figure 10.2).

Treatment

- Start with ABCs and CPR as needed. Remember to check pulse for one full minute before declaring death. "No one is dead until they're warm and dead."

- Mild cases may be treated with passive rewarming techniques including the removal of wet clothing and application of blankets, and other techniques.

- Moderate-to-severe cases require active rewarming, which includes warm humidified O_2, heated IV fluids, and peritoneal lavage. Extreme cases with cardiac arrest may benefit from cardiopulmonary bypass rewarming although this is very impractical.

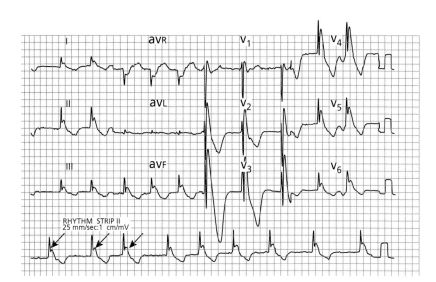

FIGURE 10.2 Hypothermia ECG showing rhythm disturbance of atrial fibrillation and slow ventricular response, prolongation of QRS, and delayed repolarization (J waves) (arrows).

Oxford Handbook of Emergency Medicine. Third edition. Wyatt JP. Illingworth RN, Grahm CA Copyright 2006. Oxford University Press.

Q 10.3

A 19-year-old male athlete comes to the ER with reports of loss of consciousness during football practice on a hot, humid day. The coach states he had been practicing vigorously and had been skipping water breaks. He was found unconscious on the sideline and was disoriented until emergency medical service (EMS) arrived minutes later. His temperature was taken rectally and found to be 41.1°C (105.9°F), and cold packs were placed in the axilla and groin on the way to the ER. On exam, his vital signs are stable and temperature is normal. He is responsive upon questioning and has damp, sweaty skin. Mini Mental Status exam is normal. Screening labs:

Na	137 mEq/L	**Urinalysis**	
K	4.1 mEq/L	Sp. grav.	1.020
Cl	102 mEq/L	Nitrate	Neg
CO_2	24 mEq/L	Leuk est	Neg
BUN	21 mg/dL	Blood	positive
Cr	1.0 mg/dL	Bili	negative
Glu	96 mg/dL	WBC	negative
AST	102 U/L	RBC	1–2 cells/hpf
ALT	98 U/L	Mucous	none
T bili	0.9 mg/dL	Casts	none
T protein	6.6 g/dL		
Alk phos	52 U/L		

What is the best course of management?

A. Administration of IV fluids in ER until urine output is assured, then release to his coach.
B. Administration of IV fluids and admission followed throughout the course by repeat lab studies.
C. Aggressive PO hydration with electrolyte solution and follow up the next day with his primary care physician.
D. Administration of IV fluids in ER until urine output is assured, then instructions to remain out of sports for the remainder of the season.
E. Admission to the ICU and administration of sodium bicarbonate.

Q 10.4

What is the most common serious complication of this patient's condition?

A. Coma and death by increased ammonia levels.
B. Sepsis from immune suppression.
C. Respiratory failure from flash pulmonary edema.
D. Stevens–Johnson reaction to proper treatment.
E. Disseminated intravascular coagulation (DIC) from hepatic and renal failure.

Heat Stroke

Symptoms

History of exposure to heat is found often in conjunction with exertion that produces severe CNS dysfunction—often loss of consciousness. Patient often has evidence of lack of thermoregulatory control such as dry, sweatless skin. Mental functioning is impaired.

Diagnosis

Physical exam: Evidence of end-organ damage may include right upper quadrant (RUQ) pain, arrhythmia, and hematuria. Always obtain temperature per rectum!

By definition, demonstration of end-organ damage is found by labs.

Labs: Transaminases often show >3× normal but may be normal at acute presentation, **creatinine kinase** elevation indicating muscle damage, increased BUN/creatinine indicating kidney damage, and urine **myoglobin** indicating saturation of kidneys. Electrolytes often show dehydration and hypernatremia, and hyperchloremia. In severe heat stroke, phosphorus and calcium levels are altered. CBC shows hemoconcentration. Coagulation profile may show increased PT/aPTT and INR indicative of liver damage. ABG for Ph and metabolic acidosis. Lactate dehydrogenase (LDH) levels may be taken early and show some correlation to short-term prognosis.

Monitor cardiac function for arrhythmias.

Watch for other problems that may develop such as fulminant hepatic failure, respiratory failure, kidney failure, DIC, and eventual brain death.

Imaging: None specifically indicated although individual organ systems may need imaging as the course progresses, that is, CXR for decreased respiratory functioning.

Treatment

- Immediate cooling with wet blankets, fans, cold water, ice packs to axilla and groin if possible.
- ICU admission.
- IV fluids (multiple boluses plus at least 2× maintenance) to increase and maintain vigorous urine output.
- Intubate if necessary.
- Treat seizures with benzodiazepines as needed.
- Manage concurrent organ damage and its effects.
- DIC may be an indication of eminent crash, be vigilant.
- In mild-to-moderate cases, hold out of sports or vigorous activity for the entire heat season. Decreased activity is warranted for the next heat season as well. A re-injury may be fatal!

TABLE 10.6 Common complications of surgery by systems

Complication	Symptoms	Associations	Management
CNS	Acute decrease in mental status, obtundation, or lack of arousal from surgery	Anesthesia effects/side effects, hypoxic brain injury, hypothermia, hypoglycemia, electrolyte disturbances	Check glucose level and correct, naloxone as needed, give O_2, check temperature and provide warmth, replete electrolytes (do not forget Mg)
Respiratory	Respiratory distress or failure, desaturation, and hypoxemia	Pulmonary embolism (PE) (thrombo, air, fat), atelectasis, pneumonia, aspiration pneumonitis, pulmonary edema, pneumonia	Oxygen, mechanical ventilation as needed, diagnosis of PE and anti-coagulation, incentive spirometer postoperative, antibiotics, and pneumonia treatment as needed
Gastrointestinal	Constipation, nausea, vomiting, bleeding, abdominal pain	Paralytic ileus, ischemia, perforation, anesthetic effects/side effects, adhesion formation, and resultant obstruction	NPO status, nasogastric (NG) tube as needed, stool softeners, antiemetics, tincture of time, or reevaluation for surgery and possible laparotomy

Complications of Surgery

See Table 10.6.

Hemorrhage Complicating Surgery

Diagnosis

Frank bleeding around surgical site or other wound area. Generally fairly obvious but may be seen as decreased blood pressure, increased heart rate, and hypovolemic shock symptoms. There may also be hiding blood in body cavities, "third spacing."

Labs: Hemoglobin/hematocrit usually would not change in the acute setting. If after surgery, a relative decrease may be seen compared to preoperative status.

Treatment

- Prophylactic prevention is the best weapon and includes stopping warfarin (Coumadin) dosing and switching to real heparin before surgery, then stopping it the day before the procedure, and stopping all aspirin/herbals/NSAIDs before surgery; also stop clopidogrel (Plavix) before surgery.

- Direct pressure on the bleeding location if obvious. Other techniques include use of bovie electrocautery, suturing the bleeding patient, and tourniquet.

- Reverse warfarin (Coumadin) effect with vitamin K if in the acute setting and if patient has good hepatic function.
- Fluids and blood products as needed.
- Treat with pressor agents as needed.

Postoperative Infection

Symptoms

Generalized fever, local pain, swelling, oozing/drainage from wound, and erythema. Patients may also exhibit symptoms of infection in places other than surgery site. The mnemonic to remember: "Wind, water, walking, wound, and wonder drugs" is the 5 W's of surgery. They stand for the sources of postoperative fever and include respiratory infection (pneumonia, atelectasis), urine or urinary tract infection (UTI), DVT or pulmonary embolism (PE), surgery site infection, or anesthetic or drug effect, respectively.

Diagnosis

Always examine the wound for signs of infection.
Labs: Urinalysis (UA) and urine culture for UTI especially after long-indwelling catheter.
Imaging: Consider CXR for pneumonia. Doppler ultrasound of the legs if suspicious.
   Draw blood cultures if still uncertain of site.

Treatment

- Usually, first-generation cephalosporin or penicillin is given intra-operation for infection prophylaxis. Consider continuing treatment after procedure if infection is highly likely (dirty wound) or confirmed. Otherwise, tailor antibiotics to specific sensitivities and recommendations for location.

Other Complications of Surgical Procedures

See Table 10.7.

Burns

Diagnosis

See Table 10.8.

TABLE 10.7 Common complications of surgery

Complication	Association/diagnosis	Treatment
Hematoma	Noninflammatory mass under the wound. Ultrasound (U/S) may be used to confirm presence of blood clot	Either watchful waiting for reabsorption if mild without adverse mass effect or open evacuation
Dehiscence	Separation of closed wound site; may be caused by necrosis of wound edges, underlying hematoma, infection, excess tension on suture line, or lack of undermining and suturing of wound	Remove sutures and recluse if uncomplicated or allow healing by secondary intention
Suture abscess	Usually small local abscess at suture site; caused by retained stitch	Incision and drainage of abscess; treat local cellulitis as indicated; remove the suture
Hypertrophic scar formation and keloid	More common in dark-skinned individuals; complication of late healing	Steroid injection, radiation therapy, dermabrasion, pressure dressings, or surgical removal and debulking

TABLE 10.8 Classification of burns

Classification	Association	Level of injury
Superficial burn	Sunburn or mild hotwater. Skin is red without blisters	Epidermis only
Superficial partial thickness burn	Often surrounded by redness with blister formation. Capillary refill is present.	Epidermis and papillary dermis. Deep dermis, hair follicles, and sweat glands are sparred.
Deep partial thickness burn	Blistering and white appearance of injury area with blister formation. Capillary refill is usually absent.	Epidermis, reticular (deep) layer of dermis. Sweat glands, hair follicles, capillaries, and nerve fibers are burned.
Full thickness	Charred, pale, painless, and leathery skin. No capillary refill. No blistering.	Through the epidermis and dermis and possibly into the subcutaneous tissues.

Determine body surface area (BSA) according to the rule of 9s:

- Face and scalp   9%
- Back   18%
- Front   18%
- Perineum   1%
- Arm each   9%
- Leg each   18%

See Figure 10.3 and Table 10.9.

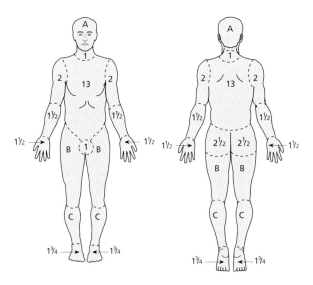

FIGURE 10.3 Lund and Browder chart. Assessing the extent of burns by the estimation of body surface area.

Oxford Handbook of Emergency Medicine. Third edition. Wyatt JP, Illingworth RN, Grahm CA. Copyright 2006. Oxford University Press.

TABLE 10.9 Relative percentage of body surface area by age.

Area	Age 1 year	Adult
A=1/2 of head	8 ½	3 ½
B=1/2 of thigh	3 ¼	4 ¾
C=1/2 of one lower leg	2 ½	3 ½

Determine if the patient is at risk for inhalational injury. Have a low threshold for treating.

Labs: Obtain screening Chem-7, CBC, albumin, calcium, ABG for pH, and UA.

Imaging: Consider CXR if pneumonia suspected.

Treatment

- Admission criteria are as follows:
  - Lightning or electrical burns.
  - Third-degree >1% estimated BSA.
  - Second-degree more than >10% estimated BSA.
  - Third-degree burn on hand, feet, face, perineum.
  - Circumferential burns.
  - Coexisting inhalational injury.
- Superficial partial thickness burns should be cooled by rinsing with cool water/saline irrigation.
- If minor, dress with Epilock or Elasto-Gel and monitor as out-patient. May recommend aloe containing OTC preparations for pain relief.

- If more serious:
  - Remove all clothing and jewelry including rings and watches that are remotely near the burned area.
  - Give O_2
  - Tetanus prophylaxis.
  - Do not apply ice to burned area.
  - Do not rupture blisters unless infected or overtly large.
  - Systemic or topical antibiotics are indicated in some second- and all third-degree burns.
  - Systemic pain relief to include opioids.
- In severe burns:
  - Place NG tube, Foley catheter, two large bore IVs.
  - IV fluids with rate > maintenance for first 24 h.
  - ECG monitoring for first 24 h.
  - Monitor electrolytes.
  - NPO status initially, then, high-protein diet.
  - Consider total parenteral nutrition (TPN) if NPO status expected >5 days.
  - Possible escharotomy if circumferential and causing breathing restriction or pseudocompartment syndrome of extremity.
  - Skin (usually split-thickness) grafting.
  - Daily debridement and redressing of wounds.
- Consultation or transfer to burn center.
- During initial resuscitation, the **Parkland formula** for fluid repletion can be used.
- LR (lactated Ringer) ml = 4 ml/kg (percentage of BSA burned), the first half should be given over the first 8 h, and the second half over the next 16 h.
- Topical preparations include silver sulfadiazine (Silvadene), silver nitrate, and mafenide (Sulfamylon).
- Important side effects of topicals include
  - Silver nitrate: May leach Na, Cl, and K out of wound and cause deficiency
  - Mafenide: Metabolic acidosis and possible renal tubular acidosis.

Q 10.5

According to the Colorado Medical Society classification of concussion, an athlete with brief, traumatic injury to the head and who suffers mild disorientation, brief amnesia of the event with complete recall returning in 2 min, and no loss of consciousness has had what grade of concussion?

A. Grade 1
B. Grade 2
C. Grade 3
D. Grade 4
E. Not able to classify based on the information given.

Concussion

Symptoms

May range from simply getting patient's "bell rung" during a sporting event to sustained loss of consciousness. Symptoms may include headache, confusion, disorientation, amnesia, loss or blurring of vision, loss of hearing, nausea, vomiting, or focal motor disturbance.

Diagnosis/Treatment

There are three main classification systems for concussion. These are those proposed by the American Academy of Neurology (AAN), Cantu et al., and the Colorado Medical Society. The most widely used is that developed by the Colorado Medical Society and are summed up in Table 10.10.

TABLE 10.10 Colorado Medical Society system of grading concussion

	Grade 1	Grade 2	Grade 3
Features	Confusion, no loss of consciousness (LOC), no postevent amnesia	Confusion, postevent amnesia, no LOC	LOC of any duration
Management	Neuro checks q. 5 min; athlete may return to play if asymptomatic for 20 min	Athlete may return to play if asymptomatic for 1 week	Athlete should be transported to a hospital emergency department; athlete may return to play 1 month after injury if asymptomatic for 2 weeks
Third	Full thickness; charred or severely disfigured appearance with or without blisters		None

Source: Guidelines for the Management of Concussion in Sports. Rev. May 1991. Denver: Colorado Medical Society.

At-the-scene examination should include mental status questioning and evaluation, complete neurologic exam (including fundoscopy), examination of the head for skull fracture, otoscopy for hemotympanum, presence of Battle's sign, or ear/nose leakage of CSF.

Imaging: If warranted, CT scan of the head for intracranial bleeding/edema or signs of mass effect or herniation. MRI may be more sensitive for diffuse and axonal injury; however, it is rarely used in the acute setting. Imaging of the cervical spine is almost always warranted and may be done by plain x-ray.

Consider hospitalization for anyone with ongoing seizures, focal neurologic signs, persistent confusion, amnesia, or without reliable, responsible party able to watch the patient for ongoing or worsening symptoms.

Answers

10.1 B. Organophosphate and carbamate poisoning are becoming favorite chemical/biologic weapons of terrorist groups, but are also used extensively in the horticulture industry. They are cholinesterase inhibitors capable of causing severe cholinergic toxicity. Antidotes consist of strong anticholinergics such as pralidoxime (2-PAM) and atropine. In this mass casualty situation, these agents and prepared, trained, and level-headed staff can significantly affect the outcome.

10.2 A. The use of metronidazole combined with alcohol produces a disulfiram-like reaction causing inhibition of aldehyde dehydrogenase. Symptoms include severe nausea/vomiting and abdominal cramps. In this case, this therapy may lead to significant symptoms if the patient decides to continue to use EtOH.

10.3 B. This patient has had a heat stroke by history of loss of consciousness, increased temperature, and evidence of end-organ damage. The clinical course is to acutely present in the early phase of heat injury and to have effects of injury worsen. This patient has had significant history of heat stroke and should be admitted with aggressive IV fluid administration and frequent repeat liver function, renal function, electrolyte, and coagulation studies. Administration of sodium bicarbonate (E) may eventually be indicated although it is not indicated with the information given.

10.4 E. Patients with severe heat stroke may have several life-threatening complications including seizure and central nervous system (CNS) involvement and hepatic/renal failure. The latter of these is one of the answers given and commonly leads to disseminated intravascular coagulation (DIC) and eventual death. If heat injury presents with significant hepatic injury, make sure the facilities can support DIC as a complication.

10.5 B. The Colorado Medical Society clinically grades concussion based on three factors: presence of loss of consciousness, post-event amnesia, and confusion. In this scenario, the patient had two of these factors without LOC, thus has suffered a grade 2 concussion.

11   Cardiovascular Diseases

Hypertension	248
End-Organ Hypertensive Effects	249
Secondary Hypertension	250
Acute Myocardial Infarction	251
Angina Pectoris	253
Pericarditis	254
Cardiomyopathy	255
Hypertrophic Cardiomyopathy	255
Congestive Heart Failure	256
Myocarditis	258
Heart Block	258
Arrhythmias	260
Atrial Fibrillation/Flutter	260
Ventricular Tachycardia	261
Ventricular Fibrillation	262
Asystole/Pulseless Electrical Activity	263
Wolff–Parkinson–White Syndrome	263
Abdominal Aortic Aneurysm	264
Peripheral Vascular Disease	265
Arterial Embolism/Thrombosis	266
Raynaud's Disease/Phenomenon	266
Superficial Thrombophlebitis	267
Venous Thrombosis	268
Varicose Veins	269
Atherosclerosis	270
Valvular Disease	270
Infectious Endocarditis	270
Congenital Heart Disease	273

Hypertension

Symptoms

Typically asymptomatic with possible exclusion of headache. Symptoms from associated conditions such as retinal disease, cerebrovascular disease, or congestive heart failure (CHF) may be present.

Diagnosis

The Seventh Report of the Joint National Committee on Prevention, Detection, Evaluation, and Treatment of High Blood Pressure (JNC 7) reported the following guidelines and treatments for hypertension.

Exam may reveal signs of left ventricular hypertrophy (LVH) including displaced point of maximal impulse (PMI) or S4. Fundoscopic exam may show AV nicking or "copper-wire" appearance of vessels (see Table 11.1).

Two separate blood pressures must be taken on separate days to constitute hypertension.

A workup should be done to exclude secondary causes of hypertension (see section on secondary hypertension). These include an ECG and urinalysis; Chem-7 including blood glucose, serum potassium, creatinine, calcium; CBC for hematocrit (Hct); and a lipid profile.

Treatment

- Goal is to reduce blood pressures to <140/90 or <130/80 in diabetic patients and renal insufficiency patients.

- Consider that some medications increase blood pressure, such as oral contraceptives (OCPs) and nonsteroidal antiinflammatory drugs (NSAIDs).

TABLE 11.1 Classifications of hypertension

Classification	BP range (mmHg)
Prehypertension	120–139/80–89
Stage I	140–159/90–99
Stage II	≥160/≥100

TABLE 11.2 Characteristics of antihypertensive classes

Medication	Special considerations	Side effects
Thiazide diuretics	First line; indicated especially in African Americans; contraindicated in gout and nephrolithiasis patients	Increased urination upon starting, gouty flares, calcium-based kidney stones
β-Blockers	Protective in ischemic heart disease; contraindicated in asthmatics	Bradycardia, alopecia, erectile dysfunction
ACEI	Indicated especially in diabetics	Cough, angioedema, hyperkalemia
ARB	Indicated as next alternative for patients intolerant of ACEI	Hyperkalemia
Calcium channel blockers		Lower extremity edema

ACEI, angiotensin-converting enzyme inhibitor; ARB, angiotensin II receptor blocker.

- If the patient's blood pressure is <20/10 mmHg from goal, lifestyle modifications can be tried first. These include weight reduction, Dietary Approaches to Stop Hypertension (DASH) diet, dietary sodium reduction, physical activity, and moderation of alcohol consumption.
- **Medications:** Best first line is a **thiazide diuretic**. Add additional medications from other classes as needed to obtain the desired effect [calcium channel blockers, β-blockers, angiotensin II receptor blockers (ARBs), α-blockers, angiotensin-converting enzyme inhibitors (ACEIs)]. Manage comorbidities as needed and control other diseases, for example, diabetics should receive an ACEI or ARB (see Table 11.2).

End-Organ Hypertensive Effects

Symptoms

Three common organ systems include cardiac, neurologic, and renal. Symptoms of LVH, including those of CHF or ischemic phenomenon. These include shortness of breath, dyspnea on exertion, cough, paroxysmal nocturnal dyspnea (PND), peripheral edema, or ascites. Ruptured brain aneurysm may produce acute focal neurologic deficits, dementia, mental status change, or sudden death. Symptoms of renal disease are often lacking until significant failure exists. General decrease in energy; possible mental status changes are sometimes presenting symptoms.

Diagnosis

If uncontrolled hypertension has existed for significant amount of time, obtain ECG for likely LVH or arrhythmias, B-type natriuretic peptide (BNP) for CHF, basic metabolic panel (BMP) for electrolytes, and BUN/creatinine [calculate creatinine clearance to estimate the glomerular filtration rate (GFR)], TSH, and UA for protein and urine microalbumin.

Imaging: Obtain chest x-ray for cardiomegaly, pulmonary edema (seen by Kerley B lines, diffuse opacities, increased vascular markings, and cephalization).

Echocardiography for ejection fraction and any possible wall motion abnormalities.

Treatment

- Control blood pressure to prevent these disorders.
- Use β-**blockers and ACEIs** to control blood pressure preferentially after damage has occurred. In CHF, spironolactone and other diuretics also show benefit. ACEIs are especially important in renal disease (although their use in renal failure is contraindicated).
- Avoid NSAIDs.

Secondary Hypertension

Symptoms

Varied since the etiology of disease is varied. Symptoms may stem from extensive differential diagnosis such as:

- Sleep apnea
- Drug induced
- Chronic kidney disease
- Primary aldosteronism
- Renovascular disease such as renal artery stenosis
- Chronic steroid therapy
- Cushing's syndrome
- Pheochromocytoma
- Coarctation of the aorta
- Thyroid or parathyroid disease
- OTC dietary supplements (e.g., ephedra, ma huang, bitter orange)
- Cocaine, amphetamines, other illicit drugs
- NSAIDs
- Cyclooxygenase-2 inhibitors.

Diagnosis

The JNC 7 recommends ECG and laboratory evaluation per the following: ECG; UA for protein; Chem-8 including blood glucose, serum potassium, creatinine, and calcium; CBC for Hct; fasting lipid profile; and optional microalbumin measurement.

If history/physical dictates, add the following:

- TSH
- Chest x-ray
- Provocative renal nuclear scans
- Selective arteriography
- Plasma/urine catecholamines
- Plasma renin
- Aortogram
- Renal biopsy
- CT scan of abdomen
- 24-h urine cortisol.

Treatment

- As appropriate for each condition after identification.
- Internal medicine or nephrology consultation may be appropriate if diagnosis not found. Do not be afraid to ask for help.

Q 11.2

A 48-year-old obese African American female presents to the ER with crushing substernal, left-sided chest pain and left shoulder numbness for the past 8 h. She is diaphoretic on interview and very anxious. ECG shows ST segment depression in the anterior lateral leads. What is the next step in management?

A. Obtain thallium imaging.
B. Start tPA therapy.
C. Start a glycoprotein IIb/IIIa inhibitor such as eptifibatide (Integrilin).
D. Give morphine, place oxygen, give aspirin, and give nitroglycerin.
E. Consult cardiology for emergent coronary catheterization.

Acute Myocardial Infarction

Symptoms

Classically, left-sided crushing chest pain that radiates down the left arm or up to the jaw. Diaphoresis, shortness of breath, nausea, or lightheadedness may be present. In the elderly or diabetics, these symptoms may or may not be present [silent myocardial infarction (MI)]. History may reveal exertion, history of angina, or risk factors such as coronary artery disease (CAD) equivalents (e.g., diabetes), male gender, African descent, smoking, significant EtOH use, hyperlipidemia (especially LDL), obesity, sedentary lifestyle, "type A" personality, or age >40 years.

Diagnosis

Exam may show signs of acute heart failure including pulmonary rales, increased jugular venous pulsation, S3, S4, or arrhythmia.

Obtain stat ECG: Look for Q waves, T-wave inversion, ST segment depression (ischemia) or elevation (infarction), new left bundle-branch block, new heart block, shifted axis, or arrhythmia (especially V-tach). Order old records and ECGs for comparison. Changes occur in contiguous leads.

Labs: On admission, obtain CBC, BMP, TSH, coagulation profile. Importantly, get cardiac enzymes, which include creatine kinase (CK), CK-MB, troponin. Cardiac enzymes should be taken q. 6–8 h ×3.

Nitroglycerin is sometimes used in diagnosis, in that if chest pain is relieved, the pain is caused by a cardiac source. This is low sensitivity, since most chest pain of any origin is relieved by nitroglycerin.

Imaging: Chest x-ray for pneumonia or dissection.

If workup is negative for acute injury, obtain fasting lipid profile and cardiac stress test (via exercise or chemical stress) and consider thallium nuclear medicine imaging. This will help risk stratify.

Treatment

- Stabilize the patient if unstable. Consider advanced cardiac life support (ACLS) protocols.
- Start IV fluids.
- Remember **MONA** (morphine, oxygen, nitroglycerin, aspirin) as first line when patient presents.
- Make NPO.
- After above are done and while labs, imaging, and ECG are pending, obtain history and physical. If clinical suspicion is high for cardiac origin, place patients on oxygen, have them chew an aspirin for antiplatelet action, start IV β-blocker for cardioprotection, ACEI for post-MI benefits, high-dose statin for plaque stabilization, and heparin or low molecular weight (LMW) heparin (Lovenox) for anticoagulation.
- If ischemia is proved ongoing (either by dynamic ECG changes or cardiac enzymes), get cardiac catheterization with balloon angioplasty at the earliest. Cardiologist will evaluate for coronary artery bypass grafting (CABG).
- Thrombolytics (tPA, streptokinase) are controversial, must be given within 6 h of symptom onset, and have many contraindications. Generally, a risky choice on the test.

- If found to be having non-ST segment elevation MI(NSTEMI), consider glycoprotein IIb/IIIa inhibitors (Integrilin, abciximab).
- After event (and found not to have had an ischemic origin to symptoms), risk stratify and place on aspirin [or clopidogrel (Plavix)]. Lower risk factors such as obesity, smoking, hypertension, and diabetes control.
- Look for post-MI complications including depression.

Angina Pectoris

Stable angina: Chronic or recurrent condition of angina with exertion.
Variant (Prinzemetal's) angina: Spasm of coronary vessels with temporary or partial occlusion resulting in angina. May be associated with cocaine use.
Unstable angina: Recent onset of angina at rest.

Symptoms

Substernal pain, pressure, tightness, heaviness, or sharp pain of relatively short duration. Diaphoresis, nausea, dyspnea, or radiation of pain or numbness down left arm or up to the jaw may be present. This feeling is not pleuritic and classically may be relieved by rest or nitroglycerin.

Diagnosis

Physical exam: S4, new murmur, rhythm, rate, or signs of heart failure should be noted.
Resting ECG often is negative, but may show signs of ischemia if unstable angina is present.
Labs: Obtain CBC for Hct, TSH, lipid profile, Chem-7 for electrolytes and glucose, in acute setting three sets of cardiac enzymes (CK, CK-MB, troponin) 6–8 hours apart to evaluate for MI.
Imaging: Chest x-ray. Consider CT of the chest if aortic dissection is thought possible.

Special Testing

Echocardiography for valvular or structural abnormality.
  Exercise stress testing to evaluate for ECG changes during cardiac stress (exercise or chemical).
  Stress echocardiography to visualize wall motion abnormalities.
  Radionuclide testing (Thallium, persantine thallium) to visualize myocardial blood flow.
  Coronary angiography to visualize and quantify degree of coronary blood vessel occlusion.

Treatment

- Aggressive management of contributing diseases such as diabetes and hypertension.
- Control of risk factors such as obesity, smoking, and hyperlipidemia.

253

TABLE 11.3 Effects of drug therapy

Agent	Effect
Intermittent short-acting (nitroglycerin) or long-acting nitrates (isosorbide di/mononitrate)	Reduce preload stress
β-Blockers	Reduce cardiac output and cardiac exercise response as well as provide cardioprotection against ischemic injury
Calcium channel blockers	Reduce myocardial contraction demands and cause vasodilation; very effective especially in spasm-associated angina
Aspirin or clopidogrel (Plavix)	Exert antiplatelet effects and inhibition of prostaglandins

- Medications (see Table 11.3).
- **Surgery:** Cardiac catheterization with balloon angioplasty or stent placement. CABG is also a possibility.

Pericarditis

Symptoms

Sudden onset retrosternal chest pain. May be pleuritic and radiate to neck or jaw. Classically relieved with leaning forward. Fever, myalgias, anorexia, pleuritic component to chest pain may be seen. History may reveal recent URI or other minor infection.

Diagnosis

Physical exam: Classic pericardial friction rub.
Labs: CBC may show increased WBCs, ESR or CRP likely increased. Investigate other causes with ANA, rheumatoid factor, etc.
Imaging: Chest x-ray may show pericardial effusion with "water bottle" appearance of heart. Chest CT may reveal constrictive thickened pericardial sac, but is rarely indicated in acute pericarditis.
ECG: Pan-elevation of ST segment. This is a classic difference from MI. If significant effusion is present, electrical alternans may be seen which is the alteration of axis of QRS between beats (rare).
Echocardiography: May show effusion or constriction. Effusion may be new or worsening.

Treatment

- NSAIDs, classically aspirin.
- Oral or IV steroids if NSAIDs ineffective.

- **Surgery:** Pericardiectomy/pericardiotomy if hemodynamic compromise. Pericardiocentesis with needle aspiration may be considered.

Cardiomyopathy

Symptoms

Symptoms parallel heart failure. Types of cardiac muscle disease include dilated, arrhythmogenic, restrictive, hypertrophic, and unclassified.

Diagnosis

Labs: Screening labs such as CBC, Chem-7 for electrolytes and renal function. Consider BNP, ESR.

Imaging: Chest x-ray for cardiac dilation or signs of pulmonary edema/congestion. Consider CT scan of chest.

ECG for increased QRS voltage indicating dilation, arrhythmia, signs of ischemia, altered axis.

Echocardiography for visualization, wall motion abnormalities, chamber dilation, or restriction.

Stress testing for reversible ischemia.

Treatment

- Treat for heart failure (see section Congestive Heart Failure).
- Consider dual chamber pacemaker to improve contractility.
- Heart transplant in severe cases is definitive although low long-term survival.

Hypertrophic Cardiomyopathy

Synonyms: Idiopathic hypertrophic subaortic stenosis and hypertrophic obstructive cardiomyopathy (HOCM).

Symptoms

Dyspnea, syncope, presyncope, angina, fatigue, or palpitations. Sudden cardiac death is the worst sudden discovery of disease. History may reveal a relatively young athlete with no prior knowledge or symptoms of heart disease.

Diagnosis

Physical exam: Harsh crescendo/decrescendo systolic murmur that lengthens with Valsalva, S4, displaced PMI.

Labs: Screening labs such as CBC, comprehensive metabolic profile (CMP), and coagulation profile are indicated, but none are diagnostic.

ECG: Increased QRS voltage suggesting LVH, nonspecific ST-T waves, Q waves in anterior and lateral leads mimicking MI, P-wave abnormalities indicating left atrial enlargement (LAE), short PR interval. AFib is a late and concerning finding.

Imaging

Chest x-ray: May show normal or increased cardiac size. Pulmonary congestion and edema are rare findings.

Echocardiography is the best initial procedure. This shows asymmetric septal hypertrophy, LVH, LAE, small ventricular chamber size, and mitral and aortic valve irregularities.

Cardiac catheterization: Reveals often patent vessels, obstruction to ventricular outflow, and abnormal diastolic ventricular filling.

Treatment

- Avoid strenuous exercise or situations.
- Medications are aimed at reducing contractility to allow for increased ventricular filling. Thus, avoid digoxin or afterload reducers such as nitrates or diuretics.
- Pacemaker placement is the standard.
- **Surgery:** Left ventricular myomectomy is recommended for severe cases, and has generally good outcome.

Congestive Heart Failure

See Figure 11.1.

Symptoms

Shortness of breath, dependent edema, ascites, dyspnea on exertion, or PND. If in acute exacerbation, look for coughing up **frothy sputum.**

Diagnosis

Physical exam: Basilar rales, pitting edema, increased PMI, and S3 gallup.
Labs: Screening CBC, Chem-7 for electrolytes (hyponatremia) and renal function, liver function tests (LFTs) for bilirubin, TSH, HIV. Obtain **BNP (B-type natriuretic peptide).** Consider cardiac enzymes.

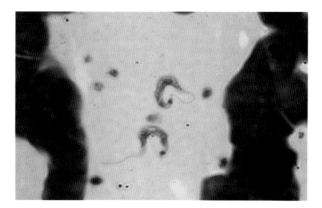

FIGURE 11.1 Chagas disease is the most common cause of congestive heart failure worldwide (although not in North America). Here are two parasites of *Trypanosoma cruzi*.

With permission Nivaldo Medeiros, MD.

Imaging: Chest x-ray may show cardiomegaly, increased vascular markings, cephalization and signs of pulmonary edema (Kerley B lines).

ECG may show increased QRS voltage indicating LVH or right ventricular hypertrophy (RVH) or arrhythmia.

Echocardiography: Best test, which may show structural abnormalities including LVH, wall motion abnormalities, and **ejection fraction**.

Radionucleotide imaging may also be used to evaluate systolic cardiac function and ejection fraction.

Cardiac catheterization to evaluate for possible narrowing of coronary vessels.

New York Heart Association Classification of CHF

Class I: Patients with no limitation of activities; they suffer no symptoms from ordinary activities.

Class II: Patients with slight, mild limitation of activity; they are comfortable with rest or with mild exertion.

Class III: Patients with marked limitation of activity; they are comfortable only at rest.

Class IV: Patients who should be at complete rest, confined to bed or chair; any physical activity brings on discomfort and symptoms occur at rest.

Treatment

- Properly control hemodynamically unstable patients.
- Place on O_2 therapy and low-sodium diet.
- Acutely, reduce extravascular fluid volume by giving diuretics (Lasix). Consider addition of metolazone (Zaroxolyn) for synergy and/or spironolactone for hypokalemia. This will often reduce respiratory problems (but has not shown decrease in mortality).
- Morphine can reduce respiratory drive and anxiety, and decreases preload.
- Vasodilators such as IV nitroglycerin may show short-term benefit by reducing preload, afterload, and systemic resistance.
- Digoxin is the classic drug to improve contractility (inotrop), but make sure there is no MI, hypertrophic cardiomyopathy, or aortic stenosis present.
- ACEIs and β-blockers show good effectiveness in decreasing mortality and are considered first line.
- Use dopamine or dobutamine for short-term improvement in hospitalized, severe cases.
- As outpatient, control risk factors such as hypertension and smoking. Low-sodium diet is critical.

Myocarditis

Symptoms

Symptoms can be variable but include chest pain, unexplained fatigue or sinus tachycardia, palpitations, symptoms of CHF, or symptoms of pericarditis. History may reveal recent URI or enteritis illness.

Diagnosis

Physical exam: S3 or S4, irregular rhythm indicating arrhythmia, murmur, or friction rub.

Lab: CBC and Chem-7 tend to show nonspecific findings. Cardiac enzyme findings may mimic MI.

ECG: Often mimics pericarditis or MI. May also show arrhythmia or heart block.

Chest x-ray: Possible cardiomegaly, increased pulmonary vasculature or pulmonary edema as in CHF.

Echocardiography: Clinically, most valuable test. May show dilated cardiomyopathy, wall motion abnormalities, characteristic appearance of myocardial tissue, valvular dysfunction or thrombi.

Cardiac MRI: May be helpful to show local cardiac muscle damage or edema.

Endocardial biopsy is the gold standard although rarely used because of inherent risk. Criteria to evaluate the biopsy are called the **Dallas criteria,** and basically outline degrees of inflammation.

Treatment

- Nonspecific and supportive care are the standard.
- Intravenous immunoglobulin (IVIG) has recently shown evidence to be helpful.
- Treat specific causes if known.
- Otherwise, provide O_2 as needed, treat CHF symptoms, and monitor course.
- In advanced cases, cardiac transplant may be considered.

Heart Block

See Tables 11.4–11.6 and Figures 11.2–11.5.

TABLE 11.4 First-degree heart block

Degree	Characteristic on ECG	Treatment
First	Prolonged PR interval (>0.2 s)	Generally none Avoid β-blockers or calcium channel blockers

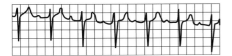

FIGURE 11.2 First-degree heart block.

Oxford Handbook of Emergency Medicine. Third edition. Wyatt JP, Illingworth RN, Graham CA. Copyright 2006. Oxford University Press.

TABLE 11.5 Second-degree heart block

Degree	Characteristic on ECG	Treatment
Second Mobitz I (Wenckebach)	Elongating PR interval until dropped QRS	Atropine and transcutaneous pacing if symptomatic acutely; consider permanent pacemaker if symptomatic chronically
Mobitz II	Consistent, predictably dropped QRS with normal PR intervals	Pacemaker placement

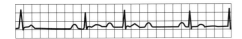

FIGURE 11.3 Mobitz type I atrioventricular (AV) block.

Oxford Handbook of Emergency Medicine. Third edition. Wyatt JP, Illingworth RN, Graham CA. Copyright 2006. Oxford University Press.

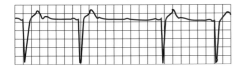

FIGURE 11.4 Mobitz type II atrioventricular (AV) block.

Oxford Handbook of Emergency Medicine. Third edition. Wyatt JP, Illingworth RN, Graham CA. Copyright 2006. Oxford University Press.

TABLE 11.6 Third-degree heart block

Degree	Characteristic on ECG	Treatment
Third	Total atrial/ventricular disassociation, P waves and QRS unrelated	Pacemaker placement

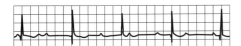

FIGURE 11.5 Third-degree heart block.

Oxford Handbook of Emergency Medicine. Third edition. Wyatt JP, Illingworth RN, Graham CA. Copyright 2006. Oxford University Press.

Arrhythmias

Q 11.3

A 72-year-old Caucasian female presents to the ER with complaints of heart pounding and feeling lightheaded for 12 h. An ECG shows atrial fibrillation with rapid ventricular response. On records review, she has been shown to have multiple previous encounters for the same typed arrhythmia over the past 5 years. While in the ER she spontaneously converts to normal sinus rhythm. How long should she be maintained on anticoagulation therapy?

A. She should not be anticoagulated.
B. 3–4 weeks.
C. 3–6 months.
D. 1 year.
E. Indefinitely.

Atrial Fibrillation/Flutter

Symptoms

Often asymptomatic but may present with palpitations, lightheadedness/presyncope, tiring easily, dyspnea on exertion, symptoms of heart failure (dependent edema, pulmonary congestion, etc.), or unexplained fatigue. Be aware of possible thrombotic events that may lead to symptoms of transient ischemic attack (TIA)/stroke. History may reveal alcohol abuse (holiday heart) or prior MI.

Diagnosis

Physical exam: Irregularly irregular rhythm.
Labs: Obtain screening Chem-7, hepatic function panel, CBC. Obtain cardiac enzymes to evaluate for MI. Order TSH.
ECG: P waves are absent. "F" waves appear like P waves, but are usually smaller and unassociated with QRS segments. QRSs are irregularly irregular and heart rate is often anywhere between 90 and 170 bpm.
Echo: Transthoracic for structural abnormalities and evaluation of heart function.

Transesophageal for possible left atrial thrombi if duration of atrial fibrillation is unknown or >48 h.

Chest x-ray for lung or cardiac abnormalities.

Consider Holter monitoring for paroxysmal atrial fibrillation.

Treatment

- If unstable, remember ACLS guidelines and perform external cardioversion.

- If stable, "control the rate or convert the rhythm." This can be done by various antiarrhythmic drugs such as β-blockers, nondihydropyridine calcium channel blockers (verapamil, diltiazem), digoxin, or amiodarone. Consensus for best agent is controversial. Diltiazem (Cardizem) is a popular choice for outpatient therapy. Electrocardioversion is also an option, but clinically rarely used.

- Anticoagulation and Cardioversion

  - Guidelines from the Seventh American College of Chest Physicians (ACCP) Consensus Conference on Antithrombotic Therapy and the American College of Cardiology (ACC) recommend that outpatients who have been in AFib for more than 48 h should receive 3–4 weeks of warfarin (Coumadin) before *and* after cardioversion. An alternative strategy supported by the American Academy of Family Practice (AAFP) and American College of Physicians (ACP) states that transesophageal echocardiography is sufficient to rule out atrial thrombi. If negative, cardioversion without preanticoagulation is safe.

  - After cardioversion, anticoagulation with warfarin (Coumadin) should be maintained for 3–4 weeks. Keep the INR between 2 and 3.

  - Chronic AFib patients should be maintained on warfarin (Coumadin) or aspirin long term.

  - Routine use of antiarrhythmic drugs for the maintenance of sinus rhythm was not shown beneficial in the large, multicenter AFFIRM (Atrial Fibrillation Follow-up Investigation of Rhythm Management) trial.

- **Surgery:** Electrical ablation procedures exist, but are rarely indicated or used.

Ventricular Tachycardia

Diagnosis

ECG

See Figure 11.6.

Three or more consecutive, wide QRS (ventricular origin) beats at a rate of 100–200 bpm. AV dissociation is the hallmark since the ventricles are beating independently of the atria.

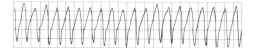

FIGURE 11.6 Ventricular tachycardia (VT) with a rate of 235 bpm.

Oxford Handbook of Clinical Medicine. Sixth edition. Longmore, M, Wilkinson, IB, Rajagopalan S. Copyright 2004. Oxford University Press.

Monomorphic—one general shape.

Polymorphic—more than one shape. When associated with prolonged Q-T and appears to revolve around a stable baseline is termed torsades de pointes.

Treatment

- If unstable, immediate synchronized cardioversion is indicated. Use standard protocol of 200 J, 200–300 J, and 360 J for monophasic defibrillator or equivalent if biphasic. Between shocks, give either amiodarone 150 mg IV over 10 min or lidocaine 0.5–0.75 mg/kg IV push.

- If stable (or while preparing for cardioversion), consider treatment with antiarrhythmics such as procainamide, lidocaine, β-blockers, magnesium, or amiodarone.

Ventricular Fibrillation

Symptoms

Since this is an unstable rhythm, patient drops to the ground and is inherently cardiovascularly unstable. **Associated with MI.**

Diagnosis

ECG: Rapid wide complex ventricular beats with no recognizable rhythm (see Figure 11.7).

Treatment

- DC cardioversion is the most effective action. Use standard protocol of 200 J, 200–300 J, and 360 J if monophasic defibrillator or equivalent if biphasic.

- Between shocks, give epinephrine 1 mg IV push or vasopressin 40 mg IV push. If unsuccessful, reattempt DC cardioversion and consider further antiarrhythmics such as amiodarone, lidocaine, and magnesium.

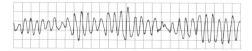

FIGURE 11.7 Ventricular fibrillation.

Oxford Handbook of Clinical Medicine. Sixth edition. Longmore, M, Wilkinson, IB, Rajagopalan S. Copyright 2004. Oxford University Press.

Asystole/Pulseless Electrical Activity

Diagnosis

ECG shows the absence of electrical activity in asystole. Make sure fine VFib is not present.

In pulseless electrical activity (PEA), uncoordinated electrical activity without the result of pulse is present. No specific arrhythmia may be identified.

Treatment

- Make sure ECG reading is accurate and the patient is unresponsive.
- Start cardiopulmonary resuscitation (CPR) and obtain IV/IO access.
- Asystole/PEA are *NOT* shockable rhythms.
- Give epinephrine 1 mg IV/IO and repeat every 3–5 min.
- Or give vasopressin 40 U IV/IO to replace first and second doses of epinephrine.
- Consider atropine 1 mg IV/IO and repeat every 3–5 min.
- For PEA, consider the H's and T's. Correct as soon as possible (see Table 11.7).

Wolff–Parkinson–White Syndrome

Symptoms

Clinically, may range from mild palpitations to syncope. Severe palpitations may also be a presenting sign. Uncommonly, further arrhythmias such as ventricular fibrillation may develop and lead to death.

Diagnosis

Wolff–Parkinson–White (WPW) is caused by conduction through an A-V accessory pathway. This may be from the atria to the ventricle, or vice versa. Commonly may proceed to **atrial fibrillation** or **ventricular fibrillation**. The manner of sudden cardiac death from WPW is atrial fibrillation,

TABLE 11.7 H's and T's often responsible for arrhythmias

H's	T's
Hypovolemia	Toxins
Hypoxia	Tamponade, cardiac
Hydrogen ion (acidosis)	Tension pneumothorax
Hypo/Hyperkalemia	Thrombosis (coronary or pulmonary)
Hypoglycemia	Trauma
Hypothermia	

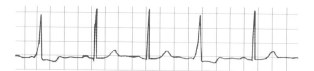

FIGURE 11.8 Wolff–Parkinson–White (WPW) syndrome with delta waves apparent in first and fourth beats. Notice how the delta wave both broadens the ventricular complex and shortens the PR interval.

Oxford Handbook of Clinical Medicine. Sixth edition. Longmore, M, Wilkinson, IB, Rajagopalan S. Copyright 2004. Oxford University Press.

which progresses to conduct rapidly through the accessory pathway leading to ventricular fib.

ECG: Characteristic short P-R interval with a **delta wave** (see Figure 11.8).

Provocation or dysrrhythmia and risk stratification can be done with electrophysiologic testing, but this is generally done by a cardiologist.

Treatment

- Immediate cardiology referral is indicated.

- Restrict vigorous physical activity and sports participation until seen by cardiologist.

- Avoid digoxin, β-blockers, and calcium channel blockers, which can slow conduction through the AV node and isolate conduction through the accessory pathway.

- **Radiofrequency ablation** of the accessory pathway is the standard.

- Drugs that may be used in the intermittently symptomatic patient are quinidine, disopyramide (Norpace), procainamide (Pronestyl), and propafenone (Rythmol).

- In asymptomatic patients without concern for further progression after workup, no therapy may be indicated.

Abdominal Aortic Aneurysm

Symptoms

Most often, asymptomatic. May present with pulsatile or vague epigastric mass or pain, urethral obstruction (and symptoms), or back pain from vertebral body erosion. The triad of **shock, abdominal pain, and pulsatile mass** suggests rupture. Obtain family history for Marfan syndrome or Ehlers–Danlos syndrome. Check blood pressure and obtain smoking and CAD risk factors. These relate directly to diagnose and treatment options.

Diagnosis

Physical exam: Palpable, pulsatile mass in the abdomen.

Imaging: Ultrasound is the initial standard. May measure unruptured aneurysm, but need to obtain CT if rupture present. CT is also the best preoperative test.

MRI is a good choice if the patient is unable to tolerate CT contrast, can wait somewhat longer for the test, and is not hemodynamically unstable.

Greater than 90% are infrarenal.

Treatment

- Control risk factors such as smoking and hypertension.

- β-blockers are the agents of choice for hypertension (HTN).

- Surgical correction is the best option, but size does matter. Indications are size greater than **5.5 cm or growth greater than 0.5 cm per 6 months**.

- For medium-sized aneurysms (3.5–5.5 cm), watchful waiting and control of risk factors are best. Serial ultrasounds are indicated every 6 months to track expansion.

- Aortic stents have recently been used, but are of uncertain benefit thus far.

Peripheral Vascular Disease

Symptoms

Intermittent claudication is the most common symptom and is pathognomonic. This is often in the lower extremities, but may occur in back and buttocks. Obtain a complete history of risk factors including atherosclerotic factors, hyperlipidemia, smoking, age, sex, and fitness level.

Diagnosis

Physical exam: Lower extremity appearance is often cold, pale, shiny, and hairless.

Ankle-brachial index (ABI): Ratio of ankle and brachial blood pressures is often abnormal. Normal is between 0.90 and 1.3.

Exercise treadmill testing with pre- and post-ABI is often used.

Segmental limb pressures may be helpful in further evaluation.

Doppler ultrasound to establish the degree of flow.

Angiography and MRA are useful but are used before surgery, not for diagnosis.

Treatment

- Control of risk factors such as smoking, hyperlipidemia, diabetes, and hypertension, are critically important.

- **Graded exercise training** is the single most effective treatment.

- Antiplatelet agents such as aspirin, dipyridamole (Persantine), and clopidogrel (Plavix) have all been shown to have some benefit. Other antiplatelet agents such as cilostazol (Pletal) and pentoxifylline (Trental) have also been used with success.

- Surgery is reserved for severe cases of larger vessels.

Arterial Embolism/Thrombosis

Symptoms

Rapid-onset extremity pain or numbness.

Diagnosis

Physical exam: Loss of pulse, redness, and swelling may be seen. Signs of complications such as compartment syndrome must be clinically considered.

Arterial Doppler ultrasound to establish flow.

Ankle-brachial index.

Angiography is not useful in diagnosis, but may play a role in preoperative imaging.

Labs: D-dimer (if positive, further testing needs to be done before test is useful), coagulation panel. Chest pain or symptoms may warrant cardiac enzymes.

ECG as indicated.

Treatment

- Oxygen.

- Pain medications as needed.

- Aspirin.

- Anticoagulation with heparin or LMW heparin (Lovenox).

- Consider thrombolytics, but make sure they are not contraindicated in patient. These include tPA and streptokinase.

Raynaud's Disease/Phenomenon

Disease: Idiopathic vasospasm of distal extremity vessels causing symptoms. Usually bilateral.

Phenomenon: Due to underlying disease or cause. Often unilateral or localized to individual digits.

Symptoms

Symptoms most often occur with exposure to cold, alcohol, or smoking. First distal extremity or digits loose sensation, turn white or have notably increased pallor. Upon warming, pain and paresthesias set in, which can be debilitating. In severe cases, may progress to atrophy of fat pads and eventual autoamputation. History may reveal similar symptoms in family members. Patient is often female and middle aged or young.

Diagnosis

Physical exam: White or pale appearance to distal digit with well-demarcated transition line in finger, loss of sensation or tenderness to distal digit. Swelling or erythema may be present after event.

Cold challenge (with immersion in cold water) may be diagnostic.

Nailfold capillary exam is suggestive of secondary causes if capillary loops appear enlarged or distorted.

Test for secondary causes and obtain ANA, TSH, ESR, CBC, coagulation profile.

Treatment

- Treat secondary causes of disease (lupus, scleroderma, etc.).

- Avoid cold exposure with gloves or insulated foot wear. Behavioral modification after symptom recognition to abort attacks with warm water, windmill arm motion, etc., may be useful.

- Medications

  - Cold weather, long-acting calcium channel blockers (nifedipine, amlodipine, etc.) have been shown effective. Aspirin or topical nitroglycerin may be added as the next step.

  - In severe cases, IV prostaglandin/prostaglandin analogs or chemical sympathectomy with lidocaine or bupivacaine may be indicated.

Q 11.4

You are consulted on a 36-year-old Native American male cancer patient being given systemic chemotherapy for lung cancer who has developed a painful area of the right upper arm. The intern on the heme/oncology service demonstrates that the patient seems to have a tender, erythematous, linear area to the right upper arm for the past 5 days. She tells you the team has been treating it as superficial thrombophlebitis, but now states the patient has developed a fever over the past 12 h and the site has gotten worse. What is the next step in management?

A. Start anticoagulation with heparin.
B. Consult surgery.
C. Start aspirin therapy.
D. Stop chemotherapy.
E. Evaluate the patient for thrombolytic therapy.

Superficial Thrombophlebitis

Symptoms

Pain, tenderness, erythema, and local swelling along the affected superficial vein. This may/may not be associated with obvious predisposing factors such as pregnancy, exogenous estrogen use, hypercoagulable state, prolonged hospital stay, prolonged IV catheter use, or saphenous cut-down procedure. If septic, may be associated with fever and signs of infection.

Diagnosis

Physical exam: Classically reveals a tender, **palpable "cord"** commonly with surrounding erythema.

Labs: Obtain CBC for WBCs to evaluate for possible septic thrombus or cellulitis, β-hCG, coagulation profile, platelet studies, protein C and S levels, antithrombin III level, ANA, factor V level, and other blood clotting disease as indicated.

Imaging: Ultrasound may be used to both confirm the presence of a superficial venous thrombosis and exclude deep venous thrombi.

Treatment

- Warm compresses, NSAIDs, and elevation are the standard treatment.
- Remove any possibly thrombosed catheters.
- Anticoagulate only if associated with deep venous thrombosis (DVT). Otherwise, it is not needed.
- Treat coagulation disorder.
- Measures against embolism are not indicated as are in DVT.
- Antibiotics and surgical exploration may be indicated if thrombus is septic.

Venous Thrombosis

Symptoms

Pain, erythema, or swelling usually in the lower extremities. History often reveals hypercoagulable state, prolonged sitting or stasis, or injury (Virchow's triad-stasis, hypercoagulable state, endothelial damage). This may include OCP use, pregnancy, hormone replacement therapy, long plane flight, smoking, recent injury, or blood clotting disorder such as protein C and S deficiency.

Diagnosis

Physical exam: May reveal positive Homans' sign (pain in calf on dorsiflexion of ankle), erythema, swelling, warmth, and tenderness of affected limb.

Labs: D-dimer is classic, but if positive simply indicates that further testing needs to be done. If negative, is fairly reliable. CBC for platelet count and Hct, coagulation profile, fibrinogen, complete metabolic panel, and urinalysis. Further testing is indicated if cause remains idiopathic and may include protein C and S levels, factor V Leiden, factor VIII level, ANA, and PSA in men older than 50 years.

Imaging: Doppler compression ultrasound is most widely used and considered most accurate, but beware that this is only reliable for clots in femoral and popliteal areas.

Contrast venography is the gold standard but involves contrast and is not the first-line test.

MRI may be a good alternative to contrast venography, but is second line to Doppler ultra sound.

Impedence plethysmography may also be used, where available, but much less common.

Clinically, consider pulmonary embolism. If suspected, do a chest CT or V/Q scan.

Treatment

- LMW heparin, enoxaparin (Lovenox) (1 mg/kg SC b.i.d.), or Heparin IV or SC should be started immediately. Enoxaparin is most convenient and avoids the excess monitoring needed with heparin. However, it is most appropriate for uncomplicated disease.

- Start warfarin (Coumadin) at the same time and overlap these by several days to allow the INR to achieve a level between 2 and 3. Then enoxaparin or heparin may be discontinued.

- Duration of warfarin (Coumadin) use varies with the level of complication of DVT. If uncomplicated and likely due to temporary coagulation defect, 3 months is adequate. If complicated with hereditary or acquired (malignancy) hypercoagulable state, surgery, need for prolonged inactivity, or pulmonary embolism, longer therapy may be required and last from 6 to 12 months to indefinite.

- Inferior vena cava (IVC) filters may be an option for those that are not candidates for anticoagulation, but do increase chances recurrent DVT.

- Thrombolytics are still being researched and are not currently recommended for the treatment of DVT.

- Remember to place all hospitalized patients on DVT prophylaxis of some sort.

Varicose Veins

Symptoms

Often noticed by patient to be unsightly, purple, tortuous veins on lower extremities. Usually nontender (although large lesions may be painful), but patient may fixate on them. Rarely inflamed or erythematous, unless overlying skin infection. Skin breaks and subsequent bleeding is rare. These may also be accompanied by telangiectasial lesions in same areas.

Diagnosis

Physical exam: Tortuous enlarged veins and telangiectasias usually of the lower extremities.

Treatment

- Prevention with support stockings and frequent breaks for those with jobs requiring long standing or foot work.

- Injection sclerotherapy with hypertonic saline or sodium tetradecyl sulfate, electrocauterization, or laser treatment is effective for telangiectasial lesions.

- **Surgery:** Vein ligation and stripping, removal with subsequent skin grafting, or stab evulsion phlebectomy is effective in management, but careful consideration of the extent of disease should be done before referral.

Atherosclerosis

Symptoms

The disease itself is asymptomatic, but complications include peripheral vascular disease, angina, MI, and stroke. Look for symptoms of each. History is important and may reveal risk factors such as diabetes, smoking, obesity, hyperlipidemia, alcoholism, or hypertension.

Diagnosis

Atherosclerosis is not directly diagnosed or necessarily tested for. Testing for risk factors of end-organ damage includes lipid levels, hypertension, markers of global inflammation, and direct end-organ damage.

Direct measurement of narrowing of vessels is tested for by carotid artery ultrasound and coronary artery catheterization when indicated.

Treatment

- Lifestyle modification to slow the progression of developing atherosclerosis is very effective. Increase activity, stop smoking, lose weight, and control diabetes.
- Medications
  - Aspirin may be used for antiplatelet effects for prophylaxis or if an atherosclerotic plaque ruptures.
  - Statins (lovastatin, simvastatin, etc.) have been shown to reduce cholesterol levels and increase HDL and thus slow the progression of the disease. Please see section on disorders of lipoid metabolism in Chapter 5 for further discussion.
- Research has shown that with significant control of risk factors, atherosclerosis can be reversed.

Valvular Disease

See Table 11.8.

Infectious Endocarditis

Symptoms

Fever, chest pain, rigors, malaise, back pain, anorexia, weight loss, conjunctival hemorrhage, painful hand or toe lesions (**Osler's nodes**), CHF symptoms, or symptoms of systemic circulation including TIA or stroke. History may include previous valve disease or irregularities or cause of bacteremia. Recent dental work or IV drug use is classic.

Diagnosis

Physical exam: New murmur with increased intensity with deep inspiration, cardiac friction rub, Osler's nodes (painful, deep, lesions on fingers and toes),

TABLE 11.8 Cardiac valvular defects

Lesion		Associations/Exam	Treatment
Mitral	Stenosis	May be caused by rheumatic heart disease Atrial fibrillation is uncommon complication **Diastolic** blowing murmur with/without opening snap	Rate control with digoxin or β-blocker as needed Anticoagulate if AFib present Antibiotic prophylaxis for dental procedures. Treat with balloon valvuloplasty or valve replacement
	Regurgitation	**Holosystolic** murmur made louder with Valsalva	Valvular repair or replacement if symptomatic or EF <60%
Mitral valve prolapse		Chest pain, anxiety, palpitations, dyspnea, and possibly panic attacks **Midsystolic click**, late **systolic** murmur	Reassurance that MVP rarely leads to cardiac problems
Aortic	Stenosis	Syncope, CHF, angina, sudden death After symptoms develop, short-term mortality is high May be associated with rheumatic heart disease if mitral also affected Harsh, **systolic** crescendo/decrescendo murmur Made softer with Valsalva	Antibiotic prophylaxis for dental procedures Valvular replacement is the standard (unless severely elderly)
	Regurgitation	Endocarditis, rheumatic fever, collagen vascular disease, aortic dissection, bicuspid aortic valve, and syphilis Look for widened pulse pressure High-pitched, **diastolic**, decrescendo murmur	Afterload reduction with nifedipine or ACEIs Valvular replacement is definitive and often best treatment

ACEIs, angiotensin-converting enzyme inhibitors; CHF, congestive heart failure; EF, ejection fraction; MVP, mitral valve prolapse.

Janeway lesions (small skin infarctions), nail bed splinter hemorrhages, and Roth spots (retinal exudates).

Blood cultures: Take three different cultures from two different sites. *Staphylococcus aureus* is the most common of bacterial causes, but culture results may be negative with the HACEK (*Haemophilus aphrophilus, Haemophilus parainfluenzae, Actinobacillus actinomycetemcomitans, Cardiobacterium hominis, Eikenella corrodens, Kingella kingae*) organisms.

Labs: CBC for WBC and Hct, ESR, CMP for screening, urinalysis for hematuria, rheumatoid factor.

Echocardiography: Transthoracic echo should be done first, but if negative obtain a transesophageal echo to look for vegetations.

Clinical tool: Duke's criteria is the classic clinical tool for diagnosing infective endocarditis (see Table 11.9).

TABLE 11.9 Duke's criteria

Criteria	Description
Minor	Positive blood cultures for infective endocarditis
	Positive echocardiogram
	New valvular regurgitation
Major	Predisposition, i.e., pre-existing valvular condition or IV drug use
	Fever (Temp >100.4°F)
	Vascular phenomena, i.e., arterial emboli, mycotic aneurysm, Janeway lesions, conjunctival hemorrhages
	Immunologic phenomena, i.e., glomerulonephritis, Osler's nodes, Roth spots, rheumatoid factor (RF) positive
	Microbiologic evidence: Positive blood culture, but not meeting a major criterion or serologic evidence of active infection with organism consistent with endocarditis

Definite infective endocarditis: Two major criteria or one major criterion and three minor criteria or five minor criteria.

Treatment

- Prevent with antibiotic prophylaxis in selected heart disease patients, obviously avoid IV drug use.

- Give oxygen.

- Start antibiotics empirically. If likely to be skin organism, start antistaphylococcal penicillin such as oxacillin or nafcillin *plus* penicillin G or, alternatively, ampicillin *plus* gentamicin. If methicillin-resistant *Staphylococcus aureus* (MRSA) is possible; replace penicillin with vancomycin. Cultures should then guide treatment. Treatment should continue for 4–6 weeks. Do not forget to check gentamicin and vancomycin peaks and troughs.

- **Surgery:** Valvular replacement may be indicated, depending on the severity of case and the presence or absence of emboli.

Q 11.5

You are evaluating a 2-month-old infant male brought to your office for a well child check. On cardiac exam, you hear a systolic "machinery"-type murmur. After an echocardiogram, you determine it is safe to treat this condition with medication. What medication below is indicated?

A. Amlodipine.
B. Indomethacin (Indocin).
C. Acetaminophen (Tylenol).
D. Propranolol (Inderal).
E. Prostaglandin E_1.

Congenital Heart Disease

See Table 11.10.

TABLE 11.10 Common congenital cardiac defects

Defect	Associations	Exam	Treatment
Ventricular septal defect	If lesion is large, Sx of CHF, frequent respiratory infections, or FTT; often close on their own; most common congenital heart defect Eisenmenger's syndrome: Pulmonary HTN → RVH → conversion to R to L shunt, causing cyanosis	Pansystolic vibratory murmur	Follow small lesions annually for closure Surgery for large lesions as soon as possible
Atrial septal defect	Often asymptomatic until adulthood. Sx of CHF are late finding of large defects. Eisenmenger's syndrome is possible late	Fixed split S2, systolic ejection murmur	Small, asymptomatic defects do not need closure Large defects may be surgically repaired Antibiotics before dental procedures
PDA	Not diagnosed due to physiologic PDA in the first few days of life Produces L to R shunt Associated with prematurity, high altitude, first trimester rubella	Machinery murmur, wide pulse pressure, bounding peripheral pulses	Eliminate possibility of other heart defects before treating Child may depend on PDA for life! Keep open with prostaglandin E1 if indicated Close with indomethacin (Indocin) or other NSAID
Coarctation of the aorta	Turner's syndrome, male sex, bicuspid aortic valve Rib notching on chest X-ray	Higher blood pressure in upper than lower extremities Diminished lower extremity pulses Systolic murmur	Surgical correction is the standard Balloon angioplasty is the possibility depending on defect
Tetralogy of Fallot	Features 1. Pulmonary stenosis 2. RVH 3. Overriding aorta 4. VSD "Tet spells"-child stops running/exercising to stop and squat Chest X-ray shows boot-shaped heart	Systolic ejection murmur, single S2 Cyanosis	If cyanotic at birth, give PGE Surgery is the standard of care, and requires several different procedures Treat tet spells with O_2, knee/chest position, morphine, and β-blockers

CHF, congestive heart failure; FTT, failure to thrive; HTN, hypertension; NSAID, nonsteroidal antiinflammatory drug; PGE, prostaglandin E; PDA, Patent duitus arteriossus; RVH, right ventricular hypertrophy; VSD, ventral septal defect.

Answers

11.1 B. Cough is a common complaint of those started on angiotensin-converting enzyme inhibitors (ACEIs) and may lead to noncompliance and otherwise "refractory" hypertension.

11.2 D. This patient presents with clinical features of acute coronary syndrome. Initial treatment should be a combination of drugs and oxygen known as "MONA," which stands for morphine, oxygen, nitroglycerin, and aspirin. Although other answers may be treatments later in the management of this patient, they are not the next step.

11.3 E. This patient has a long prior history of atrial fibrillation, thus may be called recurrent/chronic. Indefinite anticoagulation is thus indicated.

11.4 B. The treatment for septic superficial thrombophlebitis is generally with surgery, although broad-spectrum antibiotics may also have a role. Consultation is indicated in this patient.

11.5 B. This patient has the classic murmur of a patent ductus arteriosus (PDA), which are commonly found in newborns and are generally non-pathologic. If persistent, and, after echocardiogram workup, the child is not thought to depend on blood flow through it, the PDA may be closed with indomethacin (Indocin).

Croup	275
Acute Bronchitis	277
Acute Bronchiolitis	277
Pneumonia	278
Influenza	278
Chronic Obstructive Pulmonary Disease (COPD)	280
Chronic Bronchitis/Emphysema	280
Asthma	282
Pneumoconiosis	283
Malignant Neoplasm of Bronchus and Lung	285
Pulmonary Tuberculosis	287
Sarcoidosis	288
Cystic Fibrosis	289
Pulmonary Embolism	291
Pulmonary Hypertension	292
Spontaneous Pneumothorax	294
Pertussis	294
Wegener's Granulomatosis	295

Croup

Symptoms

It is often a disease of childhood; the patient presents with low-grade fever, "**barking**" or "seal-like" cough, **stridor**, fatigue, and possibly hypoxia and cyanosis in advanced cases. History may reveal recent URI.

Diagnosis

Largely a clinical diagnosis.

Physical exam: The most popular clinical tool is the Westley croup score that evaluates the level of consciousness, stridor, cyanosis, air entry, and retractions.

Labs: CBC shows that leukocytosis is common, but the test is not required. Lymphocytes may be seen in differential.

Rapid antigen testing is available in some centers.

Polymerase chain reaction (PCR) or viral culture is rarely used.

Imaging: Classic posteroanterior (PA) neck x-ray shows "**steeplechase**" sign indicating subglottic narrowing.

Order a lateral neck to exclude epiglottis.

Fiberoptic laryngoscopy if available and patient is stable.

Q 12.1

A 14-month-old male infant presents to the clinic with a mother's complaint of subjective fever, increased fussiness, poor PO intake, and "barking" cough. The child has been sick for 2 days with similar reports from the day care that the child attends. Vital signs are BP 110/86 mmHg, temperature 101.0°F (38.3°C), HR 120, RR 26, O_2 saturation 96%. On exam, the child is responsive, but with a noticeable stridor on inspiration. Lung exam is unremarkable, except for coarse upper airway sounds. PA neck x-ray does show subglottic narrowing in the upper airway. What is the next step in management?

A. Ceftriaxone (Rocephin) and IV fluids.
B. Nebulized albuterol and IV dexamethasone.
C. Nebulized epinephrine and dexamethasone.
D. Supplemental oxygen therapy alone.
E. Nebulized albuterol and inhaled fluticasone/salmeterol (Advair).

Treatment

- In mild cases, no treatment is necessary.

- Outpatient monitoring in most, inpatient monitoring in severe cases.

- Place patient on humidified oxygen.

- Racemic, nebulized epinephrine for moderate-to-severe cases. Expect improvement within 30 min.

- **Corticosteroids** are the standard treatment. These most commonly include dexamethasone or budesonide (Pulmicort) nebulized. These generally show improvement within 6 h. Oral prednisone may also be used, but adjust the dose to equal that of dexamethasone.

- Follow up in 24 h for confirmation of improvement.

Acute Bronchitis

Symptoms

Usually seen in combination with other URI-type symptoms. Symptoms consist of malaise, chilliness, mild-to-moderate fever, chest congestion, chest fullness, and cough. The most persistent of these is cough, which may be present for weeks after successful treatment.

Diagnosis

Generally, clinical assessment is all that is necessary.

Physical exam: Mild scattered rhonchi throughout bilateral lung fields, mild anterior cervical lymphadenopathy, and low-grade fever.

Labs: If significantly ill with increased temperature, prolonged illness despite treatment, or concomitant underlying disease such as chronic obstructive pulmonary disease (COPD), sputum culture and gram stain may be indicated. If done, base treatment with antibiotics on sensitivities is achieved.

Chest x-ray: May be used to exclude other common respiratory infections such as pneumonia, but will be negative with genuine bronchitis.

Treatment

- Supportive care is most effective, since the vast majority of cases are caused by viruses.
- Increasing hydration or oral guaifenesin (Robitussin) may be useful as a mucolytic.
- Steam inhalation may help for a short time.
- If cough is productive, avoid suppressing it with medication.
- Antibiotics are useful if a bacterial cause is suspected or if underlying respiratory illness exists. Use amoxicillin or azithromycin PO.

Acute Bronchiolitis

Symptoms

Most commonly caused by a virus, bronchiolitis is thought of as a wheezing, respiratory illness for children younger than 2 years. This may or may not include respiratory distress. The most common virus is respiratory syncytial virus (RSV) although others do exist. This diagnosis may be given if others such as pneumonia, foreign body, or atopy are excluded.

Diagnosis

Physical exam: Tachypnea, intercostal and subcostal retractions, and audible wheezing. The chest may appear hyperexpanded. Findings on auscultation include any combination of wheezing, prolonged expiration, crackles, or fine rales. In severe illness, signs of respiratory distress may be present including increased work of breathing and cyanosis.

Labs: Oxygen saturation may be lower than clinically suspected. CBC may show an increase in WBCs (adjust for age of patient) and often shows lymphocytic predominance. In moderate-to-severe disease, obtain an arterial blood gas (ABG).

Viral studies with direct antigen or immunofluorescence testing of serologic or nasal secretions for RSV may be useful. Viral culture or PCR is employed less because of the time course to result.

Imaging: Chest x-ray may show hyperinflation and peribronchial thickening. Patchy atelectasis with volume loss may result from airway narrowing and mucus plugging. Look for flattened diaphragms and air-bronchograms, which are indicative of disease.

Treatment

- Supportive care.

- Hospitalize in case of toxic appearance, hypoxemia, cyanosis, or moderate-to-severe respiratory distress, or if caretaker is unable to care for patient at home.

- Consider intubation and respiratory support. If required, intubate earlier rather than later.

- Give IV fluids.

- Inhaled bronchodilators (albuterol) are routinely used; however, research does not support to a strong degree. Oral bronchodilators have not been shown to be effective.

- Nebulized epinephrine has been shown to be more effective than bronchodilators, but should be tried after bronchodilators.

- Corticosteroids have not been shown to be effective in mild–moderate disease in infants and children. Younger infants, newborns, or those children with underlying lung disease may benefit from a short course.

- Antiviral therapy such as ribavirin may be effective, but should be reserved for sicker, younger patients with severe or complicating disease due to cost and impracticality.

- To help prevent flu virus-caused disease, vaccinate.

Pneumonia

See Table 12.1 and Figure 12.1.

Influenza

Symptoms

Abrupt onset of fever, severe myalgias, anorexia, sore throat, headache, stuffy nose, arthralgias, cough, fatigue, chest congestion, and malaise. Clinically distinguish from a cold or URI.

TABLE 12.1 Bacterial vs viral pneumonia

Etiology	Symptoms	Diagnosis	Treatment
Bacterial, community acquired	Moderate-to-high fever, productive cough, night sweats, chills, chest congestion, pharyngitis, wheezing, or chest pain	Leukocytosis on CBC, often with left shift on differential Elevated ESR, CRP Obtain blood culture and sputum cultures to identify organism CXR is best way to diagnose Opacity often lobar or segmental Make sure to check lateral CXR to exclude retrocardiac opacities	Treat supportively with oral hydration and routine inspiratory therapy. Oxygen if O_2 sat <93% Consider admission. Give antipyretics to suppress fever as needed Consider a mucolytic to aid break up of consolidation Antibiotics should be tailored to organism/setting, but a **macrolide** (azithromycin, clarithromycin) is often first line. Fluoroquinolone (levofloxacin) is second. Consider amoxicillin/clavulanate or cephalosporin in combination with above.
Viral	Low-grade fever, mild cough, chest congestion, general malaise, headache, or wheezing. May be relatively asymptomatic	Lymphocytosis on CBC without left shift on differential CXR may show diffuse, patchy opacities throughout lung fields	Supportive care that rarely needs admission Fluids, mucolytics, inspiratory therapy, and antipyretics Consider suppression of cough only late in disease course

CRP, C-reactive protein; CXR, Chest x-ray; ESR, erythrocyte sedimentation rate.

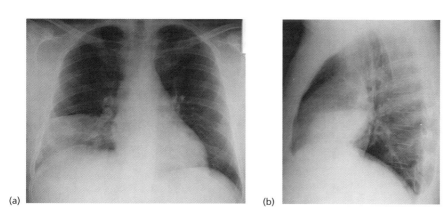

(a) (b)

FIGURE 12.1 Opacity of right middle lobe indicating infiltrate.

Oxford Handbook of Clinical Medicine. Sixth edition. Longmore M, Wilkinson IB, et al. Copyright 2004. Oxford University Press.

Diagnosis

Labs: Nasal washings and direct antigen testing are the most accurate and convenient techniques available. Several commercial testing kits are available, but only one distinguishes between influenza types A and B. Viral culture,

PCR, or antibody titers are possible, but impractical. CBC may show mildly increased leukocytes; but if significantly high, consider secondary bacterial infection.

Chest x-ray is rarely needed, but may be used if significant respiratory symptoms are present. Viral pneumonia appears as more diffuse, patchy infiltrates.

Treatment

- Supportive outpatient care is often all that is needed.
- Give nonsteroidal antiinflammatory drugs (NSAIDs) or acetaminophen.
- Antiviral agents include amantadine (Symmetrel), rimantadine (Flumadine), zanamivir (Relenza), and oseltamivir (Tamiflu). Amantadine and rimantadine are recommended for the treatment of influenza A only; zanamivir and oseltamivir work against both.
- Yearly vaccination still remains the best prevention.

Chronic Obstructive Pulmonary Disease (COPD)

Chronic Bronchitis/Emphysema

Symptoms

Chronic Bronchitis

By definition, productive cough for three consecutive months for two consecutive years. Patient may also have dry cough, wheezing, smoking history, shortness of breath, dyspnea on exertion, and acutely progressive dyspnea at rest. Classically called **blue bloaters** from the chronic, hypoxemic, and hypercapnic state, these patients often have a cyanotic appearance.

Emphysema

Look for smoking history, exposure to noxious fumes or irritants, weight loss, wheezing, shortness of breath, dyspnea on exertion, and eventual dyspnea at rest. The patients are classically referred to as **pink puffers** because of their often emaciated appearance, higher than normal respiratory rate, and acyanotic appearance. These patients may also look plethoric because of possible polycythemia secondary to chronic hypoxemia.

Diagnosis

Physical exam: Rhonchi, wheezing, with often wet-sounding cough. Increased chest volume, lower than expected diaphragm position, and prolonged expiratory phase. Pursed lip breathing may be observed along with the use of accessory muscles and retractions.

Pulmonary function tests (PFTs) show FEV1/FVC <70%, and increased total lung capacity (TLC) due to increased residual capacity. FEV1 may be normal or low.

Imaging: Chest x-ray shows hyperexpanded lung fields, possibly with superior segment bullae, flattened diaphragms, and narrowed mediastinum.

DLCO (carbon dioxide diffusing capacity) is prolonged in emphysema.

ABG may show hypercapnia, hypoxia, and decreased pH.

CBC may show mild polycythemia due to chronic hypoxemia.

Treatment

- Oxygen and smoking cessation are the only treatments shown to reduce mortality.

- Treatment guidelines come from those supported by the American College of Chest Physicians and by the Global Strategy for the Diagnosis, Management, and Prevention of Chronic Obstructive Pulmonary Disease. These groups support that β_2-agonists (albuterol), the long-acting anticholinergic tiotropium (Spiriva), and the short-acting anticholinergic ipratropium bromide (Atrovent) are the mainstays of therapy. These may be used for chronic control of symptoms and acute exacerbations. Steroids, either IV or PO, may be given and show good effect in a short course. Also in acute setting, antibiotics (macrolide or fluoroquinolone) should be given and may decrease the course of exacerbation. Theophylline or inhaled steroids mixed with a β_2-agonist (Advair) may be considered for chronic disease (but are not a choice for acute exacerbations).

- Consider bullectomy or lung volume–reducing surgery in advanced cases. Lung transplant is reserved for optimal patients with advanced but isolated disease.

- Vaccination against influenza and pneumococcal pneuomonia (Pneumovax) should be given regardless of age.

Q 12.2

A 7-year-old Caucasian male comes to your office for a routine asthma checkup. The boy is accompanied by his mother who states his asthma bothers him at most of his soccer activities and at school. The boy reports having to use his albuterol inhaler at least once per day. His mother also states he sometimes coughs at night with resulting sleep disturbance about twice per week. A records review indicates his last pulmonary function tests 4 months ago with the value of FEV1 70% predicted. Currently, he is only taking albuterol for his symptoms, but his mother asks if there is anything more you can do. What is the most likely diagnosis?

A. Mild intermittent asthma.
B. Mild persistent asthma.
C. Moderate persistent asthma.
D. Severe persistent asthma.
E. Moderate intermittent asthma.

Q 12.3

What is an example of appropriate therapy for the above diagnosis?

A. Continue albuterol PRN although prescribe the nebulized form to control nighttime symptoms.
B. Low-dose maintenance prednisone until clinical improvement is seen, then a slow taper.
C. Addition of montelukast (Singulair), zafirlukast (Accolate), or inhaled cromolyn sodium with follow-up scheduled for the next week.
D. Addition of fluticasone/salmeterol (Advair) and addition of montelukast (Singulair).

Asthma

Symptoms

Patients may have wheezing, chronic cough, decreased exercise tolerance, chest tightness, and shortness of breath. Asthma is usually diagnosed in children, but may exist at any age. Look for frequency of rescue medication usage, accompanying conditions such as **eczema** and **allergic rhinitis**, environmental triggers (smoking in home), and family history.

Diagnosis

Physical exam: Wheezing (although may be absent if airways totally constricted), prolonged expiratory phase, and tachypnea.
Labs: CBC most often normal. Differential may show eosinophilia.

Pulmonary function testing is the most accurate way of diagnosis with decreased FEV1 and peak expiratory flow (PEF). FEV1 classically improves ≥**12%** after bronchodilator administration, which demonstrates **reversibility**.

Regular PEF measurement to monitor the course of disease.

Bronchoprovocation testing (methacholine challenge) is sometimes used, which shows greater response to common bronchoconstrictor in asthmatic patients. This challenge has a high negative predictive value.
Imaging: Check chest x-ray at least once.

Consider skin allergen testing for common irritants, which may elicit trigger identification.

Consider IgA, IgG testing for congenital abnormalities (see Table 12.2).

Treatment

- In acute exacerbation, the mainstays are short-acting bronchodilators (albuterol, levalbuterol, and pirbuterol) and supplemental oxygen.

- Add ipratropium (Atrovent) for synergism as needed acutely. No benefit, however, has been proven after admission to the hospital.

- Give systemic corticosteroids (prednisone, methylprednisolone, and prednisolone); although they are not short acting, they are often helpful in the acute setting to speed recovery.

- Consider epinephrine 1:1000 or terbutaline, systemically or inhaled.

TABLE 12.2 Classification of Asthma

Degree of disease	Symptoms	Nighttime symptoms	Lung function	Recommended step for initiating treatment
Mild intermittent	Symptoms of asthma occurring two or fewer times per week	≤2 nocturnal awakenings per month due to asthma symptoms	FEV1 or PEF ≥80% predicted	Step 1
Mild persistent	Symptoms ≥2 times per week but less than once per day	≥2 times per month	FEV1 or PEF ≥80% predicted	Step 2
Moderate persistent	Daily symptoms with the need for rescue medications, exacerbations affect activity and occur ≥2 times per week	≥1 time per week	FEV1 or PEF 60%–80% predicted	Step 3
Severe persistent	Daily or continual symptoms that affect activity; frequent exacerbations	Frequent	FEV1 or PEF ≤60% predicted	Step 4 or 5

FEV1, forced expiratory volume in 1 second; PEF, peak expiratory flow.

- For severe exacerbations not responsive to initial therapy, consider IV magnesium sulfate or heliox.
- Monitor patient for at least 1 h after administration of medication to ensure effect.
- The National Asthma Education and Prevention Program, Expert Panel Report 3 (EPR 3), guidelines recommend a stepwise approach by starting with the most aggressive step and then "stepping down" to achieve control (see Table 12.3).
- Educate the patient and family with the "asthma action plan," a color-coded, written plan for medications to be taken at home.
- Avoid triggers if identified.
- Follow up the patient with best peak flow recordings at home to be able to intervene early if needed.

Pneumoconiosis

Symptoms

May be due to the inhalation of many different inorganic dusts and thus presentation varies greatly. May be asymptomatic or have severe shortness of breath, cough, weight loss, sputum production, wheezing, dyspnea on exertion, or hypoxemia. Look for a history that contains exposure to coal dust, silica, asbestos, mining, or berylliosis. Disease is worsened by smoking.

TABLE 12.3 Stepwise approach to asthma therapy for patients ≥12 years old and adults

Step	Treatment
Step 1	No daily medication needed Short-acting bronchodilator PRN
Step 2	Short-acting bronchodilator PRN Low-dose inhaled corticosteroid (combination = Advair) Consider cromolyn, nedocromil (Tilade), zafirlukast (Accolate), montelukast (Singulair), or theophylline
Step 3	Short-acting bronchodilator PRN Low- to medium-dose inhaled corticosteroid + long-acting bronchodilator Consider addition of montelukast (Singulair), zafirlukast (Accolate), theophylline, or zileuton (Zyflo)
Step 4	Short-acting bronchodilator PRN Medium-dose inhaled corticosteroid + long-acting bronchodilator, Consider addition of montelukast (Singulair), zafirlukast (Accolate), theophylline, or zileuton (Zyflo)
Step 5	Short-acting bronchodilator PRN High-dose inhaled corticosteroid + long-acting bronchodilator, AND consider addition of omalizumab (Xolair)* for those with allergies
Step 6	Short-acting bronchodilator PRN High-dose inhaled corticosteroid + long-acting bronchodilator + oral corticosteroids AND consider addition of omalizumab (Xolair)* for those with allergies

Examples:
Short-acting bronchodilator—albuterol, levalbuterol, and pirbuterol.
Long-acting bronchodilator—salmeterol (Serevent), formoterol (Foradil Aerolizer).
Inhaled corticosteroids—budesonide, beclomethasone, flunisolide, fluticasone, mometasone, triamcinolone acetonide.
Systemic corticosteroid—prednisone, methylprednisolone, prednisolone.
Advair—salmeterol/fluticasone.
*Those placed on omalizumab should be educated and closely monitored for the rare but life-threatening side effect of anaphylaxis.

Diagnosis

Physical exam: Varied presentation of rhonchi and adventitial sounds.
Labs: No definite lab tests are indicative of the disease. Rule out infectious process with proper labs.
Imaging: Chest x-ray is variable and may show patchy infiltrates throughout lung fields, hilar lymphadenopathy, miliary pattern, multiple small round opacities, or larger single opacities.

Treatment

- Prevention and avoidance is the only effective way to control disease. Otherwise, minimize symptoms.

- Supplemental oxygen as needed.

- Eventual lung transplant may be beneficial.

Q 12.4

A 79-year-old African American female presents to the inpatient ward for the evaluation of a 9-month history of apparent wasting, increasing fatigue, hemoptysis, and cough. She had a chest x-ray in the ER suggestive of a peripheral mass of the left lung. On interview, you discover she has a history of cigarette smoking, nephrolithiasis, hypothyroidism, hyperlipidemia, hypertension, and right hip fracture 4 months ago. Her vital signs are stable and she is afebrile. Physical exam shows moderate temporal wasting and decreased breath sounds in the left lung base. She has an intermittent wet cough on deep inspiration and coughs up some pinkish sputum upon exam. Screening labs from the ER are normal except for serum calcium level to 14.1 mg/dL. What is the most likely diagnosis?

A. Small cell cancer of the lung.
B. Adenocarcinoma of the lung.
C. Squamous cell carcinoma of the lung.
D. Pulmonary fat embolism.
E. Sarcoidosis of the lung.

Malignant Neoplasm of Bronchus and Lung

Several histologic types including adenocarcinoma, squamous cell, small cell, and large cell.

Symptoms

Variable symptoms depend on histologic type and location, but may include wasting, cough, **hemoptysis**, wheezing, fatigue, bone pain, fever, dysphagia, dyspnea, hoarseness (due to recurrent laryngeal nerve involvement), shortness of breath, chest pain, cachexia, loss of appetite, facial swelling, or **Horner's syndrome (ptosis, miosis, and anhydrosis)**. Symptoms may also come from paraneoplastic syndromes seen commonly with lung malignancies. History invariably reveals smoking, exposure to asbestos, radon gas, or other irritant (see Table 12.4).

Diagnosis

Physical exam: Lung exam shows dullness to percussion, rhonchi, rales, decreased breath sounds, increased tactile fremitus, or egophony. Look specifically for supraclavicular and infraclavicular lymphadenopathy.

Labs: CBC for leukocytosis or leukopenia, Chem-7 including electrolytes and calcium, obtain ionized calcium if serum calcium is elevated, phosphate, magnesium, adrenocorticotropic hormone (ACTH), thyroid hormone, parathyroid hormone, and parathyroid-related peptide. Sputum sample or bronchoscopy with or without washings are useful in centrally located cancers and may reveal histologic type.

Imaging: CXR is often the first indicator of nodule or suspicious lesion. Look for location being either central or peripheral, which may help with identification. If consolidation is seen in a single lobe or in one complete lung, consider postobstructive tumor (blocking bronchus).

CT scan is generally the next step, and is useful in telling the location and extent of disease. If positive, look for other tumors by scanning the rest of the body.

TABLE 12.4 Associated conditions with malignancy of the lung

Syndrome	Association
Eaton–Lambert syndrome	Myasthenia gravis–like syndrome that spares ocular involvement
Superior vena cava syndrome	Plethora and swelling of the face due to tumor compression of the superior vena cava
Horner syndrome	Caused by Pancoast tumor (apical, posterior lung tumor that compresses spine)
	Produces classic triad of ptosis, miosis, and anhydrosis

TABLE 12.5 Paraneoplastic syndromes associated with lung malignancy

Histologic cancer type	Classic paraneoplastic syndrome
Small cell carcinoma	Cushing's syndrome (ACTH production), hyponatremia (SIADH production)
Adenocarcinoma	Trousseau's syndrome (hypercoagulable state)
Squamous cell carcinoma	Hypercalcemia, hypophosphatemia

ACTH, adrenocorticotropic hormone; SIADH, syndrome of inappropriate antidiuretic hormone.

Bone scan may be useful in finding metastases.

Biopsy is the gold standard and may be obtained transthoracically or bronchoscopically, depending on peripheral or central location, respectively. In patients whose disease is thought to be non small cell histology and are surgical candidates, throracotomy may be used for diagnosis and treatment. In patients with suspected small cell or metastatic non-small cell cancers, a less invasive form such as thoracentesis of pleural effusion, lymph node biopsy, bronchoscopy, or transthoracic needle aspiration should be employed. In other tumors in which type and stage are less clear, the modalities available are cytologic analysis of sputum, flexible bronchoscopy, and video-assisted thoracoscopic surgery (VATS) (see Table 12.5).

Treatment

- Small cell lung cancers are usually found after the stage of metastasis, thus chemotherapy is the mainstay. Overall, small cell 5-year survival rates are, however, between 5% and 25%.

- Non-small cell lung cancers are much more commonly found before metastasis and with localized disease, thus surgical resection is often effective. Local or regional disease may be treated with radiation or chemotherapy. Distant metastases are usually treated with chemotherapy or radiation, but this is generally thought of as palliative.

Pulmonary Tuberculosis

Symptoms

Active disease: Cough, hemoptysis, fever, night sweats, weight loss, severe malaise, or pleuritic chest pain. Disseminated disease may show symptoms of distant organ system involvement. The classic example is Pott's disease, which is tuberculosis (TB) of the spine. Detailed travel history and exposure history should be done to elicit possible transmission route.

Latent disease: Asymptomatic.

Diagnosis

Physical exam: Coarse sounding lungs, rhonchi, rales, decreased breath sounds, egophony, or tactile fremitus.

Labs: Three separate sputum samples stained for acid fast bacilli (AFB) may be used to give presumptive diagnosis. Culture is available but takes 2–6 weeks for results, sensitivities take longer. Direct nucleic acid amplification does exist although used only if AFB stain is positive and <7 days treatment, very expensive. Also obtain CBC, Chem-20 for AST, ALT, bilirubin, alkaline phosphatase, serum creatinine, a platelet count, HIV, and Hep B and C. Obtain CD4 count if HIV+ (see Table 12.6).

Steroids, anergy, chemotherapy, and immunocompromised states can alter screening PPD.

Imaging: Chest x-ray is generally accepted imaging, which, in active disease, may show hilar lymphadenopathy (Ghon complex), cavitary lesions, opacity suggesting infiltrate, effusion, miliary pattern of opacities, or granulomas often in the apices. Reactivation TB tends to be in the superior, posterior lobes of the lungs. CT chest may also be used for the confirmation of disease.

If extrapulmonary disease is suspected, imaging and/or biopsies may be needed.

Treatment

- The Joint Committee of the American Thoracic Society (ATS), the Infectious Diseases Society of America (IDSA), and the

TABLE 12.6 Screening purified protein derivative (PPD) (read 48–72 h after placement)

Population	Positive Mantoux PPD skin test (induration)
HIV+ persons, chemotherapy patients, hepatitis C patients, recent exposure to active tuberculosis (TB)-infected person, or immunocompromised	≥5 mm
Exposure risk factors such as **health care workers**, immigrants, homeless, diabetics	≥10 mm
Low risk of disease	≥15 mm

Confirm positive PPD with second test before diagnosing latent TB.

Centers for Disease Control and Prevention (CDC) recommend a two-phase regimen of treatment to include an initial phase and a continuation phase. The mnemonic **RIPE** summarizes the medications: **R**ifampin, **I**soniazid (INH), **P**yrazinamide, and **E**thambutol. These should be taken according to several regimens that include therapy lasting a total of 6 months. This therapy may be focused after cultures return sensitivities, although ethambutol should be included in the focused regimen. A baseline eye and visual examination should precede the use of ethambutol, and additional vitamin B$_6$ should be given to prevent INH-associated neuropathy.

- If treating latent TB (from positive PPD), recommendations are for the regimen of INH lasting 9 months (range 6–12 months).

- Monthly monitoring of treatment and lab testing is indicated.

- Referral to infectious disease specialist may be necessary.

Sarcoidosis

Symptoms

Approximately half of patients are asymptomatic. Symptoms include cough, malaise, shortness of breath, fever, night sweats, skin lesions, Bell's palsy, and arthritis. Often this disease is multiorgan, so look for extrapulmonary involvement (skin, cardiac, hepatic, renal).

Diagnosis

Labs: CBC often shows lymphopenia, anemia, or leukopenia. Chem-20 may show increased ALT and infrequently hypercalcemia. Check urine for hypercalciuria (more common than hypercalcemia). Hypergammaglobulinemia may be seen. ACE level is often elevated (the value in using ACE level for monitoring disease is still unclear).

Imaging: Chest x-ray is most useful. **Bilateral hilar lymphadenopathy** is the key finding. CXR be used to define the stages by Scadding's classification (see Table 12.7).

CT scan is useful in demonstrating abnormalities in greater detail.

TABLE 12.7 Staging of sarcoidosis

Stage	Findings on CXR
Stage 0	Normal
Stage 1	Hilar adenopathy alone
Stage 2	Hilar adenopathy and parenchymal infiltrates
Stage 3	Parenchymal infiltrates alone
Stage 4	Pulmonary fibrosis

CXR, chest x-ray.

PFTs reveal a restrictive pattern and are useful in the following disease when done routinely.

Bronchoscopy with biopsy will demonstrate noncaseating granulomatous tissue. Bronchoalveolar lavage (BAL) may reveal characteristic CD4-positive lymphocytes.

Obtain routine EKG.

Obtain screening PPD.

Treatment

- If any treatment is necessary, **prednisone is the mainstay**. Other immunomodulating drugs such as methotrexate (Trexall), hydroxychloroquine (Plaquenil), and azathioprine may be used, but require frequent monitoring.

- Routine office visits while on prednisone and early in the disease is recommended.

- Refer patient for an ophthalmic exam.

Q 12.5

A 10-day-old infant comes to the ER with her mother complaining that the infant is not stooling since discharge from the hospital, increased fussiness, subjective fever, and fast breathing. The mother states that the infant was born by a spontaneous vaginal delivery at term without complication. She states her baby only stooled once in the hospital and has been breast-feeding since. She also was noted to feel hot over the past few days with sweating noted overnight. Her vital signs show moderate tachycardia, temperature to 103.1°F (39.5°C), RR 42, and O_2 saturation to 90%. Chest x-ray was done and shows bilateral lobar pneumonia. Appropriate antibiotics are started after blood cultures are taken. What is the most appropriate next step in management?

A. Sweat chloride test.
B. Urinalysis.
C. Stool analysis for fecal fat.
D. Chromosomal analysis.
E. Echocardiogram.

Cystic Fibrosis

Autosomally inherited defect of the *CFTR* gene producing nonfunctional sodium/chloride channels.

Symptoms

May be seen in extrapulmonary systems outside the lungs, classically, meconium ileus or intussusception, at birth. In pulmonary system, patients often have recurrent lower respiratory infections, history of multiple pneumonias, chronic cough, wheezing, dyspnea, barrel chest, tachypnea, and other infections leading to symptoms of acute illness (fever, malaise, etc.). Malabsorption due to pancreatic insufficiency may be seen as steatorrhea, abdominal pain, vitamin deficiency, malnourishment, and failure to thrive. Pancreatic problems may progress to diabetes. In adults, males have infertility secondary to aspermia and females are prone to recurrent miscarriage.

Diagnosis

Physical exam: Focal loss of breath sounds, wet-sounding cough, rhonchi, wheezing, tachypnea, or clubbing and cyanosis from hypoxemia.

Labs: Sweat chloride test (pilocarpine iontophoresis) is the gold standard [cystic fibrosis (CF) patients >60 mEq/L). Confirm test with at least two positives. Genetic testing can also be done to confirm. Obtain screening labs for other abnormalities including Chem-20 for electrolyte disorders and low albumin, CBC for acute infection or increased hematocrit. Transepithelial nasal potential difference, immunoreactive trypsin (newborn screening), fecal fat, and pancreatic enzyme secretion testing may be useful in some cases. Obtain periodic respiratory cultures in acute cases.

Imaging: Chest x-ray may show consolidation, hyperaeration, hilar adenopathy, bronchiectasis, blebs, or, rarely, pneumothorax.

Pulmonary function tests (PFTs) for comparison and reference.

Exercise testing for respiratory function.

Echocardiogram for heart function.

Vitamin A and E levels and INR to evaluate clotting function, annually.

Genetic testing of family and counseling on chances of disease/carrier state in future children.

Treatment

- Oxygen as needed. Intubate if acutely necessary.
- Give antibiotics acutely if warranted. Cover for *S. aureus* and *Pseudomonas*, as well as previously cultured bacteria per patient history. Ciprofloxacin, cephalexin (Keflex) for PO regimen or tobramycin plus ceftazidime (Fortaz), or vancomycin for IV regimen is a good choice. Aerosolized tobramycin may be used for prophylaxis (1 month on, 1 month off) if previously colonized with *Pseudomonas*.
- Chest physiotherapy (percussion).
- Therapeutic enemas or laxative therapy as needed.
- BiPAP mechanical ventilation is sometimes used for nighttime hypoxia.
- Bronchodilators if response has been demonstrated.
- Dornase alfa (DNase) is the most widely used mucolytic.
- Pancreatic enzyme replacement. Avoid high doses that may cause colonic strictures.
- Vitamin supplements to replace fat solubles (vitamin A, D, E, and K)
- Treat diabetic patients with insulin as needed.
- Annual flu vaccine.

- High salt, high protein, and high calorie diet.
- Surgery with lung transplant or other solid organ transplant may be considered in the end-stage disease.

Q 12.6

A 39-year-old female business assistant has come into the ER complaining of chest pain and mild air hunger after a recent business trip to South America. She states her prior trip was uneventful, and that she stayed in hotels between her business meetings. Her prior medical history includes idiopathic hypothyroidism and acne vulgaris. Her medications include daily vitamins, oral contraceptives, levothyroxine, and minocycline (Minocin). Her vital signs are normal except for mildly increased blood pressure and moderate tachycardia. What imaging study would most likely reveal the diagnosis?

A. Chest x-ray would show pneumonia likely acquired in South America.
B. Spiral chest CT would show PE.
C. Chest x-ray would show pulmonary fibrosis due to minocycline use.
D. Chest CT will show Ghon complex and granulomas from the tuberculosis (TB) acquired in South America.
E. Doppler ultrasound of the bilateral lower extremities would reveal the presence of DVT).

Pulmonary Embolism

Symptoms

Known as "the great masquerader," pulmonary embolism (PE) presents in many different ways. Common ones are pleuritic chest pain, shortness of breath, dyspnea, tachypnea, fever, anxiety, syncope, and hemoptysis, or the patient may be asymptomatic. May include symptoms of DVT, which are lower extremity swelling, pain, tenderness, and erythema. History may reveal Virchow's triad or associated risk factors (see Table 12.8).

Diagnosis

Physical exam: Tachypnea, tachycardia, rhonchi, rales, decreased diaphragmatic excursion. DVT may be evident by lower extremity swelling, erythema, tenderness, and positive Homans' sign (pain on dorsiflexion of foot).

TABLE 12.8 Virchow's triad

Element	Risk factor
Stasis	Plane flight, immobility due to illness, obesity
Endothelial injury	Trauma, surgery, fracture
Hypercoagulable state	Pregnancy, smoking, oral contraceptive (OCP) use, coagulation disorder, malignancy, burns

Labs: D-dimer is a popular test that may show coagulation, but is only useful if negative. If positive, D-dimer is much too nonspecific to support any diagnosis. ABG may show an increased A-a gradient or primary respiratory alkalosis.

Imaging: Spiral CT is becoming the study of choice, although it may miss small PEs in the periphery. CXR may be normal or show **Hampton's hump** (wedge-shaped infarct), **Westermark's sign** (focal oligemia), atelectasis, consolidation, prominent central arteries, pleural effusion, or elevated hemidiaphragm.

Nuclear medicine V/Q scan is helpful if results are low probability (no PE) or high probability (PE). If intermediate probability, then the patient needs further workup. When ordering V/Q scan, consider the pre-test probability of PE.

Doppler ultrasound of the legs to evaluate for DVT.

Pulmonary angiography remains the gold standard, but is invasive and expensive with a significant risk of morbidity/mortality.

ECG: Characteristic S wave in lead I, Q wave in lead III, and T wave inversion in lead III (called the S1Q3T3). May otherwise show arrhythmia or sinus tachycardia, T-wave inversion in V1–V3, right axis deviation, or right bundle-branch block.

Treatment

- Stabilize the patient as needed. Consider intubation if needed. Significant arrhythmias may be seen, thus cardiac monitoring is warranted.

- Give oxygen.

- Anticoagulate initially with heparin or low molecular weight heparin [enoxaparin (Lovenox)], then with warfarin (Coumadin). Overlap these two for a couple of days to avoid transient hypercoagulable state. Warfarin dose should be loaded, and then the dosage adjusted to achieve INR between 2 and 3. Continue warfarin for at least 6 months in the uncomplicated patient and indefinitely in the patient with ongoing risk factors or a history of multiple events.

- If patient is not a candidate for anticoagulation, consider placement of inferior vena cava (IVC) filters.

- If patient has significant hypotension, saddle embolus is suspected, and situation is dire, consider embolectomy or tissue plasminogen activator (tPA). There are many contraindications to tPA and embolectomy, which have a mortality of 30%, so only attempt in case of extreme situation.

- Place patient on "warfarin diet" if on warfarin.

- Control risk factors.

- See section on Venous Thrombosis in Chapter 11.

Pulmonary Hypertension

Primary and secondary disease types exist. Primary is generally idiopathic although it does have several subtypes; secondary is due to a myriad of different disorders too numerous to mention here. Generally, exclude secondary pulmonary hypertension (PH) before diagnosing and treating primary.

Symptoms

Fatigue, dyspnea, syncope, chest pain, palpitations, hoarseness, hemoptysis, cough, or lower extremity edema. Look for symptoms of right heart failure. History may include causative drugs (such as Fen-phen).

Diagnosis

Physical exam: Loud P2, right ventricular lift, tachypnea, murmur of tricuspid insufficiency or pulmonic insufficiency, increased jugular venous pulsations, hepatomegaly, pulmonic ejection click, right ventricular S3 or S4, or lower extremity edema.

Labs: Test for suspicious causes of secondary pulmonary hypertension (autoantibody tests, HIV, hepatic function tests). Antinuclear antibody (ANA) is positive in up one-third cases of of primary pulmonary hypertension (PPH) patients. ABG may show arterial hypoxemia, reduced diffusion capacity (DLCO), and hypocapnia.

Imaging: CXR shows enlarged central pulmonary arteries, right ventricular enlargement, or increased interstitial markings.

Doppler echocardiography may show right ventricular enlargement and valvular abnormalities including insufficiencies, and is the most accurate noninvasive way to estimate pulmonary artery pressure.

Consider V/Q scan to evaluate for causative emboli. Pulmonary angiography if V/Q scan is reasonably positive, but caution advised because of the possibility of hemodynamic collapse.

ECG: Right ventricular hypertrophy and right axis deviation, right bundle-branch block, or P wave in lead II.

Pulmonary exercise testing.

Cardiac catheterization: Catheter placement is to measure pulmonary artery pressure; hemodynamics is the gold standard and is used if Doppler echocardiography is inadequate.

Treatment

- Oxygen therapy is the only proven strategy to improve mortality.
- All types of PH should be given; other therapies for control of disease and symptoms. This includes diuretics, anticoagulation with warfarin, and exercise. Digoxin is still controversial and unproven.
- Otherwise guidelines depend on the subtype of disease. These may include vasodilators, calcium channel blockers, prostanoids, endothelin receptor antagonists, and phosphodiesterase (PDE) inhibitors (Sildenafil).
- Surgical candidates may benefit from lung transplant.

Spontaneous Pneumothorax

Symptoms

Sudden onset of pleuritic chest pain, shortness of breath, air hunger, and tachypnea. History often reveals underlying lung disease such as COPD (bullous emphysema) or CF. Rarely in airplane passengers and divers. The classic example, however, is of a young, healthy male.

Diagnosis

Physical exam: Tracheal deviation, distended neck veins, decreased/absent breath sounds over one lung field, hyperresonance/tympany to percussion, hypotension, decreased tactile fremitus, and shallow/fast breathing.
Labs: Pulse oximetry and ABG. Look for hypoxia and hypercapnia.
Imaging: CXR will reveal retracted lung with identifiable border, lung markings that do not extend to periphery, hyperlucent lung field, depressed diaphragm, and deviated trachea and shifted mediastinum (away from the affected side if tension present). Ultrasound or CT rarely used in significant trauma victims or small pneumothoraces.

Treatment

- Give oxygen.
- If you suspect tension pneumothorax by symptoms and exam, do not wait for chest x-ray. Immediately treat.
- Needle decompression by inserting large-gauge needle through inferior second intercostal space at the midclavicular line. Listen for rush of air. Place a three-way stopcock valve on it and close the valve after decompression.
- Give heavy analgesia and narcotic pain medications and insert 16–22 French **chest tube** in fourth, fifth, or sixth intercostal spaces at midaxillary line. Confirm the placement with CXR and place tube to underwater seal. Keep seal in place 24 h or until bubbles cease.
- Consider pleurodesis with talc or other agent if recurrent episodes.
- Surgery for recurrence or refractory event with thoracoscopy or VATS.

Pertussis

Symptoms

Characteristic **whooping** or "staccato" cough; cough is paroxysmal, mild fever, sore throat, rhinorrhea, anorexia, postcough inspiratory gasp, or postcough emesis.

Diagnosis

Labs: CBC for leukocytosis with marked lymphocytosis; pertussis culture on special medium or PCR is rarely used, but both are needed for definitive diagnosis. DFA (direct antigen testing) is a rapid test, although it has relatively low sensitivity/specificity.

Imaging: CXR is nonspecific and shows perihilar infiltrates, interstitial edema, or atelectasis.

Treatment

- Immunize.

- Antibiotics including macrolides. Erythromycin and azithromycin (Zithromax) are first line for children and adults. Give prophylactic doses of these antibiotics to household contacts.

- Isolate patient until ≥5 days after antibiotics.

- Hospitalize very young children/infants if necessary.

- Cough suppressant and symptomatic relief is warranted. Cough likely to persist after cure of disease.

Wegener's Granulomatosis

A multisystem autoimmune disease that classically affects the triad of **upper airway, lung**, and **kidneys.**

Symptoms

Fever, cough, arthralgias, nasal congestion, chest congestion, hemoptysis, weight loss, skin rash, epistaxis, symptoms of renal failure.

Diagnosis

Physical exam: Rhonchi, egophony, tachypnea, and cough.
Labs: CBC shows leukocytosis, anemia, and thrombocytosis. ESR is markedly elevated. Comprehensive metabolic panel (CMP) may show renal failure or renal insufficiency. Rheumatoid factor increased in 50% of cases. Urinalysis may show hematuria, cellular casts, or protein. Classic lab is **C-ANCA** (cytoplasmic antineutrophilic cytoplasmic antibody), which shows excellent specificity for this disease.
Imaging: CXR may show localized infiltrates or discrete nodular densities consistent with central necrosis and cavitation. CT chest or sinuses shows indicative findings in these areas.
Biopsy of affected kidney, lung, or mucous membrane of upper airways may show the most definitive evidence of disease.

Treatment

- Consider admission even for mild disease.

- Initially, cyclophosphamide–corticosteroid combinations should be used to induce remission. Corticosteroids should then be tapered off at 2–4 weeks. Methotrexate in mild cases or in conjunction with cyclophosphamide or corticosteroids may be used. Cyclophosphamide (Cytoxan) is most successful, but also most toxic of therapies. Monitor these patients with q. week CBCs for leukopenia and bone marrow suppression.

- Recommend high fluid intake while on cyclophosphamide.

Answers

12.1 C. This patient has several features of croup including stridor, "barking" cough, poor PO intake, and subglottic narrowing (steeplechase sign) on posteroanterior (PA) neck x-ray. Treatment for moderate-to-severe croup includes humidified oxygen, nebulized epinephrine, and systemic steroids. Inpatient monitoring may be warranted, but remains a clinical decision.

12.2 C. The frequency of symptoms occurring every day and at night combined with recent pulmonary function tests (PFTs) indicating FEV1 between 60% and 80% of predicted value places this patient in the moderate persistent classification of asthma.

12.3 D. Addition of montelukast (Singulair) and Advair is an example of appropriate therapy for moderate persistent asthma. The National Asthma Prevention and Control Program guidelines recommend a stepwise approach by starting with the most aggressive step and then "stepping down" to achieve control. The other answers given indicate either inadequate (A, C) or too aggressive (B, E) therapy.

12.4 B. This patient is exhibiting the classic commonly associated hypercalcemia seen in adenocarcinoma of the lung. Hypercalcemia commonly shows the clinical features of "bones, stones, groans, and psychotic overtones." Pertinent features in this patient is fracture and history of nephrolithiasis.

12.5 A. This patient presents with several features indicative of cystic fibrosis. She likely has meconium ileus and pneumonia due to viscous secretions. Sweat chloride skin testing is the standard diagnostic test used. The other answers, although useful, would not be the next step in management.

12.6 B. This patient likely has a pulmonary embolism. Her history of long plane flight combined with oral contraceptive use gives two elements of Virchow's triad, hypercoagulable state, and stasis. Spiral CT is commonly used for the evaluation of PE as is V/Q scan. Answer E may be used to evaluate for DVT, but would not reveal the answer to her chest symptoms.

Cancer of the Esophagus	298
Esophageal Varices	298
Dysphagia	299
Malignant Neoplasm of the Stomach	300
Peptic Ulcer Disease	300
Gastritis	301
Acute Pancreatitis	302
Malignant Neoplasm of the Pancreas	304
Gallstones	305
Primary Sclerosing Cholangitis	307
Malignant Neoplasm of the Liver	307
Benign Neoplasm of the Small Intestine	308
Appendicitis	309
Intestinal Obstruction	310
Diverticular Disease	311
Inflammatory Bowel Disease	312
Irritable Bowel Syndrome	314
Peritonitis	315
Gastrointestinal Bleeding	316
Hernia	317
Colorectal Cancer	319
Perirectal and Perianal Abscess	320
Hemorrhoids	321

Cancer of the Esophagus

Symptoms

Generally presents later in the course of disease with progressive dysphagia especially to solids, weight loss, regurgitation, aspiration, hiccups, cough, hoarseness, or anemia. Histologic type of **adenocarcinoma** is associated with a history of **Barrett's esophagus**. Risk factors include longstanding gastroesophageal reflux disease (GERD), smoking, EtOH use, achalasia, male sex, history of head/neck cancer, and age >50 years.

Diagnosis

Physical exam: Cachexia, cervical lymphadenopathy.
Labs: CBC for anemia; Chem-7 for electrolyte abnormalities. Once confirmed, evaluate the hepatic function for possible metastasis.
Esophagoscopy with biopsy or brushing is the gold standard and determines the histologic type.
Imaging: Barium swallow for stenosing lesion. CT scan for local disease and visualization. Endoscopic ultrasound is useful in determining local spread.

Treatment

- Therapy is often palliative due to advanced disease at the time of diagnosis.

- Surgery is the mainstay. Radiation may be adjunctive. Chemotherapy, stricture dilation, photocoagulation, and endoluminal stent placement are generally palliative.

- Control risk factors and maintain surveillance of those at high risk, especially with Barrett's esophagus.

Esophageal Varices

Symptoms

Painless upper GI tract bleeding may present with hematemesis, weakness, pallor, or melena. Symptoms of liver cirrhosis are commonly comorbid and may include ascites, large, hard liver, and uncommonly noticeable splenomegaly. History is commonly positive for chronic excessive EtOH consumption.

Diagnosis

Physical exam: Signs of liver sclerosis may include ascites, multiple spider angiomatas, caput medusae, jaundice, hepatomegaly, and splenomegaly.
Labs: CBC for anemia. Stool may show occult blood (beware of false negatives), PT/aPTT/INR for bleeding dyscrasia, hepatic function panel for liver damage.
Imaging: First line is esophagoscopy, which may demonstrate large, tortuous, bleeding varices often in the lower third of esophagus. May treat at the

same time if actively bleeding. Doppler sonography may demonstrate patency of large vessels. Other imaging studies include MRI, endoscopic ultrasound, or venous phase angiography.

Treatment

- Stabilize the patient if needed. Consider transfusion.
- For acute bleeding, give systemic **octreotide (Sandostatin)**.
- Endoscopy may be used to inject octreotide or vasopressin to control acute bleeding. If these fail, proceed to endoscopic **sclerotherapy** or **ligation**. Lastly, consider transjugular intrahepatic portacaval shunt (**TIPS**).
- If no acute bleeding, place patient on β-blockers, specifically propranolol (Inderal). If bleeding recurs, add isosorbide mononitrate.
- Monitor with repeat blood work and repeat endoscopies to ensure stability.
- Surgery includes TIPS, portacaval shunt placement, esophageal transection, or liver transplantation.

Dysphagia

Divided into several types including oropharyngeal or esophageal. Specific etiologies differ by adult or pediatric.

Symptoms

Take age into account. Symptoms may include choking, coughing with swallowing, weak voice, weight loss, pressure sensation in mid-chest, heartburn, or longer eating time. Obtain history of whether the symptoms worsen with solids or liquids, smoking, EtOH use, or long standing GERD.

Diagnosis

Physical exam: Evaluate for external source such as thyroid tumor. Cachexia is seen in advanced cases. In infants or newborns, attempt to pass a nasogastric (NG) tube to stomach and through the nose to evaluate for esophageal and choanal atresias.

Imaging: Barium swallow is often the first-line test. May also use esophagram, cine-esophagram, or modified cine-esophagram. CT scan helpful if tumor is suspected. Targeted testing includes esophageal manometry or 24-h pH testing. Endoscopy is often needed.

Treatment

- For structural problems, surgery is the mainstay and is effective. Tumors may be excised and radiation may help (see above).
- Neuromuscular causes (achalasia, multiple sclerosis, myasthenia gravis, etc.) may respond to underlying treatment of condition.

- Complications caused by GERD may respond to acid reducers or fundoplication surgery.
- Referral to gastroenterologist is warranted.

Malignant Neoplasm of the Stomach

Symptoms

Often asymptomatic although may present as decreased appetite, early satiety, and weight loss. Risk factors include chronic gastritis, *Helicobacter pylori* infection, and diet high in nitrates (smoked fish) and salts.

Diagnosis

Physical exam: Classically, Virchow's node (palpable supraclavicular lymphadenopathy) is present.

Labs: CBC may show anemia due to ulcerated tumor bleeding. Consider hepatic function panel and alkaline phosphatase for possible metastasis.

Imaging: Barium swallow and esophagogastroduodenoscopy (EGD) with biopsy are indicated. Evaluate other areas of the body for metastasis (often seen in the ovaries and called a Krukenberg tumor) with CT, which also provides information on staging. Consider endoscopic ultrasound if available.

Treatment

Surgery is the mainstay and may involve partial resection of the stomach. Postoperative adjuvant chemotherapy can be added. Since the disease is often advanced at presentation, prognosis is commonly poor.

Peptic Ulcer Disease

Symptoms

Gnawing, burning, epigastric pain. Belching, bloating, abdominal distention, or food intolerance may accompany. May present with nonspecific symptoms or be asymptomatic until bleeding occurs causing symptoms of anemia.

Gastric ulcer pain is classically worsened by meals.

Duodenal ulcer pain is relieved by meals with exacerbation hours later.

History may reveal nonsteroidal antiinflammatory drug (NSAID) use, smoking, *H. pylori* infection, family history of ulcers, or rarely Zollinger–Ellison (ZE) syndrome.

Diagnosis

Labs: *H. pylori* testing is essential. This can be done by urea breath test, serum antibody, stool antigen, or biopsy during endoscopy. CBC for hematocrit. Serum gastrin levels along with further workup indicated if ZE suspected.

Imaging: Endoscopy with biopsy is the gold standard. Barium meal may be an alternative and is less invasive. If rupture is suspected, obtain upright plain x-ray and evaluate for air under the diaphragm.

Treatment

- Stop NSAID use.

- Control acid environment with antacids, sucralfate, H_2 blockers [ranitidine (Zantac), famotidine (Pepcid), etc.], or proton pump inhibitors [rabeprazole (Aciphex), omeprazole (Prilosec), etc.]. Monitor for liver enzyme metabolism alteration with some H_2 blockers such as cimetidine (Tagamet). Proton pump inhibitors are generally most effective, although these must be taken every day.

- Test for and eradicate *H. pylori* with triple therapy: proton pump inhibitor + amoxicillin + clarithromycin for 14 days. Test for cure after treatment.

Gastritis

Symptoms

Nonspecific epigastric pain, burning, or discomfort, anorexia, nausea, or hiccups. History may reveal *H. pylori* diagnosis, recent viral exposure, alcohol use, or NSAID use.

Diagnosis

Physical exam: Diffuse abdominal tenderness, decreased bowel sounds, and guarding.

Labs: CBC for leukocytosis, Chem-7 for BUN and electrolyte levels, K is often low after vomiting.

Treatment

- Often supportive with antacids, H_2 blockers, and proton pump inhibitors. Misoprostol (Cytotec) may help protect gastric mucosa from damage.

- Test for and eradicate *H. pylori* infection.

Q 13.1
What factor below is a drawback to the use of the Ranson's criteria?
A. Not applicable to diabetic patients.
B. Not applicable to patients with osteoporosis and treatment with bisphosphonates.
C. Requires 24 h to apply.
D. Requires 48 h to apply.
E. Does not apply to patients with hepatic sclerosis due to alcohol exposure.

Acute Pancreatitis

Symptoms

Abdominal pain commonly in the epigastrum, right or left quadrant, which may radiate to the back or shoulder. Nausea/vomiting, anorexia, weight loss, low-grade fever, restlessness, steatorrhea, and myalgias are common. Attacks are often recurrent and related to alcohol consumption, hypertriglyceridemia, or recurrent gallstones.

Diagnosis

Several clinical prognostic scales exist for predicting mortality and severity of acute pancreatitis. The most established of these is the Ranson criteria (presented in the following text), although research has not supported its being the best scale for positive and negative predictive value. The Acute Physiology and Chronic Health Evaluation II (APACHE II) score has been shown to be more accurate in severity prediction and has the advantage of being useful before the 48-hour evaluation point that the other scales require. However, APACHE II remains cumbersome (requires addition of multiple factors and adding of point scores), which limits its practical use. Other scales include the Imrie (Glasgow) and CT severity index.

A common clinical tool is the Ranson's criteria, which predicts severity of the disease (see Table 13.1).

Physical exam: Tenderness to epigastric region, diaphoresis, mildly increased temperature, dry mucous membranes, and possibly jaundice (depending on cause). Grey Turner sign (flank discoloration) or Cullen's sign (umbilical discoloration) may herald extreme disease or rupture.

Labs: See Table 13.1. Other classic labs include lipase (most specific) and amylase (less specific), elevated bilirubin, and elevated alkaline phosphatase.

Imaging: Plain abdominal x-ray may show signs of ileus (air-fluid levels, etc.) and "sentinel loop" in the loop of bowel adjacent to inflamed pancreas.

CT scan with contrast is the test of choice. Look for pseudocyst or abscess formation. Ultrasound or MRI may also be used. Endoscopic retrograde cholangiopancreatography (ERCP) may evaluate for otherwise unseen blockage of pancreatic or common bile duct, but is less practical unless already admitted (see Figure 13.1).

Treatment

- Give aggressive IV fluid replacement until urine output is adequate.
- Make NPO immediately. This is the treatment of choice.
- Consider NG tube if vomiting.
- Pain control with IV pain medications such as meperidine (Demerol).
- Consult surgeon if indicated for the complication of pseudocyst or abscess.

TABLE 13.1 Ranson's criteria for prognosis in pancreatitis

Presentation	
Age	>55 years
WBCs	>16,000 mm³
Blood glucose	>200 mg/dL
Lactate dehydrogenase (LDH)	>350 U/L
AST	>250 U/L
48 h	
Hematocrit	Fall by ≥10%
BUN	Increase of ≥5 mg/dL despite fluids
Serum calcium	<8 mg/dL
PO₂	<60 mm/Hg
Base deficit	>4 mEq/L
Fluid sequestration	>6000 ml

One point for each factor in table.
Score 0–2: 2% mortality; score 3–4: 15% mortality; score 5–6: 40% mortality; score 7–8: 100% mortality.

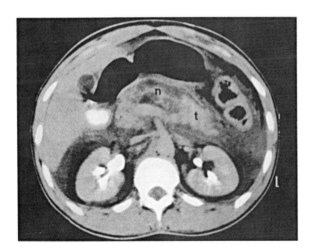

FIGURE 13.1 Acute necrotizing pancreatitis. CT shows area of necrosis (n) in the body of the pancreas that does not enhance after IV contrast material as compared with the tail (t). Also note fluid collection in the abdomen and retroperitoneum.

Copes's Early Diagnosis of the Acute Abdomen. Twentieth edition. Revised by Silen W. Copyright 2000. Oxford University Press.

- Monitor blood sugars and place on sliding scale insulin as needed.
- Maintain NPO status until pain resolves, then return to regular diet slowly.

- Prophylactic antibiotics are unproven and controversial. If started, should only be in moderate–severe disease.

- If not improving, consider CT scan and/or fine needle aspiration. Necrosis may develop.

- Chronic pancreatitis may develop, especially in those patients with recurrent acute pancreatitis. If possible, treat etiology. As exocrine and endocrine pancreatic function fail, these patients will need dietary pancreatic enzyme replacement, vitamin B_{12} replacement, and insulin therapy.

Malignant Neoplasm of the Pancreas

Symptoms

Most cancers are found at late stages and thus have advanced presentations. Pruritus, weight loss, pain, jaundice, anorexia, diabetes, referred pain to the shoulder, malnutrition, hepatomegaly, palpable mass, abdominal tenderness, or ascites. History may include occupational exposures, **smoking**, and likely race.

Diagnosis

Physical exam: Abdominal exam may reveal tenderness in epigastrium, hepatomegaly, jaundice, or mass.

Labs: CBC may show anemia. Alkaline phosphatase elevation, bilirubin level increased because of obstruction, occult blood in stool. Specific enzymes such as gastrin or insulin may be elevated. Biomarker **CA19-9** is used in pancreatic cancer, but has low sensitivity and specificity.

Imaging: Helical CT scan has high sensitivity and specificity and is currently the test of choice. Transabdominal ultrasound is also useful for screening, but not in staging. Endoscopic ultrasound is emerging as a very accurate test that shows smaller tumors. ERCP, MRI, magnetic resonance cholangiopancreatography (MRCP) also useful, and it may be possible to obtain biopsy at the time of the procedure.

Biopsy is essential whether done endoscopically or percutaneously.

Treatment

- Surgery is the only option that has been shown to decrease mortality. However, most tumors are found too late to be resectable. This may be done by the Whipple procedure (pancreaticoduodenectomy) or total pancreatectomy.

- Chemotherapy and directed radiation therapy are palliative, but may extend life. Other procedures such as celiac plexus block and biliary decompression may provide symptom relief.

Q 13.2

A 39-year-old African American female comes to the ER with complaints of fever/chills and right upper quadrant (RUQ) pain. She states these symptoms are recurrent with the association with fatty meals, although this is her most severe episode yet. Her past medical history includes recent weight loss on a proprietary diet plan, hypertriglyceridemia, and well-controlled hypertension. Her vital signs include a temperature elevated to 39.4°C (102.9°F), and physical exam reveals mild scleral icterus. What is this patient's most prominent risk factor for the most likely diagnosis?

A. Rapid weight loss.
B. Hypertriglyceridemia.
C. Antihypertensive medication.
D. Frequent fatty meal consumption.
E. Age >30 years.

Gallstones

Definitions

Cholelithiasis: Formation and presence of stones in the gallbladder.
Cholecystitis: Inflammation of the gallbladder wall, usually due to obstruction of the cystic duct by gallstones.
Choledocholithiasis: Presence or obstruction of the bile ducts by gallstones.

Symptoms

Cholelithiasis is often asymptomatic especially if stones are large and unobstructing. Choledocholithiasis often leads to cholecystitis, which presents with colicky abdominal or right upper quadrant (RUQ) pain, worsened with meals, nausea/vomiting, fever/chills, clay-colored stool, or jaundice. History may reveal 5 Fs-"Female, Fat, Forty, Fertile, and Febrile." Rapid weight loss, pregnancy, or total parenteral nutrition (TPN) use are all prominent risk factors.

- Charcot's triad—RUQ pain, jaundice, fever/chills.
- Reynold's pentad—Charcot's triad plus shock and altered mental status. Seen with suppurative **cholangitis.**

Diagnosis

Physical exam: RUQ tenderness, positive **Murphy's sign** (pain on RUQ pressure with inspiration), jaundice, and increased temperature.
Labs: CBC shows leukocytosis; comprehensive metabolic panel (CMP) shows increased bilirubin (increased direct/conjugated bili), gamma glutamyl transpeptidase (GGT), and alkaline phosphatase. Slightly elevated AST and ALT. Take blood cultures before starting antibiotics.
Imaging: Ultrasound is the classic first test for the disease. If negative but strong clinical evidence exists, obtain hepatoiminodiacetic acid (HIDA) scan. CT may also be helpful and show dilation of ducts, abscess, or pancreatitis, if present. ERCP, MRCP, or percutaneous transhepatic cholangiography (PTC) shows the status of biliary duct system and presence of stones, but is usually limited by the availability and cost (see Figures 13.2 and 13.3).

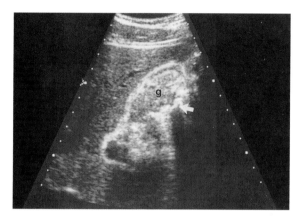

FIGURE 13.2 Ultrasound showing slightly distended gallbladder (g) with thickened wall. Variably echogenic lumen indicates the presence of debris or sludge, and presence of acoustic shadowing (arrow) is demonstrated.

Copes's Early Diagnosis of the Acute Abdomen. Twentieth edition. Revised by Silen W. Copyright 2000. Oxford University Press.

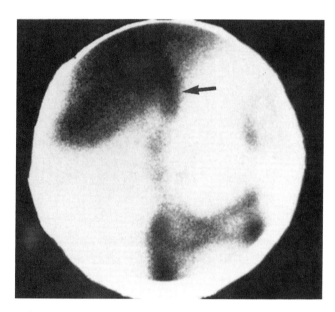

FIGURE 13.3 Normal hydroxy iminodiacetic acid (HIDA) scan virtually excluding acute cholecystitis. Note filling of the gallbladder (arrow) and excretion of the radioisotope (Technetium 99m) into the bowel.

Copes's Early Diagnosis of the Acute Abdomen. Twentieth edition. Revised by Silen W. Copyright 2000. Oxford University Press.

Treatment

- Start antibiotics, IV fluids, electrolyte repletion, and narcotic pain control.

- Antibiotics should cover gram-negative gut bacteria: piperacillin-tazobactam (Zosyn), ampicillin-sulbactam (Unasyn), or ticarcillin-clavulanate (Timentin).

- Surgery with laproscopic or open **cholecystectomy** is the most common and effective treatment. At the time of surgery, intraoperative cholangiogram should be done to evaluate for further duct stones. Surgery is often delayed for 48–72 h to wait for resolution of acute attack. In acute cholangitis (inflammation of the bile duct itself), decompressive surgery or ERCP sphincterotomy, and stent placement may be needed.

Primary Sclerosing Cholangitis

Symptoms

Often presents like RUQ pain, fever/chills, jaundice, and pruritus. History commonly reveals age <45 years, male sex, and history of inflammatory bowel disease (IBD) (especially ulcerative colitis).

Diagnosis

Physical exam: RUQ pain, positive Murphy's sign, jaundice, and increased temperature.

Labs: CBC may show leukocytosis, CMP shows elevated GGT, alkaline phosphatase, increased bilirubin (direct/conjugated). Perinuclear antineutrophil cytoplasmic antibody (p-ANCA) positive.

Liver biopsy may show characteristic "onion skin" and fibrotic appearance to tissue.

Imaging: ERCP is the test of choice and shows serial dilations/constrictions of the bile ducts "beads-on-a-string" appearance.

Treatment

- Supportive care and antibiotics for acute attacks.
- ERCP is often used for stent placement over duct constrictions, but is generally a temporary measure.
- Ursodeoxycholic acid (URSO) may reduce pruritus and have positive effects on liver tests.
- Corticosteroids, azathioprine (Imuran), penicillamine (Cuprimine), methotrexate (Trexall), and cholestyramine have all shown variable results.
- Ultimately, liver transplantation is the only cure.
- Think of **cholangiocarcinoma** that has a strong association with primary sclerosing cholangitis (PSC) and is often fatal.

Malignant Neoplasm of the Liver

Symptoms

RUQ and vague abdominal pain, weight loss, nausea/vomiting, and low-grade fever commonly in an unexplained deterioration of a stable cirrhosis patient. Paraneoplastic symptoms such as feminization, osteoarthropathy, or carcinoid syndrome may be present. History may reveal risk factors such as alcoholism, cirrhosis, hepatitis B or C, hemochromatosis, α-1-antitrypsin deficiency, NASH (nonalcoholic steatohepatitis), or exposure to vinyl chloride.

Diagnosis

Physical exam: Hepatomegaly, RUQ mass, hepatic friction rub, or bruit.

Labs: CBC may show polycythemia, CMP shows elevated calcium, low glucose, elevated AST and ALT, and other nonspecific liver function derangements. Tumor markers include **alpha-fetoprotein** (AFP >400 μg/L), des-gamma-carboxyprothrombin, GGT, and carcinoembryonic antigen (CEA).

Imaging: Ultrasound is the most widely used scan and may be used for surveillance after treatment. CT scan is important in finding extrahepatic spread. MRI shows greater detail of the tumor margins and features. Lipoidal angiography with CT is very good at delineating small tumors, and may be used for a chemotherapeutic or radioactive vehicle.

Liver biopsy with/without ultrasound or CT guidance is essential to diagnosis and may confirm histologic type.

Treatment

- Prevent disease with control of risk factors. Monitor high-risk and prior-disease patients with periodic AFP and ultrasounds.

- **Surgery** is the mainstay for primary disease. However, prognosis is still often grim due to late presentation. Liver transplant in more extensive disease can be successful.

- Palliative techniques include x-ray-guided radiofrequency ablation, alcohol injection, or chemotherapeutic embolization.

Benign Neoplasm of the Small Intestine

Several types exist including fibromas, leiomyomas, lipomas, neurofibromas, hemangiomas, or angiodysplasias.

Symptoms

Commonly asymptomatic, presentation may include vague abdominal pain, bleeding, melena, and rarely intussusception.

Diagnosis

Labs: CBC for anemia, serial stool occult testing.

Imaging: CT in large tumors.

Endoscopy with biopsy is the gold standard. Arteriography or technetium red blood scans may locate bleeding.

Treatment

- Endoscopy-assisted electrocautery, thermal obliteration, or laser phototherapy at the time of endoscopy.

- Resection is more definitive, but more radical.

Appendicitis

Symptoms

Abdominal pain classically starts in the periumbilical area, or is generalized and then localized to the right lower quadrant (RLQ). May be associated with fever, nausea/vomiting, anorexia, diaphoresis, and myalgias.

Diagnosis

Physical exam: Elevated temperature, abdominal muscle guarding, and **rebound tenderness** over McBurney's point.

- Rovsing's sign [RLQ pain on palpation of left lower quadrant (LLQ)].
- Psoas sign—pain with extension of hip.
- Obturator sign—pain with internal rotation of flexed right thigh.

Labs: CBC shows leukocytosis with left shift.

Imaging: CT scan with oral contrast is becoming the standard and may show thickened appendiceal wall, appendicolith, or surrounding fat stranding. CT is better to evaluate for abscess or other cause of pain. Ultrasound is also used although is more operator-dependent. Plain x-ray may be suggestive of appendicitis, but is not used in diagnosis.

Barium enema may show lack of filling of the appendix, but is uncommon unless another indication is present (see Figure 13.4).

Treatment

- Consult surgery for appendectomy.
- Consider giving broad-spectrum dose of fluoroquinolone and metronidazole (Flagyl) before surgery.

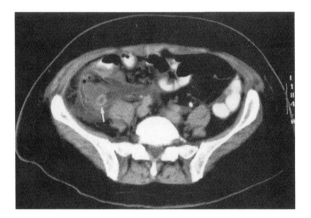

FIGURE 13.4 CT scan indicating acute appendicitis. Note thickened appendiceal wall (arrow) and surrounding "dirty fat" indicating inflammation.

Copes's Early Diagnosis of the Acute Abdomen. Twentieth edition. Revised by Silen W. Copyright 2000. Oxford University Press.

Intestinal Obstruction

Symptoms

Diffuse abdominal pain, emesis, anorexia, and obstipation. History may reveal history of no or infrequent stooling or risk factors including history of obstruction, meconium ileus, Meckel's diverticulum, volvulus, colon cancer, and recent surgery. Constipation in the elderly is a common cause.

Diagnosis

Physical exam: Distended abdomen, decreased bowel sounds or high-pitched sounds, cessation of flatus, tenderness to direct palpation. Rectal exam may reveal impaction or mass.

Labs: Screening CBC may show leukocytosis if strangulation of hernia or infectious cause is present. Hepatic function panel often shows increased bilirubin.

Imaging: Plain upright x-ray may reveal distended haustra and air-fluid levels.

Barium enema may reveal colonic obstruction or mass. Enema may be therapeutic in intussusception (see Figure 13.5).

Treatment

- Correct electrolytes.
- Consider NG tube if emesis is the significant problem.
- Attempt correction of stool impaction if this is clinically appropriate.
- Surgical consultation if other causes thought likely; these may include adhesions, volvulus, incarcerated hernia, foreign body, obstructing malignancy (amongst others).

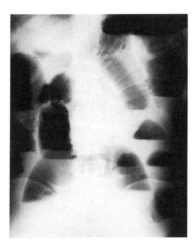

FIGURE 13.5 Erect film of bowel obstruction demonstrating multiple "step ladder–like" air-fluid levels accompanied by distended bowel.

Copes's Early Diagnosis of the Acute Abdomen. Twentieth edition. Revised by Silen W. Copyright 2000. Oxford University Press.

Diverticular Disease

Diverticulosis: Commonly right-sided intestinal wall herniation that tends to bleed because of vascular supply to location.

Diverticulitis: Inflammation and infection of commonly left-sided colonic wall herniation that tends to cause acute illness.

Symptoms

Diverticulosis often causes painless bleeding. Diverticulitis may cause abdominal pain, cramping, diarrhea, anorexia, and fever/chills. Complications include perforation, abscess, and fistula formation with symptoms including acute peritoneal signs and mass, or pneumaturia and fecaluria.

Diagnosis

Physical exam: Diverticulosis may show blood on occult testing. Diverticulitis may show LLQ tenderness, high-pitched or absent bowel sounds, or abdominal distention.

Labs: CBC shows leukocytosis in diverticulitis and low hemoglobin/hematocrit in chronic bleeding diverticulosis. Obtain blood and urine cultures.

Imaging: Diverticulosis may be seen with barium enema or colonoscopy. Bleeding sites may be evaluated with radiolabeled RBC scan or angiography. Diverticulitis is commonly demonstrated with **CT scan** with and without rectal contrast. CT is also useful in the diagnosis of abscess, perforation, or fistula formation, if present. Obtain upright chest x-ray (CXR) and abdominal x-ray to evaluate for free air in the abdomen if clinically indicated. Barium enema is less helpful in inflammatory state since uptake into diverticula is not reliable.

Colonoscopy for diverticulosis is the procedure of choice as it allows for direct therapy of bleeding at the same time.

Treatment

- High-fiber diet for prevention. Some controversy exists on trigger foods such as popcorn, strawberries, raspberries, and poppy seed muffins.

- Diverticulosis bleeding stops without therapy in a very high proportion of patients. If needed, local injection of epinephrine or electrocautery may be used. If bleeding is perfuse, consider surgical consultation.

- Diverticulitis may be treated outpatient unless complications exist. Antibiotics include ciprofloxacin (Cipro) + metronidazole (Flagyl) for 7 days.

- If abscess, perforation, or fistula is found, immediate surgical consultation is indicated.

- Recurrent attacks of uncomplicated diverticulitis are an indication for segmental bowel resection.

Inflammatory Bowel Disease

See Table 13.2 and Figures 13.6 and 13.7.

TABLE 13.2 Crohn's disease vs ulcerative colitis

Characteristic	Crohn's disease	Ulcerative colitis
Typical population	Those of Caucasian or Jewish descent; bimodal age distribution in 20s then in 50–70s	Often young women in mid-30s of Caucasian or Jewish descent
Location	Classically occurs in terminal ileum, but may arise **anywhere from the mouth to the anus**	Typically in distal colon and rectum
Clinical features	Nonbloody diarrhea, abdominal (RLQ) pain, weight loss, anorexia, low-grade fever	**Bloody diarrhea**, cramping, abdominal pain, weight loss, fatigue, bowel urgency, low-grade fever, tachycardia, and heme-positive stools
Associations	Pyoderma gangrenosum, erythema nodosum, fatty liver, iritis, episcleritis, gallstones, kidney stones, and arthritis	Primary sclerosing cholangitis, pyoderma gangrenosum, erythema nodosum, arthritis, ankylosing spondylitis, and iritis; beware of toxic megacolon (obtain x-rays)
Pathology	Transmural involvement commonly with "skip lesions"; Cobblestoning may be seen on colonoscopy; fissures or **fistula** formation common	Mucosal or submucosal involvement only; ulcers and erosions possible; barium enema may show lead-pipe colon with loss of haustra; biopsy reveals **crypt abscesses**
Labs	CBC shows normocytic-macrocytic anemia, increased ESR, normal LFTs	CBC shows normocytic anemia, increased ESR, low albumin, positive p-ANCA
Treatment	Mild cases: 5-aminosalicylic acid (5-ASA) compounds such as mesalamine (Pentasa, Asacol) and sulfasalazine (Azulfidine) +/− oral steroids	
	Moderate cases: 5-ASA compounds + oral steroids and addition of azathioprine (Azasan), 6-mercaptopurine (Purinethol), or methotrexate; consider addition of steroid enemas	
	Severe cases: Admission to hospital, NPO status, IV steroids, steroid enemas, metronidazole (Flagyl) and consider TPN; consider anti-TNF antibody infliximab (Remicade)	
	Surgery: May be helpful in ulcerative colitis, but often ineffective and possibly harmful in Crohn's disease	

ESR, erythrocyte sedimentation rate; LFTs, liver function tests; p-ANCA, perinuclear antineutrophil cytoplasmic antibody; RLQ, right lower quadrant; TNF, tumor necrosis factor; TPN, total parenteral nutrition.

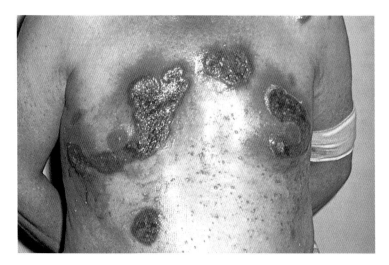

FIGURE 13.6 Pyoderma gangrenosum associated with inflammatory bowel disease.

Clinical Dermatology. Fifth edition. MacKie RM. Copyright 2003. Oxford University Press.

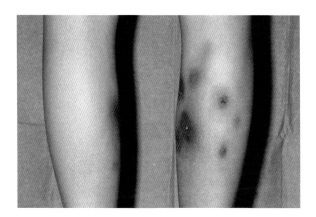

FIGURE 13.7 Erythema nodosum associated with inflammatory bowel disease.

Oxford Handbook of Clinical Medicine. Sixth edition, Longmore M, et al. Copyright 2004. Oxford University Press.

Q 13.3

A 37-year-old Caucasian female comes to your primary care office with complaints of abdominal cramps and diarrhea for the past 6 months. She states that the pain leads to frequent stooling although the discomfort is somewhat relieved by defecation. Her vital signs are normal as is her abdominal exam. Labs including thyroid-stimulating hormone (TSH), basic metabolic panel (BMP), CBC, and stool studies are normal. Plain abdominal x-ray is unremarkable. What is the most appropriate next step in management?

A. Tegaserod (Zelnorm).
B. Loperamide (Imodium) and increased dietary fiber.
C. Risperidone (Risperdal).
D. Clonazepam (Klonopin).
E. Surgical consultation.

Irritable Bowel Syndrome

Symptoms

Several subtypes include irritable bowel syndrome (IBS) with diarrhea, IBS with constipation, mixed IBS, and untypable IBS. Abdominal pain and change in bowel habits are prominent features. History often reveals coexisting anxiety or psychologic disorder, history of childhood sexual abuse, or prior autonomic nervous system abnormality.

"Red Flag" symptoms that should prompt further urgent investigation

Age of onset >50 years

Fever

Nocturnal symptoms

Blood in stools

Anemia

Weight loss >10% body weight

Profuse or large volume of diarrhea

Family history of inflammatory bowel disease or cancer

Fever

Organomegaly

Jaundice

Peritoneal signs or focal abdominal tenderness

Diagnosis

The most common criteria for clinical assessment include the **Manning criteria:**

- Pain relieved by defecation.
- More frequent stools at the onset of pain.
- Looser stools at the onset of pain.
- Visible abdominal distention.
- Passage of mucous.
- Sensation of incomplete evacuation.

Symptoms should be present for atleast 3 months before IBS is diagnosed.

Labs: Evaluate for other causes of symptoms as appropriate with stool studies (ova/parasites, fecal leukocytes, culture, etc.), serum markers for IBD, thyroid-stimulating hormone (TSH), and other tests. In IBS, these studies are generally negative.

Imaging: Evaluate for other causes and obtain plain radiograph or CT as appropriate.

Colonoscopy is often negative, but may be appropriate to eliminate other causes of the disease.

Treatment

- Detailed diet history to eliminate or reduce modifiable contributors such as high-fat diet.

- Strong physician–patient relationship is essential.

- Trial of increasing fiber in diet and increased daily exercise is reasonable. Add bulk-forming agents such as psyllium (Metamucil) or fiber supplements.

- Antispasmodics may be helpful, including dicyclomine (Bentyl), hyoscyamine (Levbid), or chlordiazepoxide-clidinium (Librax).

- Diarrheal predominant type may be treated with loperamide (Imodium) or diphenoxylate-atropine (Lomotil) after each loose stool.

- Antibiotics, rifaximin (Xifaxan) may be helpful in the diarrheal type but research is not totally conclusive.

- Serotonin receptor antagonists including alosetron (Lotronex) and tegaserod (Zelnorm) have both been shown to be somewhat effective in IBS but currently have restricted prescribing status in the United States. These should only be used in severe refractory cases because of possible side effects.

- Simethicone (Mylicon) may be helpful for bloating, and *Lactobacillus* supplements have shown subjective success.

- Tricyclic antidepressants (TCAs) such as amitriptyline (Elavil) have shown good response. Selective serotonin reuptake inhibitors (SSRIs) are still being investigated for this indication.

- Alternative therapies such as biofeedback, bowel training, herbal medications, and hypnosis have been used, although evidence showing benefit is lacking.

Peritonitis

Symptoms

Acute abdominal pain (made worse with movement), fever/chills, nausea/vomiting, constipation, and abdominal distention. History may reveal ascites from cirrhotic liver disease, penetrating injury, perforated bowel, or inflammatory intraabdominal organ disorder.

Diagnosis

Physical exam: Tenderness to palpation/percussion of all four quadrants of the abdomen (may be rebound). Tachycardia, tachypnea, and increased temperature.

Labs: CBC for leukocytosis, increased erythrocyte sedimentation rate/C-reactive protein (ESR/CRP). Obtain blood cultures. Peritoneal fluid culture is the gold standard.

Imaging: Upright CXR and abdominal x-ray are indicated for free air below the diaphragm. **CT scan** of the abdomen may show perforation site or abscess. Ultrasound may demonstrate ascites or mass.

Treatment

- IV fluids as indicated.

- Control pain with IV opioids.

- Empiric antibiotics should be started before culture results known. Ampicillin/sulbactam (Unasyn), piperacillin/tazobactam (Zosyn), or ticarcillin/clavulanate (Timentin) are good choices. Narrow spectrum according to the peritoneal culture results.

- In patients with known chronic ascites prevention of spontaneous bacterial peritonitis (SBP) with SMX-TMP DS (Bactrim, Septra) or ciprofloxacin significantly reduces episodes of disease.

Gastrointestinal Bleeding

Upper GI bleeding: Proximal to the ligament of Treitz.
Lower GI bleeding: Distal to the ligament of Treitz.

Symptoms

Regardless of the location of bleeding, patient may suffer from lightheadedness, vertigo, fatigue, orthostatic hypotension, noticeable blood loss in stools, pica, melena, or weight loss. If upper GI origin, patient is more likely to notice hematemesis, history of peptic ulcer disease (PUD), recent vomiting, or risk factors for varices. Lower GI bleeding may present with bright red blood per rectum, history of diverticulosis, hematochezia, or diarrhea. Look for historical NSAID use, EtOH use, smoking, sick contacts, or anticoagulant use.

Diagnosis

Physical exam: Pallor, tachycardia, tachypnea, or hypotension, if severe. Rectal exam and possible anoscopy are indicated to check for rectal/anal source.
Labs: CBC may show anemia, leukocytosis if infectious, thrombocytopenia. Check coagulation studies (PT/PTT/INR), and LFTs.

NG tube placement may reveal flecks of coagulated blood indicating upper GI origin.

Endoscopy, initially EGD, is the most common way to find bleeding. See individual sections for varices, Mallory–Weiss tears, and other conditions.

Radiolabeled red blood cells (99Tc-tagged RBC) scan may be used if colonoscopy is not useful. Angiography or exploratory laparoscopy are options, but only if the bleeding source is not found and brisk.

Treatment

- Apply ABCs as necessary.
- Consult surgeon as indicated.
- Vast majority of nonbrisk GI bleeding ceases without treatment. Other therapy depends on diagnosis, but may include octreotide (Sandostatin), local endoscopic injection therapy, TIPS, band ligation, β-blockers, or embolization. See individual sections for treatment modalities of different etiologies.

Hernia

Definitions

See Table 13.3.

Symptoms

Depending on the location and degree of herniation, often a bulge is felt, pain, pain on lifting, or extreme pain at bulge site or groin indicating strangulation. Males may feel fullness of scrotum or increase in scrotal size.

Diagnosis

Physical exam: The most reliable means of diagnosing a hernia is physical exam, which may reveal palpable mass, spontaneous reduction, palpable fascial defect, fullness of scrotum, or, in the case of strangulation, extreme pain on palpation with surrounding erythema and swelling.

Imaging: CT may be useful, but is often not needed (see Figure 13.8).

TABLE 13.3 Types of hernias

Hernia	Protrusion of visceral contents through fascial defect in containing wall. Often in abdomen and commonly inguinal, umbilical, ventral, femoral, or incisional
Reducible hernia	Herniation most often of visceral contents, which is either manually or spontaneously reduced
Incarcerated hernia	Herniation that is not reducible externally, but blood supply is preserved
Strangulated hernia	Herniation in which blood supply is acutely compromised causing eminent ischemia of the tissues, a surgical emergency
Indirect inguinal hernia	Herniation through the internal inguinal ring, lateral to the inferior epigastric artery
Direct inguinal hernia	Herniation through the wall of the inguinal canal, specifically through structures forming Hesselbach's triangle

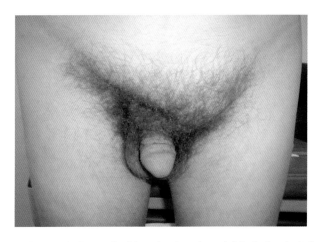

FIGURE 13.8 Inguinal hernia showing visible bulge in left inguinal region.

Courtesy: Charlie Goldberg, MD. University of California, San Diego School of Medicine, San Diego VA Medical Center.

Treatment

- Surgery is the mainstay and only effective treatment. Hernioplasty with mesh placement is the most common with simple closure of defect less common.

- If asymptomatic without danger of strangulation, may elect to not treat.

- Prevent hernias by avoiding heavy-lifting or with proper-lifting technique (avoid high intraperitoneal pressures).

Q 13.4

A 52-year-old male truck driver comes to your office for a routine health maintenance exam. His past medical history is positive for Crohn's disease, now well controlled; hyperlipidemia; hypertension (HTN); smoking; and obesity. He mainly eats on the road and infrequently sees a physician. He states his father died of colon cancer at age 47 and mother died of an MI at age 67. His two children are healthy. His vital signs are normal, and physical exam is remarkable only for moderate obesity. What is the best colon cancer screening method given below?

A. Colonoscopy every 1–3 years.
B. Colonoscopy every 5 years.
C. Colonoscopy every 10 years.
D. Flexible sigmoidoscopy every 5 years.
E. Fecal occult blood test (FOBT) annually.

Colorectal Cancer

Symptoms

Vague abdominal pain, abdominal enlargement, change in bowel habits/appearance, hematochezia/melena, weakness, anemia, or weight loss. History may indicate risk factors including:

- Colorectal cancer in first-degree relative aged <60 years or two first-degree relatives of any age.
- Family or personal history of familial adenomatous polyposis (FAP) or other genetic colon cancer disease.
- Adenomatous polyps on prior evaluations.
- Inflammatory bowel disease.
- Cancer of other areas.
- Age >50 years.

Diagnosis

The American Cancer Society recommends screening average-risk patients for colorectal cancer beginning at the age of 50 years by one of the following:

- Fecal occult blood testing (FOBT, performed on two to three consecutive stools at home. In office, single FOBT inadequate) annually.
- Flexible sigmoidoscopy every 5 years.
- Annual FOBT plus flexible sigmoidoscopy every 5 years.
- Double-contrast barium enema every 5 years.
- Colonoscopy every 10 years.

These recommendations are supported by the United States Preventive Services Task Force (USPSTF) and the American Academy of Family Physicians (AAFP).

Generally, increased-risk and high-risk patients should obtain colonoscopy every 1–3 years.

Labs: CBC for possible anemia. CEA provides disease surveillance after treatment but is not used for screening.

Imaging: As discussed earlier, best visualization is with endocoscopy (colonscopy, flexible sigmoidoscopy, or anoscopy). Virtual colonoscopy and "pill colonoscopy" are emerging technologies. CT scan may be used for staging or evaluating possible metastatic spread (see Figure 13.9).

The current staging is with the American Joint Committee on Cancer (AJCC) TNM staging system. This system uses characteristics of the Tumor, Nodal involvement, and Metastisis to classify the cancer. The Dukes criteria has historically been used for staging but has been modified and improved and is now no longer used.

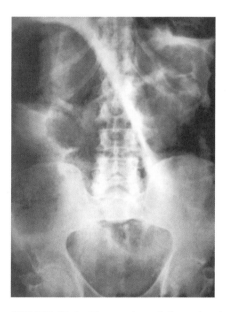

FIGURE 13.9 Obstruction of the colon by carcinoma of the sigmoid. Note massive distention of the large bowel from the cecum to the sigmoid where the obstruction was situated.

Copes's Early Diagnosis of the Acute Abdomen. Twentieth edition. Revised by Silen W. Copyright 2000. Oxford University Press.

Treatment

- Prevent with high-fiber, low-fat diet; smoking cessation; and scheduled health maintenance.
- Resection of the bowel segment and regional lymph nodes is the standard. Radiation and chemotherapy may be adjutants based on TNM stage and location (rectal and anal are more common). The classics are 5-fluorouracil (5-FU) and leucovorin.
- Refer to gastroenterologist.

Perirectal and Perianal Abscess

Symptoms

Perianal swelling, redness, tenderness, throbbing pain, pain on defecation, and possibly fever. History may reveal risk factors including IBD, injection of internal hemorrhoids, foreign objects, prolapsed hemorrhoids, and anal intercourse trauma.

Diagnosis

Physical exam: Palpable, tender, fluctuant mass of anal or rectal region.
Labs: CBC often shows leukocytosis; anemia from bleeding is uncommon.

Treatment

- Incision and drainage is the mainstay. Perianal abscesses are often treated with local anesthetic while higher abscesses require general. Iodoform packing for 24–48 h is often needed.
- Antibiotics including TMP/SMX DS (Bactrim, Septra) or ciprofloxacin/levofloxacin, *plus* metronidazole (Flagyl).
- Give stool softener for first 1–2 weeks.
- Monitor for common complication of fistula formation.

Q 13.5

A 27-year-old Caucasian female comes to your office complaining of rectal pain on defecation and feeling as if she is "sitting on a pebble." She has noticed a very tender piece of tissue protruding from her anus when cleaning herself accompanied by a scant amount of blood on the toilet paper. On anoscopy, you find an external inflamed hemorrhoid that does not appear strangulated or thrombosed, but is extremely tender. What is the best next step in management?

A. Topical antiinflammatories and sitz baths.
B. Switching to high-fiber diet.
C. Rubber band ligation.
D. Electrocaudery
E. Surgical consultation

Hemorrhoids

Symptoms

Depending on location may present with a feeling of incomplete evacuation, painless bleeding, prolapse, pruritus, palpable mass, pain associated with a thrombosed hemorrhoid, or fecal soilage. External hemorrhoids (those below the dentate line) are more sensitive and painful than internal ones. Risk factors include pregnancy, chronic constipation, liver disease, and portal hypertension.

Diagnosis

Anoscopy is the mainstay of diagnosis.

Treatment

- Prevent hemorrhoids with high-fiber diet, increased fluid intake, weight loss, and avoidance of straining.
- Topical corticosteroids, analgesics, and sitz baths for early symptom control.

- Nonoperative techniques for ablating nonthrombosed hemorrhoids include injection sclerotherapy, heat/laser coagulation, and rubber band ligation.
- Surgical excision should only be used in severe cases or thrombosis/strangulation. Effectiveness of surgery is higher than that of other techniques, but recurrence is common.

Answers

13.1 D. The Ranson's criteria is a clinical scoring system to predict mortality on the basis of the severity of pancreatitis. It, however, does require 48 h to apply.

13.2 A. This patient presents with Charcot's triad of clinical signs indicating likely cholecystitis. Risk factors include rapid weight loss, pregnancy, or recent TPN use.

13.3 B. This patient has several symptoms of diarrheal-type irritable bowel syndrome (IBS) according to the Manning criteria clinical assessment tool. For diarrheal type, loperamide (Imodium) and increased dietary fiber are the first step in treatment. Other therapies include psyllium (Metamucil), antispasmodic agents, tricyclic antidepressants (TCAs), and possibly simethicone (Mylicon). Other answers are either not suitable for diarrheal type IBS or not suitable for IBS therapy at all.

13.4 A. This patient has several risk factors including smoking, history of inflammatory bowel disease, and first-degree relative with colon cancer <60 years of age. Thus, he is at increased risk of developing colon cancer and should be screened by colonoscopy every 1–3 years.

13.5 A. For nonthrombosed, inflamed hemorrhoidal tissue, first-line treatment is topical therapy and sitz baths. High-fiber diets may prevent these, but are not effective in treatment. Other treatments listed are premature in this patient.

14 Diseases of the Kidneys and Urinary Tract

Malignant Neoplasm of the Bladder	323
Neurogenic Bladder	324
Urethritis	325
Uncomplicated Cystitis	325
Pyelonephritis	326
Enuresis	327
Malignant Neoplasm of the Kidney	327
Nephrotic Syndrome	328
Glomerulonephritis	330
Chronic Renal Failure/Insufficiency	331
Acute Renal Failure	332
Cystic Kidney Disease	334
Urinary Calculus/Renal Colic	334
Stress Incontinence in Females	335

Malignant Neoplasm of the Bladder

Transitional cell carcinomas are the vast majority of bladder cancers.

Symptoms

Often presents as asymptomatic hematuria. Urinary symptoms such as urgency, urge incontinence, frequency, nocturia, and dysuria. Abdominal pain is a late finding that may accompany local invasion and metastasis. History often reveals the patient to be a **smoker** or working in an occupation with exposure to **aniline dyes**.

Diagnosis

Labs: Urinalysis for gross and microscopic blood is the first step. Cytology should also find malignant cells in the urine. Several bladder cancer–specific biomarkers exist, but do not play a role in screening and are currently not recommended for diagnosis alone.

Imaging: Cystoscopy with biopsy is the gold standard.

Intravenous pyelogram (IVP) is useful for detecting urinary tumors outside the bladder, and should be done on anyone with suspected bladder cancer. It can show large filling defects that correlate with bladder tumors, but may miss smaller ones.

Obtain CT scan, chest x-ray, and abdominal films for staging.

Treatment

- Transurethral resection of superficial local cancers is effective. Some superficial cancers may also be amenable to instillation of mitomycin C, doxorubicin, or Bacille Calmette-Guerin (BCG).

- Deep tumors that invade into the bladder musculature may require partial or total cystectomy with diversion. Diversion will involve several options of new bladder creation often outside the body.

- Systemic chemotherapy and radiation therapy have been used in patients with deep tumor spread, although these therapies are rarely curative for metastatic disease.

Neurogenic Bladder

Symptoms

Two types:

Hypotonic (flaccid) bladder: Symptoms include painless, flaccid, distended bladder with nearly constant leaking of urine. Urinary tract infections (UTIs) are very common. History usually involves congenital or local injury to nerves supplying detrusor muscle.

Spastic (contractile) bladder: Unpredictable emptying and urge incontinence. History may include upper spinal cord damage or lesion.

Diagnosis

Labs: Check urinalysis and urine culture for UTI.

Imaging: Serial intravenous urography (IVU), ultrasound, cystography, and urethrography may be useful.

Voiding cystometrogram can check for obstruction and give some prognostic information.

Treatment

- Behavioral changes such as scheduled bathroom breaks may help in mild cases or during recovery from injury. Otherwise, it is important to distinguish between different types in order to treat.

- **For hypotonic bladder:** Indwelling or self-catheterization are treatment options. Females tend to do better with indwelling catheters than males do because of the risk of urethritis in males.

- **For spastic bladder:** Condom catheters may be used with men or external sphincterotomy in advanced cases to reduce outflow resistance.

- **Medications for either type: oxybutynin (Ditropan), darifenacin (Enablex), solifenazin (VESIcare),** and **tolterodine (Detrol)** are very effective, but are best for spastic bladder. *Watch for anticholingeric side effects in the elderly.* Several other medications including imipramine (Tofranil), hyoscyamine (Anaspaz, Cystospaz, Levbid), flavoxate (Urispas), trospium (Sanctura), and propantheline are also effective.

- α-Sympathetic blockers such as doxazosin (Cardura), prazosin (Minipress), and terazosin (Hytrin) are effective as well.

- **Surgery:** Exteriorization of the bladder or suprapubic catheterization may be needed in severe spinal cord injury or medicine refractory, extreme cases.

Urethritis

Symptoms

Dysuria is very common in both sexes. Purulent or milky, nonbloody discharge in men. Women may have dysuria, dyspareunia, vaginal discharge, or other signs of vaginitis, cervicitis, or pelvic inflammatory disease (PID). Females with uncomplicated urethritis and males should not have fever or lymphadenopathy. History may suggest other sexually transmitted diseases (STDs) or multiple sexual partners.

Diagnosis

Labs: UA and culture. Urine polymerase chain reaction (PCR) is diagnostic, but of limited availability. Culture or gram stain of discharge may reveal gonorrhea.

Urethral/cervical DNA probe for *Neisseria gonorrhoeae* and *Chlamydia* may also be useful as screening test.

Treatment

- Treat with ceftriaxone/doxycycline and azithromycin to treat both *N. gonorrhoeae* and *Chlamydia.*

- Always treat both sexual partners.

Uncomplicated Cystitis

Symptoms

Dysuria, bladder tenderness, urgency, and frequency. Fever and costovertebral angle tenderness are not part of uncomplicated cystitis.

Diagnosis

UA and urine culture—clean catch is acceptable, but catheterization is best (but impractical in many situations). Bagging in children is usually not useful because of the risk of contamination. In children, suprapubic tap may be the best option.

Urinalysis may show increased specific gravity, WBCs, bacteria, leukocyte esterase, and nitrate. Always order sensitivities with culture to guide treatment.

Treatment

- Trimethoprim/sulfamethoxazole (TMP/SMX) is still currently first line. Ciprofloxacin or gatifloxacin are also widely used. Course should be for 3 days for uncomplicated non–diabetic patients; 7–10 days for elderly, diabetic patients, or the mildly immunocompromised.

- Prophylactic treatment is sometimes given to women with recurrent and diagnosable UTIs linked to sexual intercourse before times of increased sexual activity (honeymoon).

- Asymptomatic bacteriuria in pregnancy may be treated with amoxicillin or nitrofurantoin.

Pyelonephritis

Symptoms

Fever, chills, back pain, nausea/vomiting, malaise, anorexia, headache accompanied by urinary symptoms such as frequency, urgency, incomplete voiding, and dysuria. History may reveal frequent UTIs.

Diagnosis

Physical exam: Increased temperature, costovertebral angle tenderness on percussion, and bladder pain.
Labs: CBC for leukocytosis, urinalysis may show WBCs, bacteria, casts, leukocyte esterase, or nitrates. Urine culture and sensitivities should be sent at the time of urinalysis. Send blood cultures as well.

Treatment

- Evaluate for urosepsis and make sure patient is stable.
- For severe cases, consider hospitalzation and IV antibiotics including ampicillin and gentamicin or a fluoroquinolone such as ciprofloxacin (Cipro) or levofloxacin (Levaquin).
- Mild-to-moderate cases should be placed on oral fluoroquinolones such as ciprofloxacin, moxifloxacin (Avelox), levofloxacin (Levaquin).
- Close follow-up is indicated if treated as an outpatient.
- All pregnant women with pyelonephritis should be hospitalized.

Q 14.1

The mother of a 6-year-old boy brings her son in for recurrent bedwetting. She states that he has never had a completely dry period throughout his life and that he still sleeps on a plastic mattress cover. His older and younger sisters are both sleeping dry throughout the night. The boy seems avoidant but polite. What is the first line in the treatment of this patient?

A. Desmopressin (DDAVP).
B. Imipramine (Tofranil).
C. Behavioral modification such as biofeedback and emptying bladder before bed.
D. Bedwetting alarms.
E. Reassurance that spontaneous resolution is the norm.

Enuresis

Symptoms

Loss of bladder control usually at night (nocturnal enuresis). Usually seen in children younger than 5 years, but may re-emerge in the elderly. Careful history may include behavior problems, major psychiatric trauma/disturbance, or sexual abuse. Look for symptoms of UTI.

Diagnosis

Have caregivers/patient keep a urinary diary.
Labs: UA and urine culture to evaluate for UTI.
Imaging: In children older than age 5–6 years with a history of frequent UTIs, investigate whether a structural abnormality is present. This may be done with voiding cystourethrogram (VCUG) or sonogram.

Treatment

- Reassure families of children ≤7 years of age, spontaneous resolution occurs in the vast majority of cases.

- Behavioral modification is very important in the first step. Motivational therapy, bladder training, fluid restriction before bed, late night alarms, and **enuresis alarms** are all very effective.

- Pharmocologic treatment consists of desmopressin (DDAVP) or imipramine (Tofranil) [as well as other tricyclic antidepressants (TCAs)]. DDAVP should be considered first and may also work as a short-term (e.g., summer camp) treatment if needed.

Malignant Neoplasm of the Kidney

Renal cell carcinoma is the most common primary tumor.

Symptoms

Hematuria or microhematuria is most common although advanced cases may involve flank pain, palpable mass, and fever of unknown origin.

Diagnosis

Labs: UA and renal function testing are the first labs to get. CBC may also show polycythemia due to excess erythropoietin production.

Imaging: CT scan is the best test if suspected. Ultrasound or IVP will demonstrate a mass, but suggest little about local extension. MRI shows local extension to adjacent tissue and gives further information on density, but is not the first test to order. Selective renal angiography may be done before surgery to determine local vessel involvement, but does not play a role in initial diagnosis.

Do not forget to investigate possible metastatic sites such as the lungs, liver, and brain.

Treatment

- Surgery for **nephrectomy** (with/without lymph node dissection) or partial wedge nephrectomy is the treatment of choice.

- Medications include interleukin-2 (IL-2) and other chemotherapeutic agents, but response appears erratic.

- Most tumors are fairly resistant to radiation therapy although this may be palliative in advanced cases.

Q 14.2

At what level of proteinuria is nephrotic syndrome defined?

A. >300 mg/24 h or 2+ on urine dipstick.
B. >3.0 g/24 h.
C. >3.5 g/24 h.
D. >4.0 g/24 h.
E. >5.0 g/24 h or 3+ on urine dipstick.

Nephrotic Syndrome

Symptoms

Frothy urine may be the first symptom followed by anorexia, malaise, puffy eyelids, abdominal pain, anasarca, ascites, and breathing difficulty due to pleural effusion. **Edema**, either focal or generalized, is a common physical finding.

Diagnosis

Presence of >3.5 g/24 h, albumin <3.0 g/dL, and generalized edema.

Labs: UA for the presence of protein is the first test. Urinary protein/creatinine ratio (>0.2 being concerning) should be checked. Analyze urine sediment for casts including hyaline, granular, fatty, waxy, and epithelial cells, which are typical. Test urine for lipiduria.

TABLE 14.1 Common etiologies of proteinuria

Urinary protein (g/day)	Likely source
0.15–2	Mild glomerulonephropathies, tubular proteinuria
	Overflow proteinuria
2.0–4.0	Usually glomerular
>4.0	Always glomerular

Source: Carroll MF and Temte JL. *Proteinuria in Adults: A Diagnostic Approach.* AAFP, Sep 15, 2000; vol 62; no 6.

Twenty-four hour urine protein collection is the gold standard for determining the amount of proteinuria and gives information to source of renal damage; >3.5 g/24 h is considered nephrotic range (see Table 14.1).

Check CBC for platelet levels, and coagulation profile and note clotting time may be decreased, lipids for hyperlipidemia, albumin which should be low, basic metabolic panel (BMP) for renal function (although impairment rarely seen), and sodium level for hyponatremia.

Screen for common systemic disease such as diabetes, systemic lupus erythematosus (SLE), amyloidosis, and multiple myeloma.

Treatment

- Restrict dietary protein to <1 g/kg per day with low-fat meals.
- Start an ACE inhibitor to protect the kidneys.
- Consider starting a statin for hyperlipidemia.
- **Steroids** are usually the mainstay.
- Treat hypercoagulable state with anticoagulation therapy.
- Treat edema with low-salt diet and loop diuretics such as Lasix. Add metolazone for synergism if needed.
- Diagnosis of the underlying cause and/or referral to nephrology is the best course of action.

Q 14.3

A 6-year-old Caucasian male is admitted to the pediatric ward of the hospital where you are attending. On admission, a 24-h urine collection was started and the results have just returned with a value of 3650 mg protein in the sample specimen. After conferring with your nephrology colleagues, you agree that a renal biopsy is warranted. What do you expect to find?

A. Extensive mesangial IgA and C_3 deposits on the glomerular basement membrane (GBM).
B. A "lumpy-bumpy" appearance of the GBM on immunofluorescence.
C. Linear anti-GBM antibody deposits.
D. Fusion of the epithelial cell foot processes under electron microscopy.
E. Tram-track appearance of the GBM under light microscopy.

Q 14.4

What is the preferred treatment of the most likely disease in this patient?

A. Supportive care with complete resolution expected.
B. ACE inhibitors.
C. Acetylcysteine (Mucomyst) for 2–3 weeks until proteinuria resolves.
D. High-dose steroids.
E. Steroids and cyclophosphamide combination.

Glomerulonephritis

Clinical Features

Common presentation is of "smoky-brown" urine (macroscopic hematuria), edema, oliguria, proteinuria, renal failure, and possibly hypertension. RBCs or RBC casts in the urine are a hallmark, but may not always be present (see Table 14.2).

TABLE 14.2 Common glomerulonephritis disease

Disease	Associations	Clinical features	Diagnosis	Treatment
Anti-GBM including Goodpasture's syndrome	Lung and kidney involvement; young adults	Hemoptysis, dyspnea, renal failure	Renal biopsy shows linear anti-GBM deposits; CXR shows diffuse infiltrates	Steroids, cyclophosphamide; plasma exchange therapy may be needed
Minimal change disease	Most common cause of nephrotic syndrome in **children**	Nephrotic syndrome, increased BP, renal impairment, renal NSAID damage.	Renal biopsy shows fusion of the epithelial cell foot processes on electron microscopy	**Steroids** are very effective
IgA nephropathy (Berger's disease)	**Most common cause** of GN worldwide; often young males	Gross hematuria common; attacks commonly precipitated by infection	Renal biopsy and IF shows IgA and C_3 deposits	ACE inhibitors for mild disease, cortico steroids for moderate–severe disease; 20% progress to end-stage renal disease

(continued)

TABLE 14.2 Common glomerulonephritis disease

Disease	Associations	Clinical features	Diagnosis	Treatment
Poststreptococcal glomerulonephritis	Strep throat infection often proceeds by weeks	Edema, hypertension, hematuria, oligouria, RBC casts on UA	Hematuria (casts present), proteinuria; renal biopsy shows immune deposits and "lumpy-bumpy" appearance on IF	**Supportive care**; full recovery common
Wegener's granulomatosis	Lung and kidney involvement; commonly sinus symptoms also present	Hemoptysis, dyspnea, fever, weight loss	**c-ANCA** positive	Steroids and cyclophosphamide combination; consider further immuno suppressants if needed; poor prognosis

ACE, angiotensin-converting enzyme; c-ANCA, cytoplasmic antineutrophil cytoplasmic antibody; CXR, chest x-ray; GBM, glomerular basement membrane; GN, glomerulonephritis; IF, immunofluorescence; NSAID, nonsteroidal antiinflammatory drug, UA, urinalysis.

Chronic Renal Failure/Insufficiency

Symptoms

Insufficiency is asymptomatic but it may progress to failure. Failure is also often asymptomatic but may begin with nocturia, fatigue, and decreased mental acuity with onset of uremia. If this condition progresses, the patient may experience muscular twitches, peripheral neuropathies, sensory phenomena, muscle cramps, convulsions, anorexia, stomatitis, and unpleasant taste. These symptoms progress to malnutrition and wasting, GI ulceration, bleeding, dehydration, yellow–brown skin color change, "uremic frost" (uremic crystals precipitating on skin from sweat), pruritus, osteomalacia, and further symptoms of systemic disease such as hypertensive congestive heart failure (CHF), pericarditis, and other end-organ damage.

Diagnosis

History usually reveals a cause such as hypertension or diabetes mellitus (DM). **Labs:** BMP for creatinine (often >1.5–2.0 mg/dL) and BUN. Na is often normal or only slightly abnormal. CBC will reveal normochromic/normocytic anemia and possibly thrombocytopenia. Look for increased ammonia, K, PTH, and phosphorus. Decreased vitamin D and Ca.

Arterial blood gas (ABG) will show metabolic acidosis.

Urinalysis reveals osmolarity close to that of serum (300–320 mOsm/kg) due to inability to concentrate urine. Waxy casts are common in advanced disease.

Renal biopsy is the best test for determining etiology. It may not be possible in advanced disease with small, sclerotic kidneys.

Imgaing: Ultrasound early on to evaluate the possible cause and extent of sclerosis.

Treatment

- Correct metabolic disorder, treat anemia with erythropoietin, correct vitamin deficiency, and restrict protein in the diet.

- Importantly, control glucose levels in DM patients and hypertension in hypertensive patients. These often occur together.

- **Dialysis** in advanced cases.

- Add an **ACEI** to protect kidneys in early stages. Debate exists on treatment for later stages and is contraindicated if patient has bilateral renal artery stenosis or only one kidney.

- **Surgery:** Parathyroidectomy may be indicated.

- Renal transplantation is definitive.

- Do not forget to renally dose all medications.

Q 14.5

A 44-year-old African American male presents to the ER with multiple medical problems. His past medical history is positive for alcoholism, impaired glucose tolerance, hypertension (HTN), obesity, and hyperlipidemia. His last admission was 6 months ago, and since then you notice a significant rise in his BUN and creatinine to 25 and 1.6, respectively. On exam, you note normal vital signs except for BP to 154/92. He has a 2/6 systolic murmur and 1–2+ pitting edema to dependant areas. His lungs have occasional rhonchi throughout the lung fields. The chest x-ray was reported to you as normal. What other labs should be ordered in the next step of diagnosis of his renal failure?

A. CBC for WBC count and Hct/Hb.
B. Urinalysis for protein and possible casts presence.
C. Urine sodium and urine creatinine.
D. Lactic acid level.
E. Serum osmolality.

Acute Renal Failure

See Table 14.3.

Symptoms

Rarely symptomatic, especially in the hospital. Generally, urine excretion volume is preserved, but oliguria or anuria may be seen especially with pre-renal/postrenal causes. Cola-colored urine may precede decrease in urine volume. Symptoms may progress to mental status change and metabolic derangement if extreme.

TABLE 14.3 Classification of renal failure

Etiology	Derangement
Prerenal	Most commonly dehydration; renal artery occlusion; shock
Intrinsically renal	Intrinsic renal disease or toxin. Includes NSAIDs, Wegener's, Goodpasture's, SLE, DM, polyarteritis, and ATN or glomerular injury
Postrenal	Bladder outlet obstruction such as oversized prostate, renal calculi, bladder cancer, etc.

ATN, Acute tubular necrosis; DM, diabetes mellitus; NSAID, nonsteroidal antiinflammatory drug; SLE, systemic lupus erythematosus.

Diagnosis

Order urine electrolytes and plasma electrolytes specifically sodium and creatinine. Calculate the fractional excretion of sodium (FENa).

$$FENa = \frac{UNa(PCr)}{PNa(UCr)}, U = Urine, P = Plasma.$$

<1% Prerenal, >2% intrinsically renal.

Urinalysis for proteinuria, hematuria, and osmolarity. Urinary sediment for brown granular, coarse granular, red cell, or hemoglobin casts. Cellular exam for RBCs, WBCs, epithelial cells, or eosinophils.

A 24-h urine collection for creatinine clearance and glomerular filtration rate (GFR).

Labs: Creatinine, CO_2, K, Na, Ca, ionized Ca, phosphate, BUN, uric acid, and CK. Antistreptolysin-O and complement titers, antinuclear antibody (ANA), and antinuclear cytoplasmic antibodies may be useful if the cause is not clear. BUN/creatinine ratio >15–20 supports acute renal failure (ARF).

ABG for possible modest acidosis.

Insert a Foley to evaluate for postrenal obstruction.

Ultrasound or CT of kidneys to look for possible hydronephrosis, sclerosis, nephrolithiasis, or mass.

Abdominal x-rays may be useful to find radiopaque stones.

Renal biopsy if cause is still unclear.

Treatment

- Treat the underlying cause especially if reversible.
- Start low-sodium/fat/protein diet.
- Stop all nonsteroidal antiinflammatory drugs (NSAIDs), aminoglycosides, or other offending agents. Correct metabolic and electrolyte abnormalities.
- Copious fluid replacement in severe dehydration or rhabdomyolysis may be kidney saving.
- **Dialysis with biocompatible membrane** is the definitive treatment although debate exists on when to start, how often, and for how long it should be continued.

- Consider mannitol or other diuretics for increased filtration.
- Do not forget to renally dose all medications.

Cystic Kidney Disease

Symptoms

Largely asymptomatic unless in advanced stage. When kidneys become poly-cystic or cysts become >10 cm diameter, they may contribute to lumbar back pain, abdominal pain, hematuria, recurrent UTIs, or colic due to kidney stones. In late disease, symptoms of uremia may dominate including mental status change. Rarely, symptoms of brain aneurysm may lead to findings of polycystic kidneys.

Diagnosis

Labs: Urinalysis may show mild proteinuria and hematuria. Consider urine culture for symptoms of UTI.
CBC may show elevated hematocrit.
Imaging: Intravenous pyelography findings are typical. Ultrasound and CT show a characteristic "moth-eaten" appearance of bilateral kidneys.

Obtain MRI or cerebral angiography of the brain to evaluate for berry aneurysms.

Genetic testing of family members is indicated.

Treatment

- Early detection (by age 25) is possible and may afford extra time to monitor new symptoms.
- Otherwise, treatment of hypertension and supportive care are the mainstay.
- Monitor for UTIs.
- Dialysis may be used to prolong life in later stages.
- **Surgery:** Hopeful alternative, but genetic component of disease often limits possible donors.

Urinary Calculus/Renal Colic

Symptoms

Excruciating colicky abdominal pain. Pain is described as sharp and 10/10. "Worse than having a baby." Pain may also be referred, classically to the genitals. Hematuria may be observed along with dark urine. Fever sometimes presents as UTI. Symptoms of uremia or urosepsis may be present in advanced disease.

Diagnosis

Labs: Urinalysis shows micro or gross hematuria. May be typical of UTI.
Chem-7 with calcium, ionized calcium, PTH, phosphorus, magnesium, uric acid, and creatinine.

TABLE 14.4 Treatments of urinary calculus

Treatment	Indications/associations
Extracorporeal shockwave lithotripsy (ESWL)	Stone in renal pelvis or upper 2/3rd of ureter, <2 cm, noninfected
Intracorporeal fragmentation lithotripsy (laser, electrohydraulic, pneumatic)	Used to fragment stones, which are then removed with graspers or allowed to pass
Urethroscopy with/without lithotripsy	Lower 1/3rd of ureter, normal anatomy
Percutaneous nephrolithotomy	Renal collecting system or upper 2/3rd ureter, >2 cm, ureter stricture, noncalcium stone, infection
Stenting	Upper or lower 1/3rd of ureter
Open surgery	Complex anatomy, obstruction

Imaging: The first classic test is the **KUB (kidney/ureters/bladder) plain film**. This shows most radiopaque stones. If present, intravenous pyelography is the current first-line confirmatory test. Consider spiral CT, which is becoming first line. Ultrasound may be useful, but only by experienced technicians.

If stone has passed and is captured, send it for analysis.

Treatment

- Hydration is key.
- Pain control is absolutely necessary. Use opiates including meperidine (Demerol).
- Strain urine until stone passes or 72 h after cessation of pain.
- If stone ≤5 mm, it will likely pass in <48 h.
- If stone >5 mm, see Table 14.4.

Recurrent calcium stones may respond to hydrochlorothiazide (HCTZ), uric acid stones to allopurinol (Zyloprim), and cystine stones to penicillamine (Cuprimine).

Treat underlying UTIs with TMP/SMX or levofloxacin.

Consider further metabolic and urinary workup and referral to urologist if recurrent.

Stress Incontinence in Females

Symptoms

Involuntary loss of urine, usually associated with coughing, laughing, rising from seated position, or straining. Voiding diary is useful, but generally diagnosis is made by clinical history.

Diagnosis

Physical exam: Pelvic exam may reveal rectocele, cystocele, or pelvic prolapse.

Labs: Urinalysis and urine culture for UTI.

Urodynamic testing may be useful, such as uroflowmetry, pressure flow, urethroscopy.

Cystometrogram is most useful and may show abnormal sphincter pressure or bladder dysfunction.

Treatment

- Treat underlying cause if \found.
- Avoid drugs that may aggravate symptoms such as caffeine, diuretics, anticholinergics, narcotics, calcium channel blockers, prostaglandin analogs, ACEIs, α-adrenergic blockers.
- Maintain good perineal hygiene.
- Pelvic floor (Kegel) exercises may help.
- Behavioral modifications such as biofeedback and bladder training.
- Urinary pads.
- Intermittent or indwelling catheter in extreme cases.
- Vaginal cones or pessary devices may be useful in older women. These come in multiple sizes and need individual fitting.
- Medications
  - Topical estrogen to increase urethral tone, pseudoephedrine (Sudafed) t.i.d., and imipramine (Tofranil).
  - Periurethral injection of collagen may be useful, but often requires more than one injection. Benefits are usually immediate, and this technique requires only local anesthetic.
- **Surgery:** Various bladder neck suspension and pubovaginal sling procedures exist. Refer to specialist if refractory to above treatments.

Answers

14.1 E. Since this patient is still less than 7-year-old, many sources suggest simple reassurance and monitoring of this condition for resolution. When the child is old enough (>7 years) the next most successful treatment is the use of bedwetting alarms.

14.2 C. Nephrotic range proteinuria begins at >3.5 g/day.

14.3 D. Since this is a young patient with nephrotic range proteinuria, minimal change disease (MCD) is very likely. The hallmark of MCD is the fusion of epithelial cell foot processes seen under microscopy.

14.4 D. The most effective treatment for minimal change disease remains to be high-dose steroids. Complete recovery often occurs.

14.5 C. The labs that will tell you if his renal failure is prerenal or postrenal are those used in calculating the fractional excretion of sodium (FENa). FENa $= U_{Na(PCr)}/P_{Na(UCr)}$. Generally accepted limits are: >1% prerenal, >2% intrinsically renal. Other answers may be relevant, but are not the next step.

15   Diseases of the Male Reproductive System

Breast Cancer	339
Malignant Neoplasm of the Prostate	340
Testicular Cancer	341
Prostatitis	342
Benign Prostatic Hypertrophy	342
Masses Referable to Testes	343
Testicular Torsion	344
Orchitis/Epididymitis	344
Male Infertility	345

Breast Cancer

Disease in the male comprises 1% of all breast cancers.

Symptoms

Lump often found in periareolar area. Commonly nonpainful, but may present with nipple discharge or bleeding, overlying skin changes, or pain.

Diagnosis

Imaging: Diagnostic mammogram and ultrasound. Mammogram may show calcifications such as in women.
Genetic analysis: Increased incidence of BRCA1,2.

Treatment

- Surgery including mastectomy is more common than breast-conserving therapy. Lymph node dissection is commonly done to assess involvement. Radiation and chemotherapy also play a role. Selective estrogen receptor blocker (SERB) medications, tamoxifen or raloxifene (Evista), may be used if cancer is estrogen-receptor positive.

Q 15.1

According to the United States Preventive Services Task Force (USPSTF), what is the preferred method of prostate cancer screening?

A. Prostate-specific antigen (PSA) and digital rectal exam (DRE) although no screening interval is defined.
B. PSA and DRE annually.
C. PSA and bone scan evaluation every 10 years.
D. No screening is recommended.
E. Annual PSA testing in those with previous Gleason score of >4.

Malignant Neoplasm of the Prostate

Symptoms

Commonly asymptomatic, but may present with symptoms of enlarged prostate including hesitancy, urgency, incomplete voiding, nocturia, frequency, and anuria. Ask the patient to identify lower back pain, rib pain, or other new, persistent discomfort that may potentially lead to the discovery of metastasis.

Diagnosis

Physical exam: DRE often reveals asymmetrically hard, lumpy, or firm prostate as opposed to benign prostatic hyperplasia (BPH), which is large and boggy.

Screening: Screening is a controversial subject, since early detection and current treatments have not shown to reduce morbidity or mortality. The USPSTF recommendations include the acknowledgment of PSA and DRE as being useful in detecting early prostate cancer, but they do not recommend doing such screening because of the lack of evidence of treatment benefit. The American Academy of Family Physicians (AAFP) agrees with the USPSTF. The American Cancer Society (ACS), however, states that since PSA and DRE have proven useful in cancer detection, yearly screening should start at age 50 (or age 45 in high-risk individuals). Thus, there is apparent disagreement, not in the effectiveness of detection but in the impact of the lack of benefit of treatment.

When PSA is used for screening, Table 15.1 illustrates the accepted action: PSA is also commonly used to follow prostate cancer after treatment.

When elevated PSA is found and biopsy confirms cancer, the grading is with the **Gleason score**. This scale grades the histologic appearance 1–5, the

TABLE 15.1 PSA range and interpretation

Total prostate-specific antigen (PSA) (ng/ml)	Action
<4.0	Normal, do nothing
4.0–10.0	Biopsy prostate
>10.0	Biopsy and investigate metastatic spread

lower being the most differentiated and higher the less differentiated. The score is done on the most prominent and the second most prominent appearance of abnormal cells in the biopsy. Thus, there are two scores of 1–5 added together. The total end Gleason score is then 1–10.

Imaging: After diagnosis, obtain imaging for staging and to look for metastasis. This includes radionucleotide bone scan, abdominal/pelvic CT, and intravenous pyelogram. Other less used modalities include ProstaScint scan and endorectal MRI.

Treatment

- **Transurethral radical prostatectomy (TURP)** is the most common treatment although beware the many complications including neurovascular impotence. Surgery has better long-term efficacy, but the patient's life expectancy should be taken into account.

- External beam radiation and brachytherapy (radioactive implants) are also used although are less effective than surgery for the long term. Radical prostatectomy is an alternative to TURP in select patients.

- Radiation and chemotherapy can be used for metastasis and advanced disease although overall cure rates are very low. Keep in mind the rectal consequences of radiation.

- Antiandrogen therapy is often used in advanced disease. Castration therapy may prolong survival.

Testicular Cancer

Symptoms

A mass on the testicle. Usually found by the patient, but can be found on exam. Often noticed after trauma. History of cryptorchidism that increases chances of malignancy >20 fold, which is unaffected by surgical correction.

Diagnosis

Physical exam: Hard, solid mass. Negative transillumination.
Labs: Tumor markers β-hCG and **α-fetoprotein** should be measured and may be useful in posttreatment follow-up.
Imaging: Initially ultrasound to evaluate. CT of chest, abdomen, and pelvis, and chest x-ray (CXR) are used in staging. Standard staging is with TNM system.

Treatment

Radical orchiectomy is the mainstay. Depending on the type of cancer, radiation with/without lymph node dissection is sometimes done. Chemotherapy has shown good results in some types of cancer. Prognosis is generally very good.

Q 15.2

A 21-year-old male college student comes into clinic complaining of dysuria and frequent urination. He states he has had dark urine although he denies any frank blood. He denies fever, urethral discharge, or pain with defecation. His vital signs are normal. On physical exam, he has no costovertebral angle (CVA) tenderness or bladder tenderness. Urinalysis is pertinent for increased WBC count, many bacteria, positive leukocyte esterase, and negative nitrate. Urine culture is pending. What is the best treatment for the most likely diagnosis?

A. Valacyclovir for 2 weeks.
B. Ceftriaxone ×1 in clinic.
C. Ceftriaxone and doxycycline for 2–4 weeks.
D. Ciprofloxacin for 2–4 weeks.
E. TMP/Sulfa for 3 days.

Prostatitis

Symptoms

Urinary frequency, urgency, hesitancy, dysuria, nocturia, hematuria, fevers, chills, and myalgias.

Diagnosis

Physical exam: Extremely tender prostate that may be enlarged.
Labs: Urinalysis and culture indicative of urinary tract infection (UTI). Prostate massage and culture of secretions may be done, although should only be after adequate blood levels of antibiotics are achieved to avoid bacteremia. Practically, prostate massage is rarely done in clinical practice. CBC, CRP, ESR may be indicative of infection.
Causes:

Age <35 years: *Neisseria gonorrhoeae* and *Chlamydia*.

Age >35 years or chronic disease: Enterobacteria.

Treatment

- Age <35 years → Ofloxacin or ceftriaxone + doxycycline.

- Age >35 years → Ciprofloxacin or TMP/Sulfa.

- Both therapies should be continued for 14–30 days.

Benign Prostatic Hypertrophy

Symptoms

Symptoms of bladder outlet obstruction such as difficulty starting a stream, weak stream, hesitancy, urgency, incomplete voiding, dribbling, bladder pain, stress incontinence, nocturia, and anuria. May progress to azotemia and possibly urosepsis if untreated and severe. Most often seen in the elderly or aging.

Diagnosis

Physical exam is the best way to diagnose. Symmetrically boggy prostate on DRE.

Imaging: Ultrasound may be used to estimate gland size or investigate other prostate disease.

Biopsy is not useful for diagnosis although may eliminate cancer as a possibility.

Treatment

- Acutely decompress the bladder with a Foley or suprapubic catheter.
- Long-term use **α-blockers [doxazosin (Cardura), terazosin (Hytrin), tamsulosin (Flomax), prazosin (Minipress)] and 5α-reductase inhibitors (finasteride).**
- Avoid anticholinergics, antihistamines, and narcotics.
- Surgical treatment with TURP is definitive.
- Other approaches include stents, microwave thermotherapy, high-intensity focused ultrasound thermotherapy, laser, electrovaporization, and radiofrequency vaporization, although these are rarely used.

Masses Referable to Testes

See Table 15.2.

TABLE 15.2 Testicular masses

Mass	Associations/diagnosis	Treatment
Hydrocele	Painless; no signs of inflammation; **transilluminates**; may obtain ultrasound for definitive diagnosis if needed	Observation unless growing or very large; aspiration may provide relief but can recur; surgical removal of the tunica vaginalis is the definitive treatment
Varicocele	Dilation of the pampiniform plexus (usually on the left); does not transilluminate; usually benign but may affect fertility; varies in size with standing/sitting position; exam classic for "**bag of worms**" feel	Surgical
Inguinal hernia	May be direct or indirect in relation to the inguinal canal; in extension into the scrotum, exam will reveal no cord superior to bulge (thus differentiating from other masses); can be reducible when changed to supine position; watch for possible strangulation or incarceration	Surgical (either open or laparoscopic)

Testicular Torsion

Symptoms

Acute severe testicular pain. May be referred to abdomen and cause nausea/vomiting. Typical patients are infants, toddlers, and children. Risk factors may include trauma, but most commonly are idiopathic.

Diagnosis

Phyical exam: Affected testicle may be high riding and is extremely tender. Elevating testis may relieve some pain. Opposite testis may lie horizontally instead of vertically (Angell's sign).
Imaging: Often unneeded, but ultrasound may reveal diagnosis.

Treatment

- Immediate referral to urologist for emergency surgical correction.

- While waiting, manual reduction may be attempted (although adequate analgesia is needed). Classically, turn the affected testis laterally "like opening a book."

Orchitis/Epididymitis

Symptoms

Pain and mass of the testis. Erythema, dysuria, pain with ejaculation, and symptoms of bladder outlet obstruction may be present. History may reveal recent urologic surgery, prostatitis, UTI, or recent sexually transmitted disease (STD). Exam shows erythematous, tender mass.

Diagnosis

Physical exam: Usually relieved somewhat by elevation. Rule out testicular torsion.
Labs: Urinalysis and culture. Urethral swab for *N. gonorrhoeae* and *Chlamydia*. CBC, CRP, ESR show signs of infection.
Imaging: Ultrasound may show inflammation and localize infection.
Causes:

Age <35 years: *N. gonorrhoeae* and *Chlamydia*.

Age >35 years: Enterobacteria.

Treatment

- Treat for both *N. gonorrhoeae* and *Chlamydia* if under age 35 or STD suspected:

  - Age <35 years: Ceftriaxone + doxycycline and azithromycin.

  - Age >35 years: Ciprofloxacin or levofloxacin.

- Treatment should be given for 10–14 days.

Male Infertility

Symptoms

Defined as 1 year of regular intercourse failing to produce pregnancy. Depending on the etiology, other symptoms may be present. Klinefelter's syndrome, hypogonadism, erectile dysfunction, and others.

Diagnosis

Labs: Semen analysis. This should be done twice if abnormal to confirm. Factors in a semen analysis include:

- Measurement of semen volume and pH.
- Microscopy for debris and agglutination.
- Assessment of sperm concentration, motility, and morphology.
- Sperm leukocyte count.
- Search for immature germ cells.
- Microscopic exam.

Three factors are important including concentration, motility, and morphology. Concentration is normal with at least 20 million/ml with 48 million/ml considered fertile (between these values, the patient is considered subfertile). Motility is normal if at least 50% are motile and 25% are considered rapidly progressively motile. Morphology is normal if at least 15% are seen as normal.

If the above does not elicit the diagnosis, specialized semen tests may be done and include sperm autoantibodies, biochemistry, semen culture, sperm–cervical mucous interaction, and a battery of sperm function tests (computer-aided sperm analysis, acrosome reaction, zona-free hamster oocyte penetration test, human zona pellucida–binding test, sperm chromatin, and DNA assays).

Genetic analysis may be considered and includes sex chromosome and somatic mutations testing.

Evaluate with hormonal testing to include testosterone, luteinizing hormone (LH), and follicle-stimulating hormone (FSH) to evaluate gonadal and pituitary function.

Treatment

- Treatment largely depends on the production of some amount of sperm. Otherwise, correction of underlying abnormality must be attempted. In reversible hormone-related dysfunction, treatment may include dopamine agonists for hypoprolactinemia, pulsatile gonadotropin-releasing hormone (GnRH) analogs for pituitary dysfunction, or steroids for autoantibodies. Testosterone injections may be used in hypogonadism.

- Surgery may be a viable option to treat varicocele, retrograde ejaculation, and other structural defects.

- Assistive reproductive techniques are gaining popularity and effectiveness including intracytoplasmic sperm injection (ICSI), intrauterine insemination, artificial insemination with donor semen, and *in vitro* fertilization.

Answers

15.1 D. The USPSTF has concluded that screening for early prostate cancer provides a risk to the patient's health in unneeded anxiety, biopsy, and potential complications of therapy that may not otherwise benefit the patient's health. Although it does recognize the usefulness of PSA and DRE, it does not support its use in screening. The American Cancer Society (ACS), however, does support annual screening in adult men over age 50 (or 45 if high risk) with a life expectancy >10 years.

15.2 C. This patient is under the age of 35 with symptoms consistent with prostatitis. The most frequent organisms causing this are *Neisseria gonorrhoeae* and *Chlamydia*. Treatment regimens vary, but commonly used ones are the "gut and butt" regimen, which includes ceftriaxone and doxycycline. Since coinfection is commonly present, both antibiotics are used. Other answers present either do not treat both infections or do not treat the most likely organism.

15.3 E. Three factors are important including concentration, motility, and morphology. Concentration is normal with at least 20 million/ml with 48 million/ml considered fertile (between these values, the patient is considered subfertile). Motility is normal if at least 50% are motile and 25% are considered rapidly progressively motile. Morphology is normal if at least 15% are seen as normal.

16   Diseases to the Female Reproductive System

Breast-Related Problems	348
Malignant Neoplasm of the Breast	348
Benign Neoplasm of the Breast	349
Mastitis/Breast Abscess	350
Malignant Neoplasm of the Ovary	350
Ovarian Cyst	351
Polycystic Ovarian Syndrome	352
Acute Parametritis and Pelvic Cellulitis (Pelvic Inflammatory Disease)	354
Malignant Neoplasm of the Uterus	355
Leiomyoma of Uterus	355
Endometriosis	356
Uterine Prolapse	357
Abnormal Uterine Bleeding	357
Malignant Neoplasm of the Cervix	358
Abnormal Pap Smear	359
Cervicitis/Endocervicitis	361
Malignant Neoplasm of the Vagina	362
Malignant Neoplasm of the Vulva	362
Vaginitis/Vulvovaginitis	362
Prolapse of the Vaginal Walls	363
Imperforate Hymen	364
Lichen Sclerosis (Lichen Sclerosis et Atrophicus)	364
Bartholin Cyst/Abscess	364
Dysmenorrhea	365
Premenstrual Tension/Premenstrual Dysphoric Disorder	365
Amenorrhea	366
Menopause	367
Female Infertility	368

Breast-Related Problems

Malignant Neoplasm of the Breast

Two basic types: ductal and lobular. Ductal is more common and visible on mammography. Lobular is usually incidentally discovered by biopsy of other abnormality, and is generally not visible on mammography. *In situ* lesions [ductal carcinoma *in situ* (DCIS), lobular carcinoma *in situ* (LCIS)] are those showing malignant potential but have not invaded beyond the surrounding breast duct or lobule. Sometimes referred to as "precancer," they make up the majority of malignant breast diseases.

Symptoms

Often asymptomatic, but commonly presents as a breast lump felt either by the patient or physician. Cancers are hard and mobile in surrounding tissue, but all lumps need to be investigated. Other symptoms include peau d'orange skin change (skin of the orange), regional lymphadenopathy, and nipple bleeding or nonmilky discharge. Classically, cancer occurs in upper outer quadrant (tail of Spence).

Diagnosis

Current Recommendations

Different authoritative bodies differ on the recommendations for screening especially under the age of 50. The American Medical Association (AMA), the American College of Radiology (ACR), and the American Cancer Society (ACS) all support screening with mammography and clinical breast exam (CBE) beginning at the age of 40. The American College of Obstetricians and Gynecologists (ACOG) supports screening with mammography beginning at the age of 40 and CBE beginning at the age of 19. The American Academy of Family Physicians (AAFP) recommends beginning mammography for average-risk women at the age of 50, with mammography in high-risk women beginning at the age of 40. The AAFP recommends that all women aged 40–49 years be counseled about the risks and benefits of mammography before making decisions about screening.

Organizations also differ on their recommendations for the appropriate interval for mammography. Annual mammography is recommended by AMA, ACR, and ACS. Mammography every 1–2 years is recommended by the AAFP. And finally, ACOG recommends mammography every 1–2 years for women aged 40–49 years and annually for women aged 50 and older.

If screening raises suspicion, diagnostic mammography should be performed. If positive, fine needle aspiration or excisional biopsy can be performed on palpable masses. Stereotactic biopsy can also be used to localize the lesion if not felt. Incisional biopsy and core biopsy may also be chosen.

Remember, mammography, physical exam, or aspiration cannot tell if cancer exists: **"if the rumor is tumor, tissue is the issue!"**

Treatment

Surgery: Several procedures exist and are progressively decreasing the amount of the tissue taken (see Table 16.1).

Chemotherapy: Estrogen receptor status of tumor must be assessed. Treatment for estrogen receptor–positive tumors may include selective estrogen receptor blockers (SERBs) such as tamoxifen and raloxifene (Evista). Trastuzumab (Herceptin) may also be used in HER2 receptor–positive cancers. Other traditional chemotherapy regimens can be used for metastatic or likely metastatic disease (generally postmenopausal).

Radiation: Can improve survival rates after newer breast-sparing procedures. Generally side effects are mild, but a classic one is unilateral arm lymphedema.

Benign Neoplasm of the Breast

Several types of benign breast masses including fibroadenoma, fibrocystic changes, intraductal papilloma, fat necrosis, and mammary duct ectasia. Most common, especially in younger, premenopausal women are fibroadenomas and fibrocystic change.

TABLE 16.1 Surgical treatment of breast carcinoma

Procedure	Definition/associations
Radical mastectomy (Halsted)	Complete en bloc removal of anterior chest wall including breast tissue, skin, nipple/areola, axillary lymph nodes, and pectoralis major/minor; rarely used today
Modified radical mastectomy	Removes breast tissue, skin, nipple/areola, axillary lymph nodes, and pectoralis fascia
Simple mastectomy	Removes breast tissue, nipple/areola, and skin but spares lymph nodes, muscles, and fascia; often used with radiation for DCIS, LCIS
Local excision/ lumpectomy/ segmental mastectomy	Lesion-specific removal of tumor and surrounding breast tissue; often frozen sections are used to assure clear margins in the OR; may/may not be accompanied by node dissection; appropriate for tumors <4 cm without surrounding tissue fixation, skin involvement, or fixed node involvement; often used with radiation therapy
Sentinel node biopsy	Biopsy of main lymph node(s) draining area suspicious of lesion; newest approach to avoid side effects of complete node dissection

Symptoms

Many present with breast mass, but several types present with overlying skin inflammation, bloody nipple discharge, breast enlargement, pain, and cyclic response to menstrual cycle.

Diagnosis/Treatment

Commonly, history and physical exam are used to assess the need for biopsy. Ultrasound can be used to evaluate for cystic structures and mammography if mass thought to be suspicious for malignancy. Ultimately, excision, biopsy or aspiration is the standard and is often curative depending on the type. Oral contraceptive pills (OCPs) can help symptoms by regulating periods. Nonsteroidal antiinflammatory drugs (NSAIDs) can help discomfort. Advise patient to quit smoking and caffeine use. Vitamin E and evening oil of primrose have also been used as alternative treatments.

Mastitis/Breast Abscess

Symptoms

Unilateral, swollen, warm, and extremely painful breast often with nipple retraction. Mastitis may have accompanying fever and signs of systemic infection. Potentially can progress to sepsis. Purulent nipple discharge can be present in advanced cases. Abscess may form. Both abscess and mastitis are strongly associated with breastfeeding, but may also accompany breast surgery, implants, and radiation therapy.

Diagnosis

Physical exam and history are highly suggestive.
Labs: Culture of drainage (usually shows *Staphylococcus* or *Streptococcus*), CBC shows leukocytosis.
Imaging: Ultrasound may show fluid pocket.

Treatment

Mastitis: Continue breastfeeding and give *Staphylococcus*-active **antibiotics** such as dicloxacillin or cefazolin.

Breast abscess: As with any abscess, incision and drainage (**I/D**) is mandatory. Stop breastfeeding (although continue manual milk expression) and give antibiotics such as nafcillin or oxacillin.

Malignant Neoplasm of the Ovary

Many types of tumors, including epithelial, germ cell, sex cord-stromal, unclassified, and metastatic. Epithelial are the most common tumors and the most likely to be malignant.

Krukenberg tumor—Metastasis from stomach to the ovaries.

Meigs' syndrome—Presence of ovarian tumor, ascites, and right hydrothorax. Seen in sex cord-stromal tumors.

Symptoms

Often abdominal mass is the first indication of a tumor. After advancement and tumor size increases, GI complaints, urinary frequency, dysuria, and pelvic pressure can ensue. Since the presentation is often after mass effect is felt, the stage is usually advanced at diagnosis. Risk factors include uninterrupted menstruation, late menopause, delayed childbearing, and family history/BRCA1 gene mutation. Factors that lessen risk are multiparity, breastfeeding, and hormonal birth control.

Diagnosis

Suspected by physical exam and presence of negative **pregnancy test**. Exam will show solid, fixed, nodular pelvic mass, with/without ascites or pleural effusion. **Labs: CA-125** tumor marker can be used to follow progression/regression of the disease, but is not used as screening (yet) because it is very nonspecific. Other markers such as α-fetoprotein (AFP), β-human chorionic gonadotropin (β-hCG), lactate dehydrogenase (LDH), estrogen, and testosterone can also be elevated characteristically with the subtype of malignancy. Staging is surgical and follows general TNM system. Pathology is very important to prognosis.
Imaging: Ultrasound is the mainstay of diagnosis although visible on CT/MRI.

Treatment

- **Surgery** is the first-line treatment. May include total abdominal hysterectomy/bilateral salpingoophorectomy (TAH/BSO), omentectomy, or tumor debulking.

- Some pathologic types respond well to chemotherapy and some respond well to radiation. In either case, a specialist should be involved.

Ovarian Cyst

Several types of functional cysts exist including follicular, corpus luteal, and theca luteal. Most common are the cysts that form by either the failure of follicle to rupture properly during menstruation or the failure of corpus luteum to regress normally after rupture.

Symptoms

Can be asymptomatic, but commonly cause vague lower abdominal pain. Can also cause disturbances in menstruation timing/amount and dyspareunia, and occasionally contribute to ovarian torsion.

Diagnosis

Ultrasound is the best technique to evaluate. May be suspected incidentally on other imaging of abdomen such as CT/MRI. Tumor markers are generally not useful.

Treatment

- Given chances of malignancy, treatment is based on menses state of patient. Premenarchal and postmenopausal patients need exploratory laparotomy with biopsy.

- **Observe** others for **6–8 weeks** and repeat ultrasound to the evaluation for regression. If the cyst persists without regression or is >8 cm at diagnosis, consider laparotomy and biopsy.

Q 16.1

A 27-year-old Caucasian school teacher comes to your office for the evaluation of irregular menses and months of skipped periods. She also complains of infertility despite unprotected intercourse for 1.5 years. On exam, her vital signs are normal, but you note increased fine facial hair and that she is moderately obese with BMI of 32. What is the next step in diagnosis?

A. Serum testosterone level.
B. Genetic analysis.
C. Serum luteinizing hormone (LH) and follicle-stimulating hormone (FSH) levels.
D. Ultrasound of the ovaries.
E. CT scan of abdomen with emphasis on adrenals.

Polycystic Ovarian Syndrome

Constellation of endocrinologic derangements including elevated estrogen and androgen levels, and luteinizing hormone/follicle-stimulating hormone (LH/FSH) ratio. It is thought to be due to the mechanism resulting from multiple derangements including adrenal hypersecretion of androgens, peripheral conversion of androgens to estrogens by adipose tissue, and insulin resistance. Ovaries often have multiple simple cysts.

Symptoms

Patients present with any combination of **infertility, amenorrhea, irregular menses, hirsutism, and obesity**. Physiologically, symptoms of increased androgen levels are common. Concomitantly, increased body mass index (BMI), insulin resistance, and type II diabetes are common.

Diagnosis

The National Institutes of Health (NIH) proposed guidelines to diagnose PCOS, which include:

- Menstrual irregularity due to oligo or anovulation

- Evidence of hyperandrogenism, clinical (hirsutism or male pattern balding) or biochemical (high serum androgen concentrations).

- Exclusion of other causes of hyperandrogenism and menstrual irregularity, such as congenital adrenal hyperplasia, Cushing's syndrome, androgen-secreting tumors, and hyperprolactinemia.

Labs: Labs to evaluate for hyperandrogenism include total and free testosterone level (although physiologically variable), androstenedione, and DHEA.

Labs that support PCOS but aren't evidence of hyperaldrogenism include LH/FSH ratio ≥2.5-3.0, increased serum estrone level, and decreased sex hormone binding globulin (SHBG). Testing for insulin resistance with fasting glucose or fasting glucose:insulin ratio (<4.5 supports insulin resistance) is warranted.

Labs to evaluate for other endocrinologic disorders include DHEA-S (increased in androgen-producing tumors), dexamethasone suppression test (for Cushing's syndrome), 17α-OH progesterone (increased in nonclassic adrenal hyperplasia), TSH, and prolactin.

Imaging: Ultrasound demonstrating polycystic ovaries is only required in the Rotterdam criteria for the diagnosis of PCOS. This system is thought to be accurate in diagnosis but more cumbersome because of lack of reliable ultrasonography techniques.

Q 16.2

What is the best next step in the treatment of the patient in Question Box 16.1?

A. Start a gonadotropin-releasing hormone (GnRH) agonist to regulate menses.
B. Begin oral contraceptive pills (OCPs) and advise adoption.
C. Surgical consult for weight reduction surgery.
D. Begin OCPs & metformin (Glucophage), and advise weight loss strategies.
E. Begin metformin (Glucophage) & clomiphene (Clomid), and advise weight loss strategies.

Treatment

- Consider child-bearing desire of the patient. If the patient has no desire for children, metformin (Glucophage), weight loss, and OCPs are the mainstay. If the patient has desire for children, clomiphene (Clomid), metformin (Glucophage), and weight loss.

- Weight loss alone can often be used to treat the disease.

Q 16.3

A 21-year-old African American woman comes to the ER with complaints of pain in her lower abdomen, fever, and foul-smelling vaginal discharge for the last few days. She also states she has had an increased right upper quadrant (RUQ) pain for the past 12 h, which is steadily worsening. Her vital signs are stable although her temperature is 104.0°F. She exhibits RUQ direct tenderness and positive Murphy's sign. A vaginal swab is taken for culture and DNA probe analysis. Ultrasound of abdomen is normal including gallbladder. What is the most likely cause of her RUQ pain?

A. Occult cholecystitis.
B. Ruptured appendix.
C. Ectopic pregnancy.
D. Gas pains.
E. Fitz-Hugh–Curtis syndrome.

Acute Parametritis and Pelvic Cellulitis (Pelvic Inflammatory Disease)

Commonly seen with sexually transmitted disesases (STDs), most commonly *N. gonorrhoeae* and *Chlamydia*. Major risk factor is the presence of intrauterine device (IUD).

Symptoms

Sexually active female often presents with abdominal pain, adnexal tenderness, dyspareunia, and fever. Patient may also have upper quadrant abdominal pain/vomiting/hepatic symptoms by Fitz-Hugh–Curtis mechanism (perihepatitis from infectious fluid traveling in the posterior peritoneal gutter to the hepatic membranes). Unusual vaginal discharge is often present.

Diagnosis

Physical exam: Adnexal tenderness, abdominal tenderness, **cervical motion tenderness** (Chandelier sign), and purulent cervical discharge.
Labs: Obtain pregnancy test, CBC for leukocytosis, and STD cultures or DNA probe from cervix. Consider HIV, syphilis workup.
Imaging: None specific, but in the acute setting may consider ultrasound to evaluate for ovarian torsion or abscess.

Must decide to hospitalize or not. Consider the presence of fever, degree of leukocytosis, IUD presence, adolescent patient, primigravid patient, likelihood of sepsis.

Treatment

- Always treat with more than one antibiotic.
  - **Outpatient regimen**: Ofloxacin/levofloxacin + metronidazole ×14 days _OR_ ceftriaxone IM ×1, metronidazole + doxycycline ×14 days.

- **Inpatient regimen:** Cefotetan/cefoxitin IV + doxycycline IV <u>OR</u> clindamycin IV + gentamicin IV, then doxycycline IV.
- Treat partner if STD is the etiology of infection.

Malignant Neoplasm of the Uterus

Endometrial cancer is most common.

Symptoms

Vaginal bleeding after menopause is the most common presentation and is a red flag for malignancy. Most commonly, it consists of adenocarcinoma that spreads locally or by lymphatics. Risk factors include obesity, polycystic ovarian syndrome (PCOS), nulliparity, late menopause, family history, diabetes, hypertension, estrogen-secreting malignancy, or estrogen replacement therapy without progesterone.

Diagnosis

Physical exam: Bleeding from the uterus, uncommonly a palpable mass on bimanual exam.

Imaging: Ultrasound of the uterus evaluating for endometrial stripe thickness (≤5 mm is normal). Caution: Only useful in postmenopausal women since endometrial stripe thickness varies greatly in the ovulating female. Chest x-ray may be indicated for possible metastasis.

Endometrial biopsy is the next step. If endometrial biopsy is negative but suspicion still exists, dilation and curettage (D and C) is the best test available.

Treatment

TAH with or without the removal of ovaries is the most common treatment. Radiation may be used locally if spread is suspected. Chemotherapy is not effective as primary treatment, but may be attempted if metastatic disease is present; doxorubicin (Adriamycin) or cisplatin is most common.

Leiomyoma of Uterus

Benign tumor arising from the uterine smooth muscle.

Symptoms

Often asymptomatic early in the course, but can cause menorrhagia, menometrorrhagia, pain, pressure, and urinary or bowel problems, and may complicate pregnancy.

Diagnosis

Physical bimanual exam usually provides an indication of Leiomyoma.

Imaging: Ultrasound confirms diagnosis. CT or MRI will also show them. After imaging confirms diagnosis, follow for 4–6 months to assess if they are stable or growing. Stable fibroids may be followed annually.

Treatment

- For minimally symptomatic patients, consider iron supplements, close follow-up, and/or progestin supplementation (norethindrone, medroxyprogesterone), which may reduce bleeding.

- Consider LH–releasing hormone (LHRH) agonists (nafarelin, goserelin, leuprolide) before surgery to shrink tumor as much as possible.

- Resection is the mainstay. Myomectomy or hysterectomy is the option, but have disadvantages associated with major surgery. Thus, asymptomatic stable fibroids should just be monitored without treatment.

- For younger patients, alternative surgical options include hysteroscopic or laparoscopic cautery or laser myomectomy.

Q 16.4

What important factor must be considered in the medical treatment of endometriosis?

A. Menstrual cycle length.
B. Desire to bear children.
C. Birth control option selected.
D. Thyroid state.
E. Hormonal activity of gonadal/pituitary axis.

Endometriosis

Hormone-responsive endometrial tissue outside the uterus.

Symptoms

Varied presentation, but symptoms are usually cyclic with menses. Most commonly, abdominal or pelvic **pain** of unclear etiology, dyspareunia, dysmenorrhea, pain on defecation, abdominal bloating, suprapubic pain on urination, and rarely rectal bleeding with menses. Classically, extent of disease does not correlate with the severity of symptoms.

Diagnosis

A clinical diagnosis made by detailed history and physical exam with screening labs such as CBC and Chem-7. Expect labs to be normal.

Laproscopic visualization with biopsy is the gold standard.

Treatment

- At the time of visualization, electrocautery, laser ablation, or local removal are usually tried.
- Medical treatment includes the consideration of childbearing desire.
- If the patient does not desire children, **OCPs** are the mainstay. Gonadotropin-releasing hormone (GnRH) agonists have been used, but long-term treatment (>6 months) is contraindicated because of bone mineral loss. Danazol, an antigonadotropin, can also be used, but hyperandrogenic side effects limit its use in the vast majority of patients.
- Hysterectomy (with estrogen therapy afterward) can be used as last resort.
- Pregnancy and menopause alone usually improve symptoms.

Uterine Prolapse

Uterus protruding into or through the vagina.

Symptoms

Symptoms usually seen in patients with multiple vaginal deliveries. They include pain or feeling of pelvic fullness, which worsens in upright position, dyspareunia, and backache. Patient may report the feeling of something protruding from vagina if severe.

Diagnosis

Physical exam: Imaging generally not needed. Boggy mass protruding through the vulva.

Treatment

- Generally treated conservatively with Kegel exercises, but may require the use of pessary (removable intravaginal device that provides pelvic support).
- Several surgeries exist for refractory cases including the pelvic sling and transvaginal tape. If severe, refer for surgery.

Abnormal Uterine Bleeding

Abnormalities in vaginal bleeding with respect to amount or timing.

Symptoms and Definitions

See Table 16.2.

Diagnosis

Decide if ovulatory or anovulatory based on history. Physical exam may be warranted and may reveal obvious cervical source, vaginal source, or cervical motion tenderness.

TABLE 16.2 Definitions of abnormal uterine bleeding

Oligomenorrhea	Cycle length >35 days
Polymenorrhea	Cycle length <21 days
Amenorrhea	Complete absence of menses for three cycles or 5 months (whichever is first)
Menorrhagia	Regular cycles with excessive flow or duration
Metrorrhagia	Irregular vaginal bleeding outside the normal cycle
Menometrorrhagia	Irregular cycles with excessive flow and duration
Dysfunctional uterine bleeding	A **diagnosis of exclusion** after ruling out an anatomic lesion

Labs: Do **pregnancy test** on everyone. Order CBC and coagulation profile to assess for anemia and clotting disorders.

Ovulatory bleeding: Consider hysteroscopy, ultrasound, endometrial biopsy, or D and C (gold standard).

Anovulatory bleeding: Do endocrine workup with TSH, FSH, LH, and prolactin. Consider the trial of progesterone to evaluate unopposed estrogen presence. If bleeding ceases during trial, test is positive. Proceed to ultrasound/endometrial biopsy to evaluate for endometrial hyperplasia or cancer, especially in postmenopausal woman.

Treatment

- Acute bleeding: ABCs, high-dose IV estrogen, D and C, endometrial ablation. Extreme cases may require uterine artery embolization or hysterectomy.

- Chronic treatment is generally OCPs or endometrial ablation. Clomiphene may be considered in patients who desire pregnancy.

Malignant Neoplasm of the Cervix

Symptoms

Vast majority of cases are asymptomatic and found by Pap smear. Classic presentation is of a patient with postcoital bleeding. Other symptoms may include menometrorrhagia, abnormal vaginal discharge, with possible presentation of advanced cases with obstructive uropathy, foul-smelling vaginal discharge, and pelvic pain.

Risk factors include:

- Human papillomavirus (HPV) infection (serotypes 16, 18, 31, etc.)
- Multiple sexual partners.

- Immunocompromised state.
- History of multiple STDs.
- Early onset of sexual activity.
- Tobacco use.

Diagnosis

Pap smear is the best screening tool and catches 90% of cases early on. May proceed to colposcopy with biopsies if indicated. If the entire lesion or the transformational zone cannot be visualized, a cone biopsy via loop electro-surgical excision procedure (LEEP) or cold knife may be performed.

Remember, invasion usually occurs locally and lymphatically. Death is commonly by urosepsis.

Treatment

- Can be treated at the time of colposcopy with **cryotherapy**, LEEP, or excisional biopsy.
- If advanced disease, consider hysterectomy with the removal of cervix. If invasive, lymph node dissection and staging with further imaging such as CT and MRI are indicated.
- Radiation therapy has shown benefit both pre- and post-surgically; however, it can have adverse effects on local tissues such as rectum and urinary system.
- Chemotherapy is reserved for metastatic cases, but may be considered palliative.

Q 16.5

A 31-year-old female patient comes to your office for an unrelated complaint when she states "Oh by the way, doctor, it's been over a year and a half since my last Pap smear, can we get that done today, too?" She has not previously been pregnant and all prior Pap smears have been negative. According to recent recommendations, how often should she have conventional Pap smears?

A. Annually in this age–group.
B. Biannually in this age–group.
C. Every 2–3 years.
D. Annually if she has ever had a positive Pap smear.
E. At most every 2 years if two or more risk factors exist.

Abnormal Pap Smear

Symptoms

Vast majority of patients with dysplasia are asymptomatic and found by routine screening Pap.

Diagnosis/Treatment

Different groups have slightly different recommendations on when/how often to begin screening. American College of Obstetricians and Gynecologists recommends starting within 3 years of sexual activity or age 21 and then annually until age 30. After age 30, screen every 2–3 years if the patient has had three consecutive negative Paps. The United States Preventative Services Task Force recommends at least every 3 years and makes no distinction after age 30. The American Cancer Society recommends starting within 3 years of sexual activity or age 21 and annually until age 30 if using the conventional Pap or every 2 years if with cytologic-based technique. After age 30, every 2–3 years if the patient has had three negative Paps.

Abnormal Results

See Table 16.3.

TABLE 16.3 Basics of Bethesda system of Pap smear reporting

Result	Treatment
ASC-US	See Figure 16.1
AGCs	Colposcopy
LSIL	Colposcopy/biopsies without HPV testing (since most are high-risk type). May treat with ablation or biopsy. In patients who are postmenopausal, pregnant, or adolescent, consider repeat Pap in 4–6 months without colposcopy
HSIL	Colposcopy/biopsies; if satisfactory colposcopy, consider excisional biopsy; if unsatisfactory colposcopy (incomplete visualization of transformational zone), consider cone biopsy

AGCs, atypical glandular cells; ASC-US, atypical squamous cells of undetermined significance; LSIL, low-grade squamous intraepithelial lesion; HPV, human papillomavirus; HSIL, high-grade squamous intraepithelial lesion.

Source: Adapted from American Society for Colposcopy and Cervical Pathology.

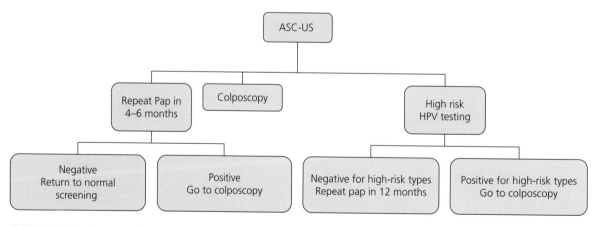

FIGURE 16.1 Suggested algorithm for the treatment of atypical squamous cells of undetermined significance (ASC-US) result on screening Pap smear.

Cervicitis/Endocervicitis

Symptoms

Pelvic pain, unusual vaginal discharge, bleeding (usually spotting), or dyspareunia. Risk factors include sexual promiscuity, low socioeconomic status, early onset of sexual activity, and nonmarried state.

Diagnosis

Diagnosis is aided by the physical exam that shows cervical motion tenderness (Chandelier sign), cervical discharge, fishy vaginal odor, or cervical bleeding.

Labs: Techniques include:

- Cervical culture.
- GC/*Chlamydia* DNA probe.
- KOH slide preparation to look for branching/budding hyphae and perform "whiff test" for bacterial vaginosis.
- Wet mount slide to look for *Trichomonades* or "clue cells."
- Viral culture of lesions.

Several different organisms may be involved including *N. gonorrhoeae*, *Chlamydia trachomatis*, herpes simplex virus (HSV), *Trichomonas*, HPV, *Mycoplasma*, and others. *N. gonorrhoeae*, *Chlamydia*, and *Trichomonas* are by far the most common.

Treatment

- Elect to treat gonorrhea and chlamydia together, since they are commonly seen in coinfection.
- Regimens vary, but memorize the classic (see Table 16.4).
- Others:
  - *Trichomonas*: Metronidazole.
  - *Gardnerella* spp.: Metronidazole.
  - HSV: Suppressive therapy with acyclovir, valacyclovir.
  - HPV: Cryotherapy, acid, electrocautery.
  - *Candida*: Fluconazole (Diflucan).
- Remember, treat the partner.

TABLE 16.4 Medication treatment for common STD's

	Classic	Alternate
Gonorrhea	Ceftriaxone IM ×1	Ciprofloxacin PO
Chlamydia	Doxycycline PO ×7 days	Azithromycin PO ×1

Malignant Neoplasm of the Vagina

Symptoms

Most commonly asymptomatic, but can present with increasing vaginal discharge, bleeding, and pruritus.

Diagnosis

Physical exam: Suspicious lesion may be seen at the time of Pap smear. Biopsies of suspicious lesions are appropriate.

Basically two types: Squamous cell carcinoma (SCC) and adenocarcinoma [seen in female offspring of women exposed to diethylstilbestrol (DES)].

Treatment

Treated according to stage. If low stage (I or II), can treat with excision, local fluorouracil (Efudex), hysterectomy, vaginectomy, or lymph node biopsy. If higher stage, radiation is generally used with/without surgery.

Malignant Neoplasm of the Vulva

Symptoms

Presentation is classically in the older woman with diabetes, hypertension, obesity, or vulvar dystrophy. Patients present with **vulvar pruritus**, pain, bleeding, or superficial mass.

Diagnosis

Direct biopsy is used for identification.

Staging is through a system by the International Federation of Gynecology and Obstetrics (FIGO) and employs TNM surgical staging methods.

Treatment

Surgical removal is mainstay. With low stage, wide excision (often vulvectomy) with regional lymphadenectomy is most common. Higher stages require the mix of excision and inguinal lymph node dissection.

Vaginitis/Vulvovaginitis

Symptoms

Vaginal pain, unusual discharge, dyspareunia, or pruritus.

Diagnosis/Treatment

Physical exam is invaluable (see Table 16.5).

TABLE 16.5 Common infections of the vulva/vagina

Cause	Diagnostic clues	Treatment
Gardnerella/ bacterial vaginosis	Clue cells on saline mount, fishy smell on KOH "whiff test"	Metronidazole; no need to treat partner
Candidiasis	Branching pseudohyphae on KOH prep, "cottage-cheese" like discharge, history of pregnancy, diabetes, or recent antibiotics	Fluconazole (Diflucan) 150 mg PO ×1; investigate the underlying cause if recurrent
Trichomonas	Wet mount reveals trichomonade organism; discharge is green, often frothy	Metronidazole; treat partner

TABLE 16.6 Definitions of vaginal prolapse

Anterior wall	Cystocele (bladder), urethrocele (urethra)
Upper postvaginal wall (rectovaginal septum)	Enterocele (bowel)
Lower postvaginal wall (rectovaginal septum)	Rectocele (rectum)
Cardinal ligaments	Uterine prolapse

Prolapse of the Vaginal Walls

Damage or weakening of any of the network of muscles and ligaments, which make up the vaginal vault (see Table 16.6).

Symptoms

Pelvic pressure, backache, dyspareunia; urinary symptoms such as incontinence, frequency, hesitancy, recurrent infection; or rectal symptoms such as constipation, painful defecation, and incomplete defecation. Vaginal atrophy from lack of estrogen is often seen.

Diagnosis

Primarily diagnosed by physical exam and visualization of the defect. Correlate with history.

Treatment

- Strengthening of pelvic muscles is essential. Kegel excercises and possibly weighted vaginal cones can be used.
- If atrophic vagina, give estrogen cream.
- Nonsurgical removable pessaries are often effective to support the internal vaginal walls.
- Last resort is surgery and includes hysterectomy, anterior/posterior colporrhaphy, and several types of sling and suspension techniques.

Imperforate Hymen

Symptoms

Classically, an adolescent girl with no history of menses who presents with cyclic abdominal pain.

Diagnosis

Physical exam shows intact hymen that may or may not be bulging from the vagina.

Treatment

Hymenotomy is the treatment, but should be done in sterile fashion. Give much assurance to the patient.

Lichen Sclerosis (Lichen Sclerosis et Atrophicus)

Symptoms

Commonly seen in postmenopausal women without hormone replacement therapy (HRT), and caused by the lack of estrogen effect on vulva. Presents with thinning of the local tissues, drying of vagina, dysuria, dyspareunia, vulvodynia, and pruritus.

Diagnosis

Physical exam: Atrophy of the vulvae and vaginal mucosa.
   Since it is difficult to rule out malignancy, biopsy is needed.

Treatment

Topical hydrocortisone 1% cream for acute symptoms and local hormone cream (testosterone 2%) to build up tissues. Vitamin A ointment also has been used with limited efficacy. May need to escalate to intralesional steroids for stubborn cases. Topical estrogen cream may also help symptoms.

Bartholin Cyst/Abscess

Bartholin glands reside at 4 and 8 o'clock positions of the opening of the vagina. Sometimes the ducts can become clogged and normal lubricating secretions may build up forming a cyst. Infection of this fluid becomes an abscess.

Symptoms

Cystic bump on the inside of vaginal opening. If abscess has formed, patient may have excruciating pain, dyspareunia, and local irritation.

Diagnosis

Physical exam: May confirm by ultrasound but not necessary in the vast majority of cases.

Treatment

- For simple cyst of 1–2 cm in size, conservative treatment with repeated sitz baths is appropriate. Spontaneous regression is the norm.

- For abscesses, I/D is the mainstay. Culture any fluid expressed. Pack the abscess and change daily. Alternatively, treatment may consist of "marsupialization" of the cavity, which basically indicates sewing the two lips of the incision open and allowing to close after healing becomes apparent. Thus, there is no closed space for recurrence of the infection. Placement of a "Word" catheter is an alternative to marsupialization and consists of a sewing a specifically designed drain in the abscess cavity. Give antibiotics based on culture results.

Dysmenorrhea

Symptoms

Cyclic abdominal cramping and lower abdominal pain that occurs in relation to menses. Begins in days preceding menses. Not related to GI or other disturbances. History reveals strong correlation to menses, and physical exam generally shows no further abnormalities to point toward other physical defects.

Diagnosis

Imaging: May rule out gynecologic abnormalities with ultrasound. Dysmenorrhea is often difficult to separate from endometriosis.

Treatment

- Mainstay of therapy is NSAIDs and Tylenol.
- Hormonal birth control often better regulates menses and thus provides relief.

Premenstrual Tension/Premenstrual Dysphoric Disorder

Symptoms

Symptoms of dysmenorrhea and related headache, bloating, breast tenderness, back/abdominal pain, irritability, and fatigue. In case of encompassing premenstrual dysphoric disorder, emotional lability, depression, impairment of social and work relationships, anxiety, and possible suicidal ideations.

Diagnosis

History and relation of symptoms to menstrual cycle. Important to consider the degree of effect of symptoms on life activities.

Treatment

- Often SSRIs are effective and comprise adequate treatment. Fluoxetine (Prozac) and sertraline (Zoloft) are the mainstays, and may be given continuously or only during luteal phase. Start with low dose and titrate up. Tricyclic antidepressants (TCAs) such as clomipramine (Anafranil) and nortriptyline (Pamelor) have also proved effective. Otherwise, partially effective treatment such as calcium replacement, vitamin B_6 in moderate doses, NSAIDs/Tylenol, vitamin E, spironolactone, danazol, and evening oil of primrose (alternative treatment) may help reduce symptoms.

- Always screen for suicidal ideations.

Amenorrhea

Symptoms

Primary: Absence of menses in females older than 16 years.
Secondary: Cessation of menses for ≥ 3 cycles or 6 months (whichever comes first).

Diagnosis

Labs: β-hCG. Then obtain TSH, prolactin level to evaluate hypothalamic pathways.

If primary, evaluate for the existence of uterus and ovaries, then for patent vagina, and then for sexual maturation and secondary sexual characteristics such as breast development. If all is normal, work up for secondary amenorrhea, (see Figure 16.2). If abnormal, consider karyotype or anatomic abnormality.

If secondary, do a **progestin challenge** (progestin 10 mg PO ×7–10 days after which monitor for withdrawal bleeding; thus the test result is negative because of appropriate response). Then follow the algorithm shown in Figure 16.2.

Treatment

- Treat the underlying cause.
- Correct thyroid dysfunction, give bromocriptine (Parlodel) in case of prolactin dysfunction. For ovarian failure, consider OCPs to regulate endometrial shedding. Clomiphene (Clomid) may be used to induce ovulation if pregnancy is desired. Treat PCOS as above. For women with hypothalamic dysfunction, GnRH analogs have been used for ovulation. Refer eating disorders to psychiatrist.

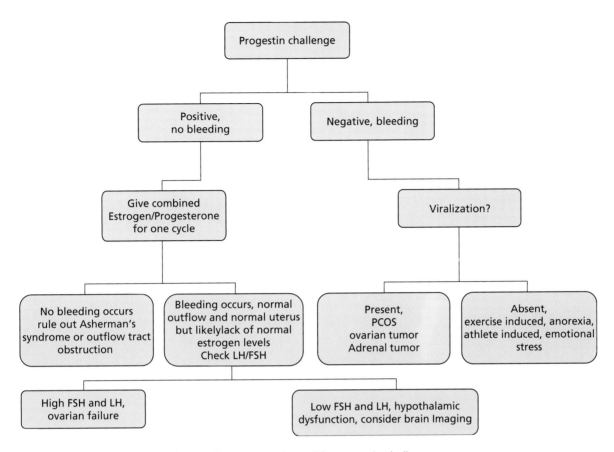

FIGURE 16.2 Investigation of secondary amenorrhea with progestin challenge.

Menopause

Symptoms

Symptom onset is usually in the perimenopausal period defined as age 48–52 with a mean age of onset of 50–51. Hot flashes are generally the first symptom noticed, but are often accompanied by fatigue, irritability, insomnia, depression, memory loss, headache, anxiety, vaginal dryness, labial atrophy, and, by definition, cessation of menses. If these symptoms occur before age 40, investigation of cause should be completed.

Diagnosis

Diagnosis is based on the history of 12 months of amenorrhea in perimenopausal period (in the absence of other medical reasons for amenorrhea).

Common practice is to test for FSH, which is usually high in ovarian failure. It is a myth that FSH is of any value during the perimenapausal period. In this period, the production of FSH is physiologically far too variable to be relied upon as an indicator of menopause. However, it may be of use in younger patients to investigate premature ovarian failure. **Menopause is currently a clinical diagnosis.**

Treatment

- A recent very large, multicenter, long-term study, **The Women's Health Initiative**, recently suggested the adverse effects of HRT. Particularly, combined estrogen/progesterone therapy, which produced dramatic increases in cardiovascular effects such as heart disease and stroke, as well as breast cancer rates. The estrogen-only arm showed increased risk of stroke and deep vein thrombosis (DVT). The study supported the theories of hormone therapy protecting from osteoporosis and lessening of symptoms attributable to menopause. Several limitations of the study exist, however, not the least of which was that the results and adverse events were seen only with 4 or more years of HRT. Further investigations are ongoing.

- Therapies that may help symptoms are many, but include short-term HRT (unproven), clonidine, SSRIs, SSNRIs, and vitamin E. Herbal remedies have been tried and show anecdotal evidence including black cohosh and soy-containing foods (presumably for phytoestrogen content).

- For protection against osteoporosis, place most patients on a bisphosphonate such as alendronate (Fosamax), risedronate (Actonel), or ibandronate (Boniva); or calcitonin, as well as on supplementation of calcium and vitamin D. Weight-bearing exercise is also an effective lifestyle change.

- Control risk factors for heart disease and stroke.

Female Infertility

Symptoms

Defined as the inability to conceive after 12 months of regular unprotected sexual intercourse.

Diagnosis

Assess **ovulation status**. Keep a diary of menstrual cycles and predicted ovulation. Evaluation of basal body temperature may be taken to assess the timing and predict most fertile days. Patient should take oral temperature as soon as she awakens every day and graph on paper. A rise of only tenths of degrees should be noted in luteal phase and thus reveal the time of ovulation.
Labs: TSH/prolactin should be taken to rule out the related disorders. LH/FSH can be assessed to determine if PCOS is present (ratio >2:1 suggests PCOS).

Assess other areas of the upper genital tract. History and physical must direct the physician to investigate other disorders such as endometriosis, scarring s/p pelvic inflammatory disease (PID), scarring s/p IUD, fibroids, Asherman's syndrome, and anatomic abnormalities.

Hysterosalpingogram may be considered to evaluate for scarring of the tubes/uterus. Asherman's syndrome can be ruled out. This also evaluates for anatomic abnormalities, including fallopian tube agenesis, bicornate uterus, fibroids, and foreign body.

Endometrial biopsy may be done to assess the viability of stroma and endometrial lining. Pelvic ultrasound at the correct time in cycle may be done to assess the thickness of endometrial lining. Cervical mucous studies may be indicated to assess density and functionality.

Treatment

- Depending on the problem, different solutions are needed.
- Timing may be adjusted if this is the problem.
- Clomiphene citrate (Clomid) for the induction of ovulation. However, consider the side effects including multiple gestation.
- GnRH analogs to regulate FSH/LH production and encourage ovulation.
- Surgery with ligature of adhesions or removal of fibroids.
- Implantation therapy may be tried in the receptive uterus as a last resort.

Answers

16.1 C. Diagnosis of polycystic ovary syndrome (PCOS) involves both the assessment of clinical risk factors and the laboratory evaluation. Risk factors include amenorrhea, infertility, menstrual irregularities, hirsutism, and obesity. Lab evaluation will further show increased LH/FSH ratio of >2:1. Answer D is no longer a requirement for PCOS diagnosis.

16.2 E. Treatment of polycystic ovarian syndrome (PCOS) requires knowledge of desired fertility. The question implies that the patient is trying to get pregnant, thus treatment should be aimed at both PCOS and infertility. Clomiphene (Clomid) will induce ovulation for infertility, and metformin (Glucophage) and weight loss will treat the underlying physiology of PCOS.

16.3 E. Fitz-Hugh–Curtis syndrome is a mechanism of irritation of the perihepatic membranes by peritoneal fluid from a remote source, often associated with pelvic inflammatory disease (PID). The fluid travels in the posterior peritoneal gutter to contact the perihepatic membranes and cause irritation and other symptoms. Lab evaluation may reveal elevated aspartate transaminase (AST) and alanine transaminase (ALT). Other answers given are possible causes of pain, but are less likely in the setting of her likely PID.

(continued)

Answers

16.4 B. The medical treatment of endometriosis varies greatly by the desire of the patient to bear children. Oral contraceptive pills (OCPs) are the mainstay of therapy if fertility is undesired. Pregnancy itself often decreases the symptoms to some degree. Other treatments include gonadotropin-releasing hormone (GnRH) agonists and danazol, with varying degrees of success. Laproscopic techniques are also used commonly as surgical options.

16.5 C. ACOG (American College of Obstetricians and Gynecologists) recommends starting within 3 years of sexual activity or age 21 and then annually until age 30. After age 30, screen every 2–3 years if the patient has had three consecutive negative Paps. The USPSTF (United States Preventative Services Task Force) recommends at least every 3 years and makes no distinction after age 30. The ACS (American Cancer Society) recommends starting within 3 years of sexual activity or age 21 and annually until age 30 if using the conventional Pap, or every 2 years if with cytologic-based technique. After age 30, every 2–3 years if the patient has had three negative Paps.

Supervision of Normal Pregnancy	371
Delivery and Labor with Minor or No Complications	372
Postpartum Hemorrhage	376
Chorioamnionitis	377
Intrapartum Group B *Streptococcus*	378
Postpartum Fever	379
Complications of Labor and Delivery	379
Shoulder Dystocia	380
Cesarean Delivery	380
Pregnancy Loss	381
Gestational Diabetes Mellitus	383
Preeclampsia/Eclampsia	385
Chromosomal Anomalies	387
Multiple Fetuses	388
Single Liveborn Before Admission to Hospital	388

Supervision of Normal Pregnancy

Maintenance Schedule

Start visits at 6–8 weeks and have the patient return every 4–6 weeks until 36 weeks, and then every 1–2 weeks until delivery (see Table 17.1).

TABLE 17.1 Commonly accepted maintenance schedule for normal pregnancy

At every visit	Assess weight gain
	Auscultate fetal heart tones
	Screen fundal height
	Screen for HTN
	Breastfeeding education
	Assess flu shot status if in season
	Counsel on family planning
	Screen for domestic abuse
	Educate regarding preterm labor
	Tobacco/EtOH screening
Weeks 6–8	Blood type and Rh factor
	Rubella titer
	Varicella
	Hepatitis B
	Syphilis with RPR
	Urinalysis/urine culture
	HIV testing
	Sickle cell carrier screen
	Tetanus booster if needed
	Flu shot if indicated
Weeks 10–12	Screening Pap smear
	Testing for gonorrhea/chlamydia
	Test for cystic fibrosis
Weeks 16–20	Triple screen (estriol, β-hCG, MSAFP) or quadruple screen (estriol, β-hCG, MSAFP, inhibin A)
	Routine ultrasound
Week 28	Gestational diabetes screen (50 g GTT)
	Iron supplements if needed
	Rh-negative patients receive RhoGAM
Week 36	Culture for group B strep
	Assess fetal position with Leopold's maneuvers and/or ultrasound
Week 41	Induction and augmentation if not contraindicated
	Biweekly nonstress tests

hCG, human chorionic gonadotropin; HTN, hypertension; GTT, glucose tolerance test; MSAFP, maternal serum α-fetoprotein; RPR, rapid plasma reagin.

Delivery and Labor with Minor or No Complications

Symptoms

Contractions can be felt differently for many women. Some are felt as back pain, and some with lower abdominal pressure. Most patients feel contractions as tightening or pain in the lower abdomen. Patients may also describe rupture of membranes (ROMs) with anywhere from a rush to a trickle of amniotic fluid leakage. Subjectively, labor can be subtle.

Diagnosis/Treatment

Labor is defined as uterine contractions with cervical change. Commonly assessed by physical exam for elements shown in Table 17.2. These are commonly followed throughout labor to assess progress.

Bishop score is a scale that adds cervical consistency and cervical position to the elements provided in Table 17.2.

Progression follows the stages shown in Table 17.3.

External monitoring includes uterine contraction monitor and continuous fetal heart rate monitor. Reading fetal strips is much like reading ECGs; it is an art. Here are the basics:

- **Reactivity:** Baseline between 110 and 160 bpm with good variability. This means at least two accelerations above baseline of at least 15 bpm lasting 15 s.

- **Early deceleration:** Mirrors contractions. Caused by increased vagal tone secondary to head compression (see Figure 17.1).

- **Variable deceleration:** Deceleration uncorrelated to contraction that drops fairly precipitously, then sharply returns to baseline. Caused by umbilical cord compression and is of concern (see Figure 17.2).

TABLE 17.2 Elements of the cervical exam

Cervical dilation	Measured in centimeters (0–10 cm). Minimal dilation is referred to as "closed" or "fingertip" and 10 cm is "Complete."
Cervical effacement	Percentage of thinning of the cervix
Station	Assesses position of head in relation to the ischial spines, estimated in centimeters: −5 (superior to spines) to 0 to +5 (inferior to spines). Station may also be measured from −3 to 0 to +3 based on thirds of the distance of the pelvic inlet and relative to the ischial spines. Both systems are estimates and both are widely used

TABLE 17.3 Stages of labor

Stage	Definition/association
Stage 1	Latent: Dilation of 0 to 3–4 cm. Longest lasting stage that may be 6–12 h
	Active: Dilation of 3–4 cm to complete (10 cm). Nulliparous should maintain ≥1.2 cm/h dilation. Multiparous, ≥1.5 cm/h
Stage II	From complete dilation to delivery. If it lasts longer than 2 h in nulliparous or 1 h in multiparous it is considered prolonged (add 1 h to this if epidural given)
Stage III	Delivery of infant to delivery of placenta

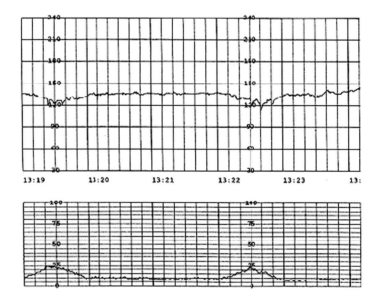

FIGURE 17.1

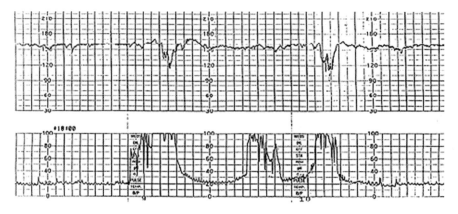

FIGURE 17.2

- **Late deceleration:** Deceleration that starts and ends after beginning and ending of contractions, respectively. This is the result of uteroplacental insufficiency and is very worrisome. Repeated lates may indicate need for cesarean (see Figure 17.3).

Delivery occurs after completion of dilation and is usually with controlled pushing by mother.

The cardinal movements are **engagement, descent, flexion, internal rotation, extension, external rotation (restitution), and expulsion.** From the physician's point of view, controlling the descent and supporting the perineum may help control any lacerations that may occur. Episiotomy can also be used if more room is needed. Shoulder dystocia cannot be relieved by episiotomy.

Types of lacerations:

- First degree—Through the skin or mucosa.

- Second degree—Extending to and involving the perineal body.

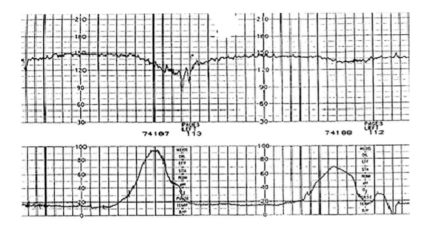

FIGURE 17.3

- Third degree—Extending through the anal sphincter.
- Fourth degree—Extending through the anal mucosa into the rectum.

Repair with absorbable suture.

Follow-up: Generally new mothers should stay in the hospital for at least 36–48 h. Diminishing lochia and pain should be noted with absence of prolonged fever (although some increased temperature is normal with delivery). Pelvic rest should be advised for 6 weeks and nonestrogen birth control should be prescribed.

Research shows that breastfeeding is best for both mother and child.

Q 17.1

A 28-year-old female G2P1 comes into the labor and delivery deck at 39 + 2 weeks in active labor. She has not been seen regularly but luckily has had several visits to your partner's clinic. In a quick record review, you note she has hypothyroidism, asthma, acne, and a history of a 3800 g of infant born via vaginal delivery. Her delivery progresses through the second stage of labor producing a vigorous infant boy. The placenta follows the baby after 12 min but you note a small trickle of blood that will not seem to stop. What is the first step in management of this patient's condition?

A. Manual fundal sweep maneuver.
B. Fundal massage.
C. Give methylergonovine (Methergine).
D. Give carboprost tromethamine (Hemabate).
E. Direct pressure to the posterior vaginal wall.

Postpartum Hemorrhage

Symptoms

Blood loss often just after delivery of the fetus or placenta. By definition, <24 h from delivery is early-onset postpartum hemorrhage (PPH) and that >24 h is late-onset. The patient may exhibit signs of lightheadedness, weakness, fatigue (overt), or orthostatic hypotension. Risk factors include overdistention of uterus (multiple fetuses, polyhydramnios), coagulation disorders, exhausted myometrium, chorioamnionitis, placental abnormalities (previa, accreta, and abruption), forceps delivery, and others. After delivery, PPH is associated with Sheehan's syndrome.

Diagnosis

Physical exam: Pale, clammy skin. Vital signs may show increased heart rate. In extreme cases, decreased blood pressure (nonorthostatic) (see Table 17.4).
Labs: Predelivery CBC will give good hematocrit baseline; postdelivery CBC will show change.

Common causes of PPH include:

- Uterine atony.
- Cervical lacerations.
- Vaginal lacerations.
- Retained products of conception (POCs).
- Uterine inversion.
- Uterine rupture.
- Placenta accreta.

TABLE 17.4 Classification of postpartum hemorrhage

Delivery type	Estimated blood loss
Vaginal delivery	>500 ml
Cesarean delivery	>1000 ml

Q 17.2

In continuing with the case from question 17.1, you note a boggy uterus that does not respond to the first course of action. What further treatment is contraindicated in this patient?

A. Misoprostol (Cytotec).
B. Carboprost tromethamine (Hemabate).
C. Methylergonovine(Methergine).
D. Oxytocin.
E. Phenylephrine.

TABLE 17.5 Characteristics of common PPH medications

Agent	Associations
Oxytocin	Increases uterine smooth muscle contraction
Methylergonovine (Methergine)	Contraindicated in hypertension
Carboprost tromethamine (Hemabate)	Contraindicated in asthma patients. Diarrhea is a common side effect
Misoprostol (Cytotec)	Dose varies but generally 800–1000 µg rectally

Treatment

- If patient is unstable, use volume expansion agents and treat possible hypovolemic shock. Consider blood products if needed.

- If PPH in association with delivery, the most common cause is uterine atony. For this etiology, start fundal massage and consider the treatments shown in Table 17.5.

- If cervical or vaginal lacerations are present, surgical repair is required.

- Retained POCs may be treated with manual uterine sweep maneuvers or dilatation and curettage (DandC) if persistent.

- Extreme measures include uterine artery embolization or emergent hysterectomy.

Chorioamnionitis

Infection of the amniotic fluid and membranes surrounding the fetus.

Symptoms

Intrapartum fever with no other obvious source. This is often associated with fetal or maternal tachycardia, uterine tenderness, foul-smelling amniotic fluid, and leukocytosis. Risk factors include prolonged ROMs, untreated vaginal infection including group B *Streptococcus* (GBS), and multiple exams during labor.

Diagnosis

Most commonly, a clinical diagnosis by increased temperature, maternal or fetal tachycardia, and uterine tenderness.

Labs: The gold standard is amniotic fluid culture. Other amniotic fluid studies, including Gram stain, glucose concentration, white blood cell concentration, leukocyte esterase level, and measurement of cytokines [e.g., interleukin-6 (IL-6)], ceramide lactoside, or short-chain organic acids, have been used in several studies but sensitivity and specificity are still lacking at this time. CBC shows leukocytosis.

Treatment

Treatment with broad-spectrum antibiotics is the standard. Commonly, ampicillin/gentamicin covers for typical bacteria very effectively. Alternatively, clindamycin may be used. Regimens commonly vary. Continue treatment until patient is >24 h afebrile.

Intrapartum Group B *Streptococcus*

Symptoms

Most commonly asymptomatic but may present during pregnancy as urinary tract infection, pyelonephritis, chorioamnionitis, bacteremia, or postpartum endomyometritis. After delivery, neonate is at risk for signs/symptoms of sepsis, bacteremia, or respiratory distress.

Diagnosis

Prepartum risk factor assessment is often done to determine need for intrapartum antibiotic prophylaxis (IAP). Some main risk factors requiring prophylaxis during labor include previous child with invasive GBS infection, GBS bacteriuria during current pregnancy, unknown GBS status during current pregnancy, and labor <37 weeks.

Labs: Commonly, screening cultures of vagina/rectum are taken at 35–37 weeks' gestation. If positive, sensitivities should be done to find the most potent antibiotic for prophylaxis (especially if penicillin-allergic patient).

Treatment

- Penicillin G is the classic first line for prophylaxis. Ampicillin may also be used as first line. Loading doses are used in both cases followed by q. 4-h dosing. Most common practice in the United States is to consider the patient "adequately treated" if ≥ 4 h pass between first dose and delivery of infant. Penicillin-allergic patients should receive clindamycin or erythromycin IV.

- No treatment after delivery is warranted for the mother.

- Standard of care of the infant varies with locale. However, "adequate treatment" status indicates a low level of acuity and concern for further lab investigation of the infant. Most institutions regard infants born to adequately treated mothers virtually equivalent to those born to GBS-negative mothers. Infants born to mothers who are not adequately treated often have blood cultures and CBC with differential [for immature to total (I/T) ratio] drawn to determine risk of GBS sepsis. See section Neonatal Sepsis in Chapter 18.

Postpartum Fever

See Table 17.6.

TABLE 17.6 Seven Ws of postpartum fever

Substance	Treatment
Womb	Endomyometritis
Wind	Atelectasis, pneumonia, PE
Water	Urinary tract infection
Walking	DVT
Wound	Incision, lacerations, hematoma
Weaning	Breast engorgement, mastitis, breast abscess
Wonder drugs	Drug fever

DVT, deep venous thrombosis; PE, pulmonary embolism.

Complications of Labor and Delivery

Definitions

See Table 17.7.

TABLE 17.7 Complications of labor and delivery

Term	Definitions	Diagnosis/associations	Treatment
Premature rupture of membranes (PROM)	Rupture of amniotic membranes before onset of labor	Physical exam to include sterile speculum. Test cervical secretions for nitrazine paper positivity, pooling in post vagina, ferning under microscope	If >36 weeks, induce and augment labor, <36 weeks, antibiotics, steroids, and bed rest
Preterm rupture of membranes	Rupture of amniotic membranes before 37 weeks gestation	Signs as above. By definition, labor is progressing	If >36 weeks, deliver baby. <36 weeks, consider steroids, and deliver
Prolonged rupture of membranes	Ruptured or suspected rupture >18 h	Signs as above. Monitor closely for development of chorioamnionitis	Start antibiotics (ampicillin or pencillin)
Postterm pregnancy	Pregnancy >42 weeks	Complications from macrosomia are increased	Induction and augmentation with special attention to possible complications. Usually offered at 41 weeks gestation to avoid complications

Shoulder Dystocia

Shoulder entrapment during delivery when attempted passage of fetus through birth canal.

Symptoms

Arrest of descent of the fetus during labor. Note ineffective contractions and pushing. The "turtle" sign refers to the head retracting back up the birth canal after a contraction/push.

Diagnosis

Clinical diagnosis at the time of delivery.

Treatment

Several maneuvers are outlined in Table 17.8 and should be performed in the order of appearance shown in the table.

Cesarean Delivery

Know the indications for cesarean section; shown in Table 17.9.

TABLE 17.8 Steps to perform (in the order presented in table) when shoulder dystocia occurs

Maneuver	Definition
McRobert's	Elevation of legs and extreme flexion of hips. Have assistant help with pushing back the mother's knees
Suprapubic pressure	Sharp pressure just superior to pubic symphysis. Meant to dislodge fetal anterior shoulder
Episiotomy	May be cut at any point in delivery to make room for operator's hands
Rubin's	Pressure to the accessible shoulder to push it toward the anterior chest which decreases the bisacromial diameter
Wood's screw	Pressure behind the posterior shoulder to try to turn the infant and dislodge the anterior shoulder. "Screwing the baby out"
Delivery of post arm	Decreases diameter of shoulder
Intentional fracture of clavicle/ humerus	Decreases bisacromial diameter. Associated with good postnatal outcomes
Zavanelli's	Pushing the head and fetus back into the birth canal and performing a stat cesarean section

TABLE 17.9 Indications for cesarean section

Maternal/fetal	Maternal	Fetal	Placental
• Cephalopelvic disproportion (CPD) • Failed induction	• Eclampsia/severe preeclampsia • Eervical cancer • Prior cesarean section (C/S) • Prior uterine rupture • Prior myomectomy • Fibroids • Ovarian tumor	• Nonreassuring fetal monitoring • Bradycardia • Absence of fetal heart tones (FHTs) • Loss of fetal heart variability • Scalp pH <7.20 • Cord prolapse • Fetal malpresentation • Multiple gestation • Hydrocephalus • Ostiogenesis imperfecta • U/S confirmed fetal weight >4500 gms	• Placenta previa • Placental abruption

Q 17.3

An 18-year-old female G1P0 comes to your clinic 6 weeks after a positive pregnancy test with "period-like" vaginal bleeding. Her vital signs are stable and a vaginal exam demonstrates a cervix at 4 cm dilation. An office ultrasound reveals fetal material without heart activity. What is the diagnosis?

A. Blighted ovum.
B. Missed abortion.
C. Inevitable abortion.
D. Incomplete abortion.
E. Threatened abortion.

Pregnancy Loss

Symptoms

See Table 17.10.

Diagnosis

Diagnosis made by history of bleeding or expulsion of POCs coupled with physical exam and assessment of cervical dilation. Other signs may include low symphysis–fundal height for gestational age.

Labs: Before 10 weeks, serial quantitative β-hCG's may be obtained (which should approximately double every 48 h in viable pregnancy). These may show less than doubling in 48-h period indicating nonviable pregnancy or very high results indicating molar pregnancy.

TABLE 17.10 Definitions of pregnancy loss

Term	Definition
Abortus	Fetal loss <20 weeks, 500 g, or 25 cm
Complete abortion	Complete expulsion of all products of conception (POCs)
Incomplete abortion	Partial expulsion of POCs
Inevitable abortion	Bleeding and cervical dilation without expulsion of any POCs
Threatened abortion	Any uterine bleeding before 20 weeks WITHOUT cervical dilation or expulsion of POCs
Missed abortion	Death of fetus without expulsion of any POCs or cervical dilation

Imaging: Doppler ultrasound often does not register a fetal heart beat, which should lead to a pelvic or vaginal ultrasound that shows no heart beat or ectopic pregnancy.

Treatment

- Initially stabilize the patient, then pelvic/vaginal ultrasound is appropriate.
- Treatment, then, depends on type of abortion. Complete abortions may be followed for temperature elevation or signs of infection. Incomplete abortions may be allowed to be completed on their own or a dilation and evacuation (D and E) can also be done, although this is more commonly done for inevitable or missed abortion after significant amount of time has passed. Any recovered POCs should be sent for genetic analysis. Threatened abortions should be followed closely for cessation of bleeding and placed on strict "nil per vagina" status. Rh-immunglobulin, RhoGAM, should be given to all women with vaginal bleeding who are Rh-negative.

Second Trimester

Treatment is as above but with consideration of later pregnancies (~16–24 weeks) the cervical ripening and induction of labor may be tried before D and E. Care should be taken to make sure all POCs are expelled. The possibilities of preterm labor or cervical incompetency should then be assessed and may be treated with future pregnancies.

Q 17.4

A term 32-year-old G3P2 comes to the labor and delivery deck in active labor. She is fully dilated and wants to start pushing. A quick records review reveals the complication of gestational diabetes White classification A2. What two complications does this predispose the fetus to during and after delivery?

A. Velamentous cord insertion and cerebral edema.
B. Shoulder dystocia and cephalohematoma.
C. Ventricular septal defect and reflex hypoglycemia.
D. Shoulder dystocia and reflexive hypoglycemia.
E. Arrest of descent and Erb's palsy.

Gestational Diabetes Mellitus

Symptoms

Generally asymptomatic but may present with classic symptoms of diabetes mellitus (DM) including fatigue, weight loss, polyuria, and polydipsia.

Complications

Maternal

- Polyhydramnios
- Preeclampsia
- Miscarriage
- Infection
- PPH
- Diabetic emergencies such as hypoglycemia, ketoacidosis, diabetic coma.

Fetal

- Macrosomia
- Shoulder dystocia
- Erb's palsy
- Delayed organ maturation
- Reflexive postpartum hypoglycemia
- Congenital malformations including cardiovascular defects, neural tube defects, caudal regression syndrome, situs inversus
- Intrauterine growth restriction (IUGR)

Diagnosis

Found most often with screening test at 24–28 weeks gestation. After screening with 1-h glucose tolerance test (GTT) is positive, confirmation must be made with 3-h GTT (see Tables 17.11 and 17.12).

TABLE 17.11 One-hour glucose tolerance test (after 50 g glucose load)

Test	Normal range
Fasting	<105 mg/dL
1 h	<140 mg/dL

TABLE 17.12 Three-hour glucose tolerance test (after 100 g glucose load)

Test	Normal range
Fasting	<105 mg/dL
1 h	<190 mg/dL
2 h	<165 mg/dL
3 h	<145 mg/dL

Two or more of these levels must be abnormal to diagnose gestational diabetes mellitus (GDM).

TABLE 17.13 Partial White classification of gestational DM

Type	Description
Class A$_1$	GDM; diet controlled
Class A$_2$	GDM; insulin controlled

GDM, gestational diabetes mellitus.

White Classification System of Gestational Diabetes Mellitus

See Table 17.13.

Treatment

- Tight glycemic control is required during pregnancy to reduce complications and birth defects. With class A$_1$, diet can be used to regulate glucose but frequent monitoring must be maintained. In class A$_2$, regular and NPH insulin are used to keep levels in control. Most oral hypoglycemics are contraindicated because of potential teratogenic effects.

- **Prenatal care changes:** After 30 weeks, monitor fetal well-being q. 4–6 weeks by nonstress tests or biophysical profiles. Consider induction at 38–40 weeks to avoid complications of larger babies. Ultrasound confirmed fetal weight more than 4500 g is an indication for cesarean section.

- After delivery, gestational diabetes mellitus (GDM) patients usually do not require insulin. However, since 25%–35% will go on to have nongestational DM in the subsequent 5 years; a 6-week postpartum GTT is usually done. Of those with GDM ~50% will develop the disease in future pregnancies.

Q 17.5

All of the following are relevant laboratory studies in the preeclamptic patient EXCEPT:

A. Lactate dehydrogenase (LDH).
B. Platelets.
C. Hematocrit.
D. Serum albumin.
E. Serum calcium.

Preeclampsia/Eclampsia

Disorder of unknown etiology, although generalized arteriolar constriction plays a role.

Symptoms

Distinction is made between degrees of preeclampsia—mild and severe. Symptoms are few for mild disease, but may include increased edema (not required for diagnosis) often occurring in the hands and face. Severe preeclampsia may include oliguria of <500 mL in 24 h, cerebral or visual disturbances, pulmonary edema, cyanosis, right upper quadrant (RUQ) pain, or fetal growth restriction. Risk factors include: Primigravida, maternal extremes of age, African American origin, chronic hypertension, multiple gestation, and family history of first-degree female relative with preeclampsia/eclampsia.

Eclampsia: Presence of grand mal seizure activity not attributable to other causes. Most often associated with preeclampsia but sometimes occurs *de novo*.

HELLP syndrome: Form of severe preeclampsia that involves *H*emolysis, *E*levated *L*iver enzymes, and *L*ow *P*latelets—memorize this mnemonic. Often accompanied with headache, scotoma, RUQ pain, and oliguria.

Diagnosis

The diagnosis relies on presence of proteinuria and high blood pressure (see Table 17.14). For strict definitions, the levels in table are all that is required.

Severe preeclampsia may also be diagnosed after fulfilling the mild criteria plus any of the following: oliguria of <400 ml/24 h, pulmonary edema, RUQ pain, headache, scotoma, abnormal liver function tests (LFTs), thrombocytopenia, or IUGR.

TABLE 17.14 Classification of preeclampsia

Preeclampsia	Blood pressure guidelines*	Proteinuria†
Mild	>140/90	>300 mg/24 h or 1–2 + urine dipstick
Severe	>160/110	>5 g/24 h or 3–4 + urine dipstick

Source: Diagnosis and Management of Preeclampsia and Eclampsia. Washington (DC): American College of Obstetricians and Gynecologists (ACOG); 2002 Jan. 9 p. (ACOG practice bulletin; no. 33).

* BP must be taken on two different occasions at least 6 h apart.

† Dipstick urine measurements must be on two samples taken 4 h apart.

There is no single lab that will diagnose, but these will provide surveillance of disease:

- CBC for hemoglobin or hematocrit, platelet count.
- Urine assessment of protein (24 h is better than dipstick).
- Serum creatinine.
- Serum uric acid.
- Liver transaminases (AST/ALT).
- Lactate dehydrogenase.
- Coagulation profile (PT, aPTT, INR).
- Serum albumin.
- Blood smear.

Treatment

- Delivery is definitive treatment for preeclampsia/eclampsia.
- **Mild:** Outpatient bed rest and frequent follow-up may be practiced by some, others may choose to monitor with hospital admission. Blood pressure monitoring as well as strict symptom surveillance should be started. Consider atenolol as needed.
- **Severe:** Observation as inpatient. Ultrasound, nonstress test, biophysical profile, and above labs should be done. Bed rest should be in the left lateral decubitus position. Seizure prophylaxes with magnesium sulfate is indicated, but start low and monitor levels closely. This may control blood pressure alone. If further lowering of BP is needed, consider hydralazine or labetalol IV. If pregnancy is after 36 weeks, consider induction and augmentation of labor.
- If eclamptic or severe preeclamptic strongly consider cesarean section.
- Magnesium sulfate should be continued for 12–24 h after delivery. The patient should still be monitored for symptoms of HELLP syndrome.

Q 17.6

A 21-year-old G1P0 37 + 6 week female comes to the labor and delivery deck in the latent phase of the first stage of labor. Her past obstetric history is unremarkable. On exam, you notice moderate extremity edema, which also seems to involve the face. Her vital signs show BP 142/93, HR 97, RR 18, temperature 98.6°F. Intake labs are sent and include a urine dipstick for protein which shows 1+ protein. She complains to you of a recent headache, right side pain, and "missing" a spot in her vision. What therapy should be started below to avoid any unnecessary complications?

A. Iron supplementation.
B. Lorazepam (Ativan).
C. Folate supplementation.
D. Magnesium sulfate.
E. Hydralazine.

Chromosomal Anomalies

Occurs with increased frequency at increased maternal age. After age 35, sharp increase in incidence of malformations.

Symptoms

Abnormalities of amniotic fluid volume (polyhydramnios or oligohydramnios), decreased fetal movement, or abnormal fetal heart rate. See Table 17.15 for postnatal signs/symptoms of disease.

TABLE 17.15 Chromosomal anomalies and their common associations

Term	Definitions
Disorder	Associations
Down syndrome (Trisomy 21)	At birth may have hypotonia, transverse palmar crease, low set ears, absent philtrum, wide spaced eyes. May also find congenital cardiac defects [ventricular septal defect (VSD)], leukemia, duodenal atresia, and early Alzheimer's disease
Edward syndrome (Trisomy 18)	Females > males, mental retardation, small size, small head, hypoplastic mandible, low set ears, **clenched fist with index finger overlapping third and fourth digits**
Patau syndrome (Trisomy 13)	Mental retardation, apnea, deafness, myelomeningocele, cleft lip/palate, **rocker bottom feet**
Turner's syndrome (XO female)	Nuchal lymphedema, short stature, **webbed neck**, widely spaced nipples, **primary amenorrhea**, lack of breast development, **coarctiation of aorta**, horseshoe kidney
Klinefelter's syndrome (XXY male)	Usually silent until adulthood. Slightly decreased IQ, **infertility, microtestes**, gynecomastia, tall stature
Cri-du-chat (deletion of short arm of chromosome 5)	Mental retardation and cry sounding high pitched "like a cat"

Diagnosis

Triple test [estriol, maternal serum α-fetoprotein (MSAFP), and β-hCG] or quadruple test (estriol, MSAFP, β-hCG, inhibin A) , amniocentesis, chorionic villous sampling. The triple/quadruple screen is part of routine labs in many practices, but remember, it gives only a probability of anomaly. When child is born a karotype and genetic testing can be done.

Treatment

- Genetic counseling/testing of parents relating to future pregnancies.
- Follow-up should be close and with multiple specialists depending on anomaly. Heart, lungs, renal, respiratory, and GI systems should be monitored or tested for dysfunction.

Multiple Fetuses

Symptoms

Mothers at advanced ages or using ovulation induction are found with increased rates of multiple gestations. Symptoms may include increased symphysis–fundal height for gestational age, rapid enlargement of uterus, excessive weight gain. Mothers have more complications during pregnancy such as preeclampsia/eclampsia, GDM, cervical incompetence, placenta previa, anemia, PPH, and preterm labor. Risks to fetus include twin–twin transfusions, small for gestational age, and malpresentation.

Diagnosis

Physical exam: Doppler fetal heart rate and physical exam may suggest multiple fetuses.
Imaging: Ultrasound is, however, the best way to diagnose.
Labs: Increased β-hCG and MSAFP are commonly present.

Treatment

Referral to specialist is mandatory. Close monitoring of pregnancy is indicated. Preterm labor is very common. Greater than twins is usually delivered by cesarean section. Perinatologists should be available and on hand. In twins, vaginal delivery may be attempted but if either is breech, take to cesarean section.

Single Liveborn Before Admission to Hospital

Patient delivers child before arriving at hospital or skilled care.

Stabilize patient and child. Obtain records if possible; give prophylactic antibiotics to mother and child. Inspect and repair any lacerations to mother. Obtain screening labs including HIV, syphilis, and hep B. Get chest x-ray and obtain sepsis labs on baby. Assist mother and child through this traumatic event.

Answers

17.1 B. The most common cause of postpartum hemorrhage is uterine atony. The first step in treating utrine atony is fundal massage. Afterwhich, medications should be tried.

17.2 B. Carboprost tromethamine (Hemabate) is a synthetic prostaglandin which stimulates smooth muscle contraction, thus is contraindicated in asthmatics.

17.3 C. The presence of bleeding and cervical dilation as well as the finding of fetal material in the uterus points to inevitable abortion.

17.4 D. Gestational diabetes mellitus (GDM) mothers have a propensity toward large for gestational age or macrosomic babies. Shoulder dystocia is a complication that may occur if the child is too large for the pelvic opening. As well, reflexive hypoglycemia may occur due to the infant's usual overproduction of insulin due to mother's excess blood glucose. When the child is born and the hyperglycemic maternal blood is withdrawn, fetal overproduction of insulin drives the baby's blood sugar down.

17.5 E. Relevant laboratory studies include: CBC for hemoglobin, hematocrit, and platelet count, urine assessment of protein (24 h is better than dipstick), serum creatinine, serum uric acid, liver transaminases (AST/ALT), lactate dehydrogenase, coagulation profile (PT, aPTT, INR), serum albumin, and blood smear.

17.6 D. This patient is suffering from severe preeclampsia by fulfilling the minor mild preeclampsia guidelines for blood pressure and urine protein and she is also having symptoms of right upper quadrant (RUQ) pain, and scotomata. Magnesium sulfate provides prophylaxis against seizures, which is the next progression of the condition.

Conditions Originating in the Perinatal Period	391
Congenital Anomalies	391
Intrauterine Growth Retardation	393
Postterm Infant	393
Birth Trauma	394
Respiratory Problems After Birth	394
Respiratory Distress Syndrome (Hyaline Membrane Disease)	394
Meconium Aspiration	395
Pneumomediastinum/Pneumothorax	396
Transient Tachypnea of the Newborn	397
Neonatal Sepsis	398
Hemolytic Disease due to Rh Isoimmunization	398
Perinatal Jaundice	399
Feeding Problems in Newborns	400

Conditions Originating in the Perinatal Period

Congenital Anomalies

See Table 18.1.

TABLE 18.1 Common congenital anomalies

Anomaly	Associations/diagnosis	Treatment
Cleft lip/palate	Abnormal development of labial groove. Poor feeding and recurrent otitis media	Surgical repair
Gastroschisis	Intestines extrude outside the abdominal wall—**WITHOUT** surrounding membrane. Often **polyhydramnios** during pregnancy	Nasogastric (NG) tube to suction. Sterile gauze dressing with immediate primary surgical closure. May require staged procedures
Omphalocele	Intestines extrude outside the abdominal wall—**WITH** surrounding membrane	Staged surgical repair
Tracheoesophageal fistula	Different types but most common ends in blind esophageal pouch. Presents with severe feeding problems and copious oral secretions	Suction of pouch and surgical repair
Diaphragmatic hernia	Abdominal cavity contents herniated through diaphragm into pleural cavity. Respiratory distress and **scaphoid abdomen**; >95% on left side	Intubation to improve ventilation. Surgical repair
Hirschsprung's disease	Absence of ganglion cells in one specific area intestinal wall. Leading to constriction of bowel. Abdominal distention and vomiting	Diversion with colostomy until >6 months old, then resection of segment with reanastomosis
Choanal atresia	Cyanosis when feeding, which is relieved by crying. Inability to pass an NG tube is pathopneumonic	Surgery

Q 18.1

A male infant is born to a homeless African American female at unknown gestational age. The mother is known to be a polysubstance abuser and has several positive results from a urine drug screen. She did not have prenatal care during pregnancy. What factor below would indicate the poorest prognosis for growth of the infant?

A. Breastfeeding.
B. Asymmetric growth restriction.
C. Symmetric growth restriction.
D. Refusal to vaccinate.
E. Selection of a formula without iron.

Intrauterine Growth Retardation

Symptoms

Associated with smoking, high blood pressure/preeclampsia, EtOH use, narcotic or amphetamine use, infections including cytomegalovirus, rubella and *Toxoplasma gondii*, placental insufficiency, genetic factors, and inadequate calorie intake in pregnancy.

Diagnosis

Physical exam: Often large discrepancy in fundal height for gestational age (after 20 weeks).

Imaging: Ultrasound is the gold standard. May need level II ultrasound to confirm.

Key points to look for are symmetric versus asymmetric growth restriction.

- **Asymmetric** often occurs with placental problems or malnutrition states. Head is relatively spared from abnormal growth and is apparent later in pregnancy. Associated with better prognosis and "catch-up" growth postpartum.

- **Symmetric** often occurs with congenital infection or genetic problems. Head is symmetrically included in abnormal growth. Poorer prognosis for normal growth after birth.

Treatment

Largely depends on the cause. For asymmetric growth restriction, proper nutrition, and close, frequent followup are warranted. For symmetric growth restriction, investigation of possible causes is needed and treatment should be aimed at etiology. Often, prevention and good prenatal care is the best approach.

Postterm Infant

Symptoms

Any infant born after 42 weeks gestation. Main risk is of being hypoglycemic or macrosomic with accompanying risks. This can include birth trauma, that is, shoulder dystocia, Erb's palsy, and other conditions.

Diagnosis

Establish dates of pregnancy.
Check for birth trauma and hypoglycemia.
Meconium aspiration is more common with later pregnancy.

Treatment

Prevention with induction and augmentation of labor should be offered and discussed at 41 weeks' gestation.

Q 18.2

A G2P1 Caucasian female at 39 + 4/7 weeks gestation has given birth to a 3750 gm male infant via vacuum-assisted vaginal delivery. The birth was complicated only by three "pop offs" of the vacuum extractor but otherwise was uncomplicated. You are consulted to evaluate the child for newborn exam. Vital signs are within normal limits. Head is atraumatic with moderate skull molding. A boggy, dark area is noted on the top most area of the head with limitations of extension by normal underlying skull sutures. Otherwise, the exam is normal. What laboratory value below will likely be found abnormal in the neonatal period?

A. White blood cell count.
B. Serum sodium levels.
C. Serum iron levels.
D. Serum glucose levels.
E. Bilirubin levels.

Birth Trauma

See Table 18.2.
See Chapter 17, shoulder dystocia section.

Respiratory Problems After Birth

Respiratory Distress Syndrome (Hyaline Membrane Disease)

Respiratory distress due to lack of mature surfactant in lungs.

Symptoms

Newborn with nasal flaring, cyanosis, grunting, or substernal retractions (accessory muscle use for respiration). Usually difficult to calm and fussy.

TABLE 18.2 Common birth traumas

Trauma	Diagnosis/associations	Treatment
Cephalohematoma	Subperiosteal hemorrhage **limited by skull sutures**. Often associated with vacuum delivery. Exam will differentiate from other trauma such as subgaleal hemorrhage	None necessary. May cause hyperbilirubinemia from blood breakdown as it resolves. Rarely can show calcifications
Subgaleal hemorrhage	Trauma to subgaleal vessels and is an emergency. **Crosses the skull sutures**. Felt as a generalized boggy scalp	Surgical evacuation of blood
Erb's palsy	Upper brachial plexus (C5–C6) injury. Adduction/internal rotation of shoulder with pronation of wrist. "Waiter's tip" position	Bracing close to body and monitoring for likely improvement
Klumpke's palsy	Lower brachial plexus (C7–T1) injury. Paralysis of the hand and wrist. May be in "claw hand" position	Bracing and passive physical therapy. Likely improvement

Diagnosis

Physical exam: Crackles throughout lung fields, low O_2 saturation, and high breathing rate.

Labs: Arterial blood gas (ABG) shows low PO_2 and high PCO_2.

Imaging: Stat portable chest x-ray (CXR) often shows diffuse "ground glass" appearance indicating atelectasis. Air bronchograms often present (see Figure 18.1).

Treatment

- Start with oxygen therapy through "blow by." Quickly move to "oxyhood" therapy (sometimes called oxygen tent) over baby's head to improve delivery of oxygen. Consider positive pressure ventilation or intubation and mechanical ventilation. Transfer to the neonatal ICU. Artificial surfactant, beractant (Survanta), given through endotracheal tube is the gold standard.

- If risk factors such as prematurity and gestational diabetes mellitus (GDM) exist, prevention is with steroids before delivery.

Meconium Aspiration

A pneumonitis, not pneumonia.

Symptoms

Newborn with nasal flaring, cyanosis, grunting, or substernal retractions (accessory muscle use for respiration). Usually difficult to calm and fussy. Exam often reveals prominent crackles throughout lungs. If air trapping occurs from proximal bronchial obstruction, "barrel chest" appearance may result. Look for signs of tension pneumothorax.

Diagnosis

Often born with meconium-stained amniotic fluid. Obtain O_2 saturation and breathing rate.

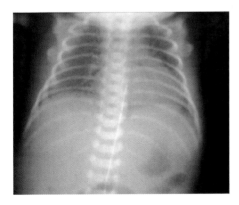

FIGURE 18.1 Chest radiograph showing typical appearance of neonatal respiratory distress syndrome (RDS).

Courtesy: Michael D'Alessandro, with permission, 2007.

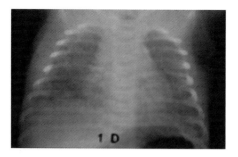

FIGURE 18.2 Typical chest x-ray of neonatal meconium aspiration. Meconium aspiration.

Courtesy: Michael D'Alessandro, with permission, 2007.

Labs: ABG shows low PO_2 and high PCO_2.

Imaging: Stat portable CXR often shows diffuse opacities in lungs or atelectasis. Should *not* show consolidation (see Figure 18.2).

Treatment

In delivery room, DeLee suctioning may be used to clear nose, mouth, and pharynx. If baby has not cried yet when transferred to resuscitation team, consider suctioning below the vocal cords with an endotracheal tube (not DeLee suction). If baby has cried, simply clear the fluid from mouth, nose, and pharynx with suction. Passing a nasogastric (NG) tube and suctioning the contents of the stomach may also act to decompress the pleural cavity. If baby still exhibits signs of respiratory distress, start oxygen therapy. Consider positive pressure ventilation or intubation and mechanical ventilation.

Pneumomediastinum/Pneumothorax

Symptoms

Signs of respiratory distress and tachypnea. May have loss of lung sounds in one field on exam. History may have positive pressure ventilation or mechanical ventilation after birth. Exam may reveal anterior superior subdermal emphysema.

Diagnosis

Physical exam: Low O_2 saturation, high breathing rate, and clinically in respiratory distress. Transillumination may reveal "flash" of light at end of expiratory cycle indicating abnormality.

Labs: ABG may show low PO_2 and high PCO_2.

Imaging: CXR shows increased, sharp heart border and lack of vascular markings extending to sides of lung fields.

Treatment

If infant is in otherwise unresponsive respiratory distress, a chest tube may be placed. If oxygenating well (with or without O_2 supplement) defect may be observed and followed without treatment. The vast majority resolve on their own.

Transient Tachypnea of the Newborn

Symptoms

Fast breathing and fussiness. Often seen in term or near-term infants.

Diagnosis

Physical exam: Low O_2 saturation, mild respiratory distress symptoms of nasal flaring, subcostal retractions, grunting, tachypnea, and possibly cyanosis.
Labs: ABG may show low PO_2, high PCO_2.
Imaging: CXR will show hyperinflated lungs with streaky perihilar markings, giving the appearance of a **shaggy heart border** with clear lung peripheries.

Treatment

- Oxygen support therapy. Intubation and mechanical ventilation are rarely needed.

- Duration is usually 12–24 h but may last as long as 72 h.

Q 18.3

A term female infant born to a G3P2 female ~24 h ago is noticed by nursing to have an increased respiratory rate and low temperature. The child appears to be small for gestational age. You are consulted and after examining the patient you order laboratory studies which are shown below:

WBC 20.9 × 1000 mm³.
Hemoglobin 18.2 g/dl.
Hematocrit 54.9%.
Platelet 242 × 1000/m³.

Diff:
Segmented neutrophil 45%.
Band form 18%.
Lymphocyte 15%.
Monocyte 10%.
C-reactive protein (CRP) 0.3 mg/dL.

Blood cultures pending.

What is the most concerning laboratory finding above?

A. Increased white blood cell count.
B. Increased immature to mature (I/M) ratio of neutrophil forms.
C. Increased band form neutrophils.
D. Increased immature to total (I/T) ratio of neutrophil forms.
E. Increased CRP.

Q 18.4

After talking to the obstetrician and clarifying the mother's history, you find she had very uncertain dating criteria for the pregnancy. If clinical improvement does not occur and the patient continues to do poorly, what is the next step in management for the most likely cause of disease?

A. Antibiotics which include ampicillin and gentamicin.
B. Artificial surfactant instillation.
C. Steroid therapy.
D. A 10% dextrose IV solution for the baby.
E. Chest tube placement.

Neonatal Sepsis

Symptoms

Respiratory distress (tachypnea, grunting, subcostal retractions, nasal flaring, etc.), temperature instability (more often lower than normal temp rather than fever), and low blood glucose. Risk factor assessment may reveal prolonged rupture of membranes (PROM) or maternal group B strep infection.

Diagnosis

Labs: Obtain CRP, blood cultures, and CBC with manual differential. Expect absolute white count to be elevated. With manual differential, calculate the I/T ratio:

$$\frac{I}{T} = \frac{Immature}{Total} = \frac{Bands}{Bands + segs + other\ immature\ cells}$$

Normal is <2–2.5. If >2.5, this indicates a sign of sepsis.
Imaging: CXR. Look for opacity indicative of pneumonia.

Treatment

- Move baby to warmer conditions to support body temperature.
- Start antibiotics. Classically, ampicillin and gentamicin.
- Obtain peripheral IV access and consider starting fluids.
- Monitor with periodic heel stick glucoses and repeat labs in 6–12 h.
- Monitor closely.

Hemolytic Disease due to Rh Isoimmunization

Erythroblastosis fetalis: The increased production of erythroblasts of the fetus in response to destruction and hemolysis by maternal antibodies.
Hydrops fetalis: A condition of severe hemolytic disease from maternal antibodies. Not compatible with life.

Symptoms

Rh negative mother has had previous exposure to Rh-positive blood, either in previous pregnancy or other exposures. Pregnancy may be associated with polyhydramnios or history of previous miscarriage or still born. Newborn may range from fairly asymptomatic to pale, with scalp edema, cardiomegaly, hepatomegaly, pleural effusions, and ascites. Often babies continue to develop jaundice secondary to hemolytic antibodies.

Diagnosis

Labs: Before birth, amniotic fluid sampling for bilirubin levels may help determine whether and to what degree hemolytic disease has affected the newborn. At birth, cord blood sample must be taken to determine fetal blood type. Do direct Coombs test and bilirubin level on this blood. If Coombs is positive, obtain fetal hemoglobin/hematocrit and reticulocyte count.

Treatment

- For mild cases, may range from no treatment with close followup to regular transfusion. For moderate-to-severe disease, **exchange transfusion** is indicated. This may be done early with partial exchange or later with double exchange depending on severity of hemolysis. Phototherapy may decrease fetal bilirubin levels transiently but is not the treatment for the hemolytic disease. Also correct acidosis and accompanying disorders, for example, heart failure.

- Transfer to the neonatal ICU.

- Remember to give mother RhoGAM to the mother at 72 h postpartum.

Perinatal Jaundice

See Table 18.3.

Symptoms

Yellow appearance to the skin and eyes. Jaundice tends to occur from the head down.

Diagnosis

Physical exam: May approximate the degree of jaundice by correlation of the anatomic level of jaundice with level of bilirubin. This is only an approximation.

Labs: Obtain total, indirect (unconjugated), and direct (conjugated) bilirubin levels from serum. Physiologically bilirubin levels should peak in the range of 12–15 mg/dL at day 2–5 and may be associated with mild jaundice. Higher levels or jaundice appearing <24 h of life are always pathologic. Otherwise bilirubin levels are compared to established nomograms to determine levels appropriate for time after birth. If abnormal, obtain a second level and

TABLE 18.3 Jaundice in the newborn

Disorder	Associations	Treatment
Physiologic	Mild jaundice appearing in term or preterm infants with levels peaking at 2–5 days and not exceeding 15 mg/dL	Phototherapy
Breast milk jaundice	Occurring in breastfed infants and usually peaking at ~20 mg/dL at 2–3 weeks of age	Treatment is to switch to bottle feeding and monitor for resolution
Illness	Infection and sepsis, hypothyroidism, liver toxicity, cystic fibrosis, and others may induce a hyperbilirubin state	Correct the disorder
Hemolysis due to maternal Rh antibodies	May present as erythroblastosis fetalis or milder form of hemolysis	See above for treatment
Metabolic derangement	Immaturity or genetic disorder of hepatic conjugating enzymes. May include Crigler–Najjar, Gilbert syndrome, or Dubin–Johnson syndrome	Phototherapy or none
Biliary atresia	May be accompanied by grayish, clay-colored stools	Treat with surgery
Medications	Sulfa drugs	Stop offending agent
Kernicterus	Often billirubin levels >25 mg/dL (although may occur lower if comorbidity present). Clinically may have spasticity, seizures, lethargy, and other neurologic signs	Neurologic damage often permanent. Prevention is key. Prompt phototherapy and exchange transfusion is treatment

calculate the hourly rate of rise. A linear relationship may then be assumed and used to extrapolate possible rise in bilirubin in future (although a linear relationship admittedly does not exist). Follow increased levels of bilirubin until they trend downward.

Treatment

- May depend on degree of hyperbilirubinemia. Mild-to-moderate disease may be treated with phototherapy "bili-lights." This conjugates bilirubin through the skin.

- Severe cases may be taken to neonatal ICU for exchange transfusion.

Feeding Problems in Newborns

Symptoms

Excessive fussiness, spitting up, lethargy, or lack of suck reflex.

Diagnosis

Difficulty feeding often involves common problems such as breastfeeding difficulties and milk allergy. If breastfed, observe mother and child breastfeeding; make sure latch is correct and beneficial as this is the most common breastfeeding problem. Milk allergy is suspected and diagnosis is supported if feeding problems resolve after switch to soy-based formula. Other allergies can be discovered after switch to hypoallergenic formula.

Initial milk from mother is colostrum and should be replaced with normal breast milk after ~3 days of breastfeeding postpartum.

Remember, <10% weight loss in newborns is normal. Return to birth weight is expected by the second week of life.

Treatment

- In case of breastfeeding problems, consider breastfeeding training by licensed, experienced breastfeeding nurse.

- For milk or formula allergy, switch to soy or hypoallergenic formula. Remember to choose iron-fortified formula.

Answers

18.1 C. Symmetric growth restriction of the baby indicates the poorest prognosis for catch-up growth in the future.

18.2 E. This patient likely has a cephalohematoma by the presence of the risk factor of vacuum extraction at delivery and suggestive exam showing limitation of bogginess by skull sutures. Associated bilirubin levels often increase when the cephalohematoma begins to break down hemolyse. This may clinically be seen as jaundice.

18.3 D. In neonates the best interpretation of the CBC and differential is done with the I/T ratio, which in this child is elevated at 0.29 (18/63). This is an increased ratio indicating possible septic process.

18.4 B. This patient now has the possible risk factor of prematurity, which should lead you to consider respiratory distress syndrome (hyaline membrane disease). Respiratory distress syndrome (RDS) is the lack of mature lung surfactant for which the treatment is instillation of artificial surfactant into the lungs. Other answers given either do not treat this most likely condition, or are inappropriate therapy.

19   Statistics/Ethics/Health Maintenance

Statistics	404
Sensitivity	405
Specificity	405
Positive Predictive Value	405
Negative Predictive Value	405
Incidence	405
Prevalence	405
Relative Risk	406
Odds Ratio	406
Absolute Risk Reduction	406
Relative Risk Reduction	406
ARR Versus RRR Example	407
Number Needed to Treat	407
p-Value	407
Confidence Interval	407
Error Types	407
Study Design	408
Cohort	408
Case Control	408
Cross-sectional Prevalence Survey	408
Randomized Control Trial	408
Meta-analysis	408
Ethics	408
Withdrawal of Care	408
Euthanasia	409
Physician-Assisted Suicide	409
Advanced Directive	409
Health Care Power of Attorney	409
Restraints	409
Involuntary Hold	409
Competence	409
Informed Consent	410
Health Care of Minors (Age <18 years)	410
Health Maintenance	410
Vaccinations	410
Cancer Screening	410
Cervical Cancer	410
Breast Cancer	411

Prostate Cancer	412
Colorectal Cancer	412
Drugs of Abuse	413
Smoking Cessation	413

Statistics

Q 19.1

A research technology company is testing a new UV light device for accurately telling malignant versus benign lesions on the surface of skin using reflected UV light. The device is tested using 1000 volunteers from Southern California. Suspicious skin lesions are identified in an objective manner and placed under the device for readings. The device is removed and the lesion biopsied, which is considered the gold standard. Results are reported as positive or negative and compared with the biopsy result (positive being any cancer, any stage/grade). The results are as follows:

Light device:		Biopsy:	
Positive	570	Positive	660
Negative	430	Negative	340
		False positive	90
		False negative	30

What is the sensitivity of the test?

A. 0.95
B. 0.86
C. 0.82
D. 0.93
E. 1.00

Q 19.2

What is the positive predictive value of the test?

A. 0.95
B. 0.86
C. 0.82
D. 0.93
E. 1.00

TABLE 19.1 2 × 2 table of outcomes based on disease presence and results of test

	Disease	No disease
Positive test	A	B
Negative test	C	D

Sensitivity

Sensitivity is the probability that a person with a certain disease will have a positive test result. Basically, sensitivity is a measure of how well a test will show a positive result when the disease is present. High sensitivity is desirable for a screening test (See Table 19.1).

$$\text{Sensitivity} = A/(A + C).$$

Specificity

Specificity is the probability that a person without the disease will have a negative test result. Basically, specificity is the measure of how well a test will show a negative result when the disease is not present. High specificity is desirable for a confirmatory test.

$$\text{Specificity} = D/(B + D).$$

Positive Predictive Value

Positive predictive value (PPV) is the probability that a person with a positive test result has the disease. Basically, PPV is a measure of how much you can rely on a positive result to actually be positive.

$$\text{PPV} = A/(A + B).$$

Negative Predictive Value

Negative predictive value (NPV) is the probability that a person with a negative test result does not have the disease. Basically, NPV is a measure of how much you can rely on a negative result to actually be negative.

$$\text{NPV} = D/(C+D).$$

Incidence

Incidence is the number of new cases of disease per specified number of a general population per specified unit of time. Thus, a new disease may have an incidence of 1/100,000 people per year.

Prevalence

Prevalence is the number of cases, new or old, present in a population at one (usually now) point in time. Thus, a disease may have a prevalence of 2.5/100,000 people in the United States.

Q 19.3

A medical epidemiologist at the local state university wants to conduct a research project involving the relationship between exposure to asbestos ore mining and development of mesothelioma lung cancer in the mine workers. He is able to find a group of workers, now retired from the mine, and have them complete a questionnaire regarding their health since working in the mines. Data is collected and statistical analysis completed. What results below may be calculated?

A. Relative risk ratio since this is a cross sectional study.
B. Relative risk ratio since this is a retrospective study.
C. Odds ratio (OR) since this is a prospective study.
D. OR since this is a retrospective study.
E. Neither OR nor relative risk ratio since this is a survey study.

TABLE 19.2 2 × 2 table of outcomes based on exposure and disease development

	Disease develops	No disease
Exposure	a	b
No exposure	c	d

Relative Risk

Relative risk (RR) compares the chance of a given disease in the group exposed to the particular risk factor with the chance of disease in those not exposed to the risk factor. Seen in prospective or experimental studies (See Table 19.2).

$$RR = \frac{[a/(a+b)]}{[c/(c+d)]}$$

Odds Ratio

OR describes the odds of exposure to a given risk factor in individuals with the disease compared to those without the disease. Used in retrospective studies.

$$OR = ad/bc$$

Absolute Risk Reduction

Absolute risk reduction (ARR) is a measure of risk reduction in the treated group as compared to the placebo group. Basically, the change in risk in the treated group as measured on the same scale to the untreated group. Used in randomized control trials.

$$ARR = \text{untreated group risk} - \text{treated group risk.}$$

Relative Risk Reduction

Relative risk reduction (RRR) is a measure of risk reduction in the treated group as a percentage of the untreated group risk. Used in randomized control trials.

$$RRR = (\text{untreated group risk} - \text{treated group risk})/\text{untreated group risk.}$$

ARR Versus RRR Example

A large population of smokers is enrolled in a multicentric study to measure the effect of a new cancer-preventing medication called Cancergon on the incidence of lung cancer. Smokers are followed up for a total of 10 years while they continue to smoke. The placebo group is given a sugar pill and the treatment group is given Cancergon, both once a day. The experimental groups are followed up throughout the study period, and the placebo group was found to have developed cancer at a rate of 5%. The treated group was found to have developed cancer at a rate of 3%. The absolute risk reduction of Cancergon is $5 - 3 = 2\%$. The relative risk reduction of Cancergon is $2/5 = 0.4 = 40\%$. For obvious reasons, many pharmaceutical companies express results of their trials in relative risk reductions.

Number Needed to Treat

Number needed to treat (NNT) is the number of individuals needed to treat in order to save one life.

$$NNT = 1/ARR.$$

p-Value

A p-value is the expression of the chance that an observed outcome is the product of random chance alone. A p-value of <0.05 (accepted value for statistical significance) means that the observed outcome has a $<5\%$ chance that it was a random occurrence.

Confidence Interval

Confidence interval (CI) expresses the certainty that the result of the study is real or a random chance. The percentage is the reciprocal of p-value. Used with RR or OR, CI states the percentage chance the observed RR or OR is within the interval stated.

Error Types

Type 1 error: Rejection of the null hypothesis when it is true—an arrogant error.

Type 2 error: Acceptance of the null hypothesis when it is not true—a humble error.

Study Design

Cohort

Selects a large population and divides it into groups based on exposure to a given risk factor. Generally, this population is observed **prospectively** and the development of disease is recorded. May be retrospective in some cases. RR is calculated. Disadvantages include cost and time.

Case Control

Selects a population with a particular disease and looks **retrospectively** to evaluate presence or absence of a given risk factor. OR is calculated. Good for rare diseases but must be retrospective.

Cross-sectional Prevalence Survey

Looks at a given population for presence of disease and risk factors. A causative link cannot be established for disease and risk factors. Takes place at one point in time.

Randomized Control Trial

A study in which subjects are randomly assigned to placebo or treatment groups, intervention is given over a specified time interval, and effects are recorded. The gold standard amongst study designs. Double blinded refers to the situation in which both experimenter and subject are unaware of which group, placebo or treatment, the subjects belong to (of course a key does exist). Single blind refers to blinding of only the subjects. Disadvantages include cost, time, and risks to subjects.

Meta-analysis

Analysis of past studies in regard to a particular clinical question. Basically, the pooling of much research on a particular subject in an attempt to consolidate a higher *N*-number and derive an answer closer to actual truth. A study of studies.

Ethics

Withdrawal of Care

The withdrawal or stoppage of medical care upon the request or presumed will of the patient. The person holding health care power of attorney may make this decision for the patient.

Euthanasia

The active administration of lethal means to end the patient's life, usually in an attempt to end suffering or prolonged illness. Euthanasia is done in the presumed best interest of the patient.

Physician-Assisted Suicide

The assistance of the physician to commit active suicide by the patient. Physician-assisted suicide (PAS) is completed at the expressed request of the patient. The only state it is legal in is Oregon.

Advanced Directive

A document reviewed and signed by the patient to direct their end-of-life decisions. They vary in details but consist of a written document stating the limitations of desired interventions during a life-threatening event or situation. These include Do-Not-Resuscitate and Do-Not-Intubate orders.

Health Care Power of Attorney

A designated or defaulted representative who is trusted by the patient to make competent end-of-life decisions on the patient's behalf. This is usually specifically designated in a legal document. However, upon the patient's incapacitation, it is often defaulted to the next of kin (spouse, children, etc.). If an advanced directive does not exist, the holder of the health care power of attorney is legally able to make end-of-life decisions.

Restraints

Use of chemical or physical restraints may be employed by the physician (usually attending only) on the basis of the patient's physical danger to themselves or others. A written "restraint note" detailing the indication, use, limitations of use, and time of expiration is required to be placed on the medical record on a daily basis in most states. Details and timing vary by state.

Involuntary Hold

The involuntary admission or committal of patients due to the belief of the physician they are in danger of being harm to themselves or others. The laws regarding involuntary hold (IH) vary by state; however, hold without court involvement is usually allowed for 48–72 h. After this period, a court hearing must be convened to further hold the patient against their will.

Competence

A judgment or legal distinction regarding patients' comprehension and ability to understand their current health care situation. This also implies the ability to make sound, rational decisions in their own best interest. The physician is often called upon to judge competence, which should be done by interview regarding both general issues and their current situation. The extreme classic case is that a depressed, suicidal patient should not be considered competent to choose whether he or she should be allowed to die or not.

Informed Consent

The relaying of information to the patients from the physician regarding their health care. This has several aspects, which include diagnosis, prognosis without treatment, prognosis with treatment, detailed proposed treatment, alternative treatments, and risks/benefits of the proposed treatment. Informed consent may be granted only if the patient is deemed competent; otherwise it must be discussed with the patient's holder of health care power of attorney.

Health Care of Minors (Age <18 years)

Minors may give informed consent and be treated as adults in specific situations, although specific laws vary by state. These situations include pregnancy; birth control; sexually transmitted diseases (STDs); and the patient being married, being legally emancipated from guardians, raising children, living independently, or serving in the Armed Forces. Never delay emergent care of a minor for lack of parental consent.

Health Maintenance

Vaccinations

Current recommendations include vaccination for the following diseases: Hep A and B, diphtheria, tetanus, pertussis, *Haemophilus influenzae* type B (Hib), polio, measles, mumps, rubella, varicella, herpes zoster, *Meningococcus*, *Pneumonococcus*, rotavirus, and human papillomavirus (HPV). Individual safety and allergy contraindications vary. Requirements for children upon entry to school vary by state. Immunocompromised patients should never receive a live virus vaccine. Pregnant patients should not receive measles mumps rubella (MMR), varicella, herpes zoster, or HPV vaccine.

See http://www.cdc.gov/vaccines for more information.

An outline of vaccines and times for vaccination is given in Table 19.3.

Cancer Screening

Cervical Cancer

Different groups have slightly different recommendations on when/how often to begin screening. American College of Obstetricians and Gynecologists (ACOG) recommends starting within 3 years of sexual activity or age 21 and then annually until age 30. After age 30, screen every 2–3 years if the patient has had three consecutive negative Paps. The United States Preventative Services Task Force (USPSTF) recommends at least every 3 years and makes

TABLE 19.3 Recommended vaccination schedule

Vaccine	Recommended schedule
Hep B	Birth, 1–2, 6–18 months
Diphtheria–tetanus–acellular pertussis (DTaP)	2, 4, 6, 15–18 months, 4–6 years
Haemophilus influenzae type B (Hib) no need for expansion here	2, 4, 6, 12–18 months
Inactivated poliovirus (IPV)	2, 4, 6–18 months, 4–6 years
Pneumococcal conjugate vaccine (PCV)	2, 4, 6, 12–15 months
Measles-mumps-rubella (MMR)*	12–15 months, 4–6 years
Varicella*	12–15 months, 4–6 years
Hep A	12–23, 18–41 months
Influenza	>6 months
Meningococcal conjugate	11–12 years
Human papillomavirus (HPV)	11–12 years (+ 2 months, then +6 months)
Rotavirus*	2, 4, 6 months
Herpes zoster	60 years
Pneumococcal polysaccharide vaccine (PPV)	≥65 years

* Live virus vaccines.

no distinction after age 30. The American Cancer Society (ACS) recommends starting within 3 years of sexual activity or age 21 and annually until age 30 if using the conventional Pap or every 2 years if with cytologic-based technique. After age 30, every 2–3 years if the patient has had three negative Paps.

Breast Cancer

Screening: Different recommending bodies differ on recommendations for screening especially under the age of 50. The American Medical Association (AMA), the American College of Radiology (ACR), and the ACS all support screening with mammography and clinical breast exam (CBE) beginning at age 40. ACOG supports screening with mammography beginning at age 40 and CBE beginning at age 19. The American Academy of Family Physicians (AAFP) recommends beginning mammography for average-risk women at age 50, with mammography in high-risk women beginning at age 40. The AAFP recommends that all women aged 40–49 be counseled about the risks and benefits of mammography before making decisions about screening.

Organizations also differ on their recommendations for the appropriate interval for mammography. Annual mammography is recommended by

AMA, ACR, and ACS. Mammography every 1–2 years is recommended by the AAFP. And finally, ACOG recommends mammography every 1–2 years for women aged 40–49 and annually for women aged 50 and older.

Prostate Cancer

Screening is a controversial subject because early detection and current treatments have not shown to reduce morbidity and mortality. The USPSTF recommendations include acknowledgment of prostate-specific antigen (PSA) and digital rectal exam (DRE) as being useful in detecting early prostate cancer but does not recommend doing such screening because of lack of evidence of benefit. The AAFP agrees with the USPSTF. The ACS, however, states that since PSA and DRE have proven useful in cancer detection, yearly screening should start at age 50 (or age 45 in high-risk individuals). Thus, there is apparent disagreement, not in the effectiveness of detection, but the impact of the lack of benefit of treatment.

Colorectal Cancer

The ACS recommends screening average-risk patients for colorectal cancer beginning at age 50 years by one of the following:

- Fecal occult blood testing (FOBT, performed on two to three consecutive stools at home; in office, single FOBT is inadequate) annually.
- Flexible sigmoidoscopy every 5 years.
- Annual FOBT plus flexible sigmoidoscopy every 5 years.
- Double-contrast barium enema every 5 years.
- Colonoscopy every 10 years.

These recommendations are supported by the USPSTF and AAFP.

Increased-risk and high-risk patients generally should obtain colonoscopy every 1–3 years.

Q 19.5

Which of the following street drugs does not have a recognized withdrawal syndrome?

A. Cocaine.
B. Lysergic acid diethylamide (LSD).
C. Phencyclidine hydrochloride (PCP).
D. Opioids.
E. Amphetamines.

Drugs of Abuse

See Table 19.4.

Smoking Cessation

Smoking cessation includes several stages. Treatment may be tailored to the individual stage. These include:

Precontemplative: Inquire whether the patients would like to quit smoking. If not, remind them of the health effects and offer literature for assistance.

Contemplative: Patients agree or want to quit, but not within a specified time table. Counsel them further on benefits of quitting and reassure of techniques to quit, and pharmacologic and social support.

Action: Plan on date of last cigarette/chew, and provide counseling, group classes, or behavioral therapies to assist. Assess suitability for pharmacologic assistance. These include:

- Nicotine replacement techniques—gum, patch, lozenges, inhaler, etc. These techniques encourage the patient to get used to an

TABLE 19.4 Common street drugs

Illicit drug	Intoxication	Withdrawal syndrome	Treatment
Opioids (heroin, Rx pain meds)	Central nervous system (CNS) depression, pupillary constriction, respiratory depression, constipation	Yes	Naloxone (Narcan) acutely
Amphetamines (Crystal, speed, crank)	Psychomotor agitation, tachycardia, pupillary dilation, paranoia, sudden death	Yes	Haloperidol (Haldol) or other antipsychotics; benzodiazepines acutely as needed
Phencyclidine hydrochloride (PCP)	Belligerence, psychosis, violence, vertical/horizontal nystagmus	Yes	Benzodiazepines acutely; Haloperidol may be useful to calm patient
Lysergic acid diethylamide (LSD, Acid)	Hallucinations, delusions, pupillary dilation	No	Benzodiazepines acutely
Marijuana (Pot, grass)	Euphoria, impaired judgment, dry mouth, increased appetite conjunctival injection, paranoia	No	Isolation from drug
Cocaine (Crack, etc)	Euphoria, insomnia, impulsive behavior, arrhythmia, cerebral infarct, paranoid ideation, weight loss	Yes	Benzodiazepines and antipsychotics acutely; clonidine, amantadine, carbamazepine may decrease cravings

alternate form of delivery of the same addiction. Then, a slow taper off will provide the end nicotine. Do not underdose, especially in the beginning.

- Bupropion (Zyban)—reduces the urge to continue smoking. Initially, this technique is harder to quit with but suppresses the urge to quit after acute phase.

- Combination therapy may be effective in those with strong addictions.

- Varenicline (Chantix) is another option and consists of a partial nicotine agonist effect.

Maintenance: Close follow-up and/or social support groups have shown higher success rates in this stage. Consider addition or dosage elevation if needed.

Relapse: Identify trigger barriers, assess strategies, and formulate another plan for quitting.

Answers

UV device	Cancer	No cancer
Positive test	570	90
Negative test	30	430

19.1 A. Sensitivity equals $570/(570 + 30) = 0.95$.

19.2 B. Positive predictive value (PPV) equals $570/(570 + 90) = 0.86$.

19.3 D. Since this research will be one of the finding disease in a group exposed to a certain risk factor, it is a retrospective study. Odds ratio may be calculated in retrospective studies.

19.4 C. p-value is, by definition, the chance the observed outcome occurs by the chance alone.

19.5 B. LSD has no recognized withdrawal syndrome although patients at the end of their high may experience depressive symptoms or apathy.

Index

Note: Page numbers in *italics* refer to figures and tables.

Abdominal aortic
aneurysm, 264–265
Abdominal injury, 234–235
Abnormal Pap smear, 359–360
Bethesda system of, *360*
Abnormal uterine
bleeding, 357–358, *358*
Abortus, *382*
Abrasion, corneal, 74–75
Abscess, 364–365
bartholin, 364–365
brain, 14
breast, 350
perianal, 320–321
perirectal, 320–321
peritonsillar, 83
skin, 145
Absolute risk reduction (ARR), 406
vs RRR, 407
Acne vulgaris, 141–142
Acquired immune deficiency
syndrome (AIDS), 190–192
Acrochordons, *153*
Actinic keratosis, 148, 153, *154*
Acute bronchiolitis, 277–278
Acute bronchitis, 277
Acute myocardial
infarction, 251–253
Acute pancreatitis, 302–304
Ranson's criteria for, 302, *303*
Acute parametritis, 354–355
Acute Physiology and Chronic
Health Evaluation II
(APACHE II) score
acute pancreatitis, 302
Acute renal failure, 332–334
classification of, *333*
Addisonian crisis, 105
Addison's disease, 104–105
Adenocarcinoma, *286*, 298
Adenoma

toxic, 96
Adenovirus, 212–213
Adjustment disorder, 46
Adrenal gland, disorders
Addison's disease, 104–105
Cushing's syndrome, 103–104
hyperaldosteronism and Conn's
syndrome, 105–106
pheochromocytoma, 107
Adrenocorticotropic hormone
(ACTH)
dependant causes, 103
independent causes, 103
Advanced directive, 409
Agoraphobia, panic disorder in, 42
Akathisia, 60
Alcoholic hallucinosis, *57*
Alcohol withdrawal, 57–58
Allergic rhinitis, 84, 282
α-Fetoprotein, 341
Alzheimer's disease, 15–16
Amaurosis fugax, transient
ischemic attack, in, 28
Amblyopia, strabismus related, 73
Amenorrhea, *358*, 366, *367*
American Academy of Family
Physicians (AAFP), 79, 319,
340, 348, 411, 412
American Academy of Pediatrics
(AAP), 79
American Cancer Society
(ACS), 319, 340, 348, 360,
411, 412
American College of Cardiology
(ACC), 261
American College of Chest
Physicians (ACCP), 261, 281
American College of Obstetricians
and Gynecologists
(ACOG), 348, 360, 410,
411, 412

American College of Physicians
(ACP), 261
American College of Radiology
(ACR), 348, 411, 412
American College of Rheumatology
(ACR), 160, 163
American Diabetic Association
(ADA), 97
American Medical Association
(AMA), 348, 411, 412
Amphetamines, *59*, *413*
Amyotrophic lateral sclerosis
(Lou Gehrig's disease), 18
Anaplastic thyroid cancer, 92
Anemias, 129
macrocytic, 130
folate/vitamin B_{12}
deficiency, 130
microcytic, 129
iron deficiency anemia, 129
lead poisoning, 129
thalassemia, 129
normocytic, 129–130
acute blood loss, 129
anemia of chronic
disease, 129
G6PD deficiency, 130
sickle cell, 130–132
acute chest syndrome, 130
aplastic crisis, 130
Aneurysm, abdominal
aortic, 264–265
Angina pectoris, 253–254
Anhydrosis, 285
Animal Bite
infection prophylaxis, 241
rabies, 10–11
Anion gap, diabetic
ketoacidosis, 99, 100
Ankle-brachial index (ABI), 265
Ankle sprain, 181–182

Ankylosing spondylitis, 174–175
Ann-Arbor staging system,
  lymphoma, 124
Anorexia nervosa, 51
Anterior cruciate ligament
  (ACL) tear, *165*
Anterior wall, vaginal
  prolapse of, *363*
Anticholinergic medications
  intranasal, allergic rhinitis, *84*
  overdose, 228
  Parkinson's disease, 17
Anticholinesterase inhibitors
  Alzheimer's disease, 15
Anti-GBM syndrome, *330*
Antihistamines
  allergic rhinitis, *84*
Antihypertensive classes
  characteristics of, *249*
Antinuclear antibody (ANA),
  systemic lupus
  erythematosus, *161*
Antisocial disorder, *60*
Anxiety disorder, 43–44
Apnea test, brain death in, 37
Apolipoprotein E gene
  Alzheimer's disease, 15
Appendicitis, 309
Arrhythmias
  asystole/pulseless electrical
    activity, 263
  atrial fibrillation/flutter,
    260–261
    hyperthyroidism, 95
  ventricular fibrillation, 262
  ventricular tachycardia, 261–262
  Wolff–Parkinson–White
    syndrome (WPW), 263–264
Arterial embolism, 266
Arterial thrombosis, 266
Arthritis
  infective, 179–180
  osteo, 182–183
  rheumatoid, 162–164
Asthma, 282–283, *284*
  classification of, *283*
Astigmatism, *68*
Asystole/pulseless electrical
  activity, 263
Ataxia-telangiectasia, immune
  deficiency, *120*
Atherosclerosis, 270
Atrial fibrillation, 260–261
Atrial flutter, 260–261
Atrial septal defect, *273*

Attention deficit disorder
  (ADD), 52
Attention deficit hyperactivity
  disorder (ADHD), 52
Autistic disorder, 54
Avoidant disorder, *60*

Babinski sign
  multiple sclerosis, 17
Bacterial vaginosis, of
  vulva/vagina, *363*
Bacterial vs viral pneumonia, *279*
Barium enema, intestinal
  obstruction, 310
Barium swallow study,
  dysphagia, 299
Barrett's esophagus, 298
Bartholin cyst, 364–365
Basal cell carcinoma, 149–150
Behavioral disorders, *52*
Bence Jones proteins, multiple
  myeloma, 125
Benign neoplasm
  of breast, 349–350
  of small intestine, 308
Benign prostatic
  hypertrophy, 342–343
Benign skin lesions, *153–155*
Bereavement, 46
β-Human chorionic gonadotropin
  (β-hCG), 341
Biceps tendonitis, *166*
Bilateral hilar
  lymphadenopathy, 288
Biliary atresia, perinatal
  jaundice, *400*
Bipolar disorders, 48–49
Birth, and delivery, 371
Birth trauma, *394*
Bishop score, labor and
  delivery, 373
Bisphosphonates, osteoporosis, 173
  hypercalcemia, 126
Bites, 226
Bladder
  hypotonic (flaccid), 324
  malignant neoplasm of, 323–324
  neurogenic, 324–325
  spastic (contractile), 324, 325
Blastomycosis, *205*
Bleeding. *See* Hemorrhage
Blepharitis, *71*
Blue bloaters, 280
Body dysmorphic disorder, *50*
Body surface area (BSA), *242, 243*

Borderline disorder, *60*
Boxer's fracture, *178*
Brain abscess, 14
Brain cancer, 33
Brain death, 36–37
BRCA 1,2
  breast cancer, 339
Breast
  benign neoplasm of, 349–350
    carcinoma, surgical
      treatment of, 349
    malignant neoplasm of, 348–349
Breast abscess, 350
Breast cancer, 339, 411–412
Breast feeding
  feeding problems in
    newborn, 400–401
  jaundice, *400*
Brief psychotic disorder, *43*
Bronchiolitis
  acute, 277–278
Bronchitis
  acute, 277
  chronic, 280–281
Bronchus
  malignant neoplasm of, 285–286
Bulimia nervosa, 51
Burns, 241–244
Bursitis, 167

CA-125, ovarian cancer, 351
Café-au-lait macules,
  neurofibromatosis, 157
Caffeine withdrawal, headache, 33
Calcium, metabolism of, *115*
Calculus, urinary, 334–335, *335*
Caloric response reflex, brain
  death in, 37
Campylobacter infections,
  intestinal, *186*
C-ANCA (cytoplasmic
  antineutrophilic
  cytoplasmic antibody), 295
Cancer
  basal cell, 149–150
  bladder, 323–324
  brain, 33
  breast, 339, 411–412
  bronchus, 285–286, *286*
  cervical, 410–411
  colorectal, 319–320, 412
  of esophagus, 298
  hepatic, 308
  kidney, 327–328
  laryngeal, 88–89

lip, 89
liver, 307–308
lung, 285–286, *286*
oral cavity, 89
pancreas, 304–305
pharyngeal, 89
prostate, 412
  malignant neoplasm
    of, 340–341
skin, melanoma, 150–152
smoking cessation, 413–414
squamous cell, 148–149, *286*
stomach, 300
testicular, 341
uterine, 355
Candidiasis, 140–141, 204–205
  of vulva/vagina, *363*
Carbamazepine (Tegretol)
  trigeminal neuralgia, 23
Cardinal ligaments, vaginal
    prolapse of, *363*
Cardinal movements of
    delivery, 374
Cardiomyopathy, 255
  hypertrophic, 255–256
Cardiovascular diseases, 247–273
Carotid stenosis, transient ischemic
    attack (TIA), *29*
Carotid endarterectomy, transient
    ischemic attack (TIA), 29
Case control, 408
Cataracts, 68
Cat scratch disease, 211–212
Cauda equina syndrome, 176
Cavities, dental. *See* Dental caries
Cellulitis, 143–144, *144*
  orbital, 72–73
  pelvic, 354–355
Centers for Disease Control and
    Prevention (CDC)
  HIV infection, 190
  pulmonary tuberculosis, 288
Central nervous system (CNS)
  degenerative/hereditary
    diseases of, 15–37
  infectious diseases of, 8–15
Central pontine myelinolysis
  hyponatremia, 117
Central retinal artery occlusion, *65*
Central retinal vein occlusion, *65*
Cephalohematoma, *394*
Cerebral palsy, 22–23
Cerebrospinal fluid (CSF)
  encephalitis, 12
  meningitis, 12

Cervical cancer, 410–411
Cervical exam, labor and
    delivery, *373*
Cervical motion tenderness
  cervicitis, 361
  pelvic inflammatory disease, 354
Cervicitis, 361
Cervix
  malignant neoplasm of, 358–359
Cesarean delivery, 380, *381*
Chancroid, *204*
Charcoal, activated, poisoning, 228
Charcot's triad, 305
Chest tube
  spontaneous pneumothorax, 294
  pneumothorax, 296
Chicken pox, 195
Childbirth, 371–389
Childhood exanthems, *200–201*
Chlamydia, *204*
  urethritis, 325
Choanal atresia, *392*
Cholangiocarcinoma, 307
Cholangitis, 307
Cholecystectomy, 305
Cholecystitis, 305
Choledocholithiasis, 305
Cholelithiasis, 305
Cholesteatoma, 80
Cholesterol, hyper
  HDL, *112*
  LDL, *113*
  total, 112
Chorioamnionitis, 377–378
Chromosomal anomalies,
    387–388, *387*
Chronic bronchitis, 280–281
Chronic obstructive pulmonary
    disease (COPD), 280–281
Chronic renal failure/insufficiency,
    331–332
Clavicle fracture, *179*
Cleft lip/palate, *392*
Clostridium difficile, intestinal
    infection, *186*
Cluster, headache, *33*
Coarctation of aorta, *273*
Cocaine, 59, 413
Coccidioidomycosis, *205*
Cohort, 408
Colchicine, gout use in, 114
Collagen vascular diseases, *171*
Colle's fracture, *178*
Colorectal cancer, 319–320, 412
Coma, 35–36

Common cold. *See* Rhinovirus
Competence, 409–410
Complete abortion, *382*
Complex regional pain
    syndrome, 18–19
Computer case simulation
    (CCS), 3
  real time vs simulated time
    control screen, 4
    final order, 5
    history, 3–4
    initial order, 4–5
    physical, 4
    respond appropriate, 5
Concussion, 245–246
Conduct disorder, *52*
Confidence interval (CI), 407
Congenital anomalies, *392*
Congenital heart disease, *273*
Congestive heart failure,
    256–257
  New York Heart Association
    classification of, 257
Cognitive behavioral therapy
    (CBT), 43, 44, 45, 49, 51
Conjunctivitis, 70
Conn's syndrome, 105–106
Conversion disorder, *50*
Corneal abrasion, 74–75
Coronary heart disease
    equivalents, *112*, 113
Cosyntropin stimulation test,
    Addison's disease, 105
Cotton wool spots, diabetes in, 63
Cranial injury, 233–234
Creutzfeldt–Jakob disease, 10
Cri-du-chat, *387*
Crohn's disease
  vs ulcerative colitis, *312*
Cross-sectional prevalence
    survey, 408
Croup, 275–276
Cryptorchidism, testicular
    cancer, 341
Cullen's sign, pancreatitis, 302
Cushing's syndrome, 103–104
Cyst, bartholin, 364–365
Cystic fibrosis, 289–291
Cystic kidney disease, 334
Cystitis, uncomplicated, 325–326
Cytomegalic inclusion disease, 212

Dacryostenosis, *71*
Deafness. *See* Hearing loss
Death, brain, 36–37

Deceleration, fetal heart rate, labor and delivery
early, 373
late, 374
variable, 373
Decongestants
allergic rhinitis, *84*
Deep venous thrombosis. *See* Venous thrombosis
Dehiscence, surgery complication, *242*
Delirium, 32
Delirium tremens, *57*
Delivery
and labor. *See also* Childbirth
complications of, *379*, 385–386
with minor or no complications, 372–375
Dementia, 55–56
Alzheimer's disease, 15
Creutzfeldt-Jakob disease, 10
Dental caries, 87–88
Dependent disorder, *60*
Depressants, *229*
Depressive episodes/disorders, 47–48
Dermatology, 139–158
Dermatomyositis, *170*
Dermatophytosis, 203
Developmental musculoskeletal deformities, *173*
Deviated nasal septum, *85*
Dexamethasone suppression test, Cushing's syndrome, 104
Diabetes insipidus, 102
Diabetes mellitus, 97–100
diabetic ketoacidosis, 98–100
gestational, 383–385
ophthalmic manifestations of, 63–64
Diagnostic peritoneal lavage (DPL), internal injuries, *235*
Dialysis
renal failure, 333
Diaphragmatic hernia, 392
Diethylstilbestrol (DES), vaginal cancer, 362
DiGeorge syndrome (Thymic aplasia), immune deficiency, *120*
Diplopia, 68
Direct inguinal hernia, *317*
Disc herniation, intervertebral, 175–176
Dislocation, shoulder *166*

anterior, 165
Disseminated intravascular coagulation (DIC), 135
Diverticular disease, 311
Diverticulitis, 311
Diverticulosis, 311
Dix-Hallpike maneuver
vertiginous disorders, 81
Dopamine, Parkinson's disease in, 17
Down syndrome, *387*
mental retardation, 20
Drugs of abuse, 413
Drusen deposits, macular degeneration in, 64
Duke's criteria
endocarditis, 271, *272*
colorectal cancer, 319
Duplex ultrasonography, 28
Dysfunctional uterine bleeding, *358*
Dysmenorrhea, 365
Dysphagia, 299–300
Dystocia, shoulder, 380, *380*

Ear, foreign body in, *227*
Eaton–Lambert syndrome, *286*
Eclampsia, 385, 386. *See also* Preeclampsia
Eczema, 282
Edrophonium (Tensilon) test, myasthenia gravis, 25
Edward syndrome, *387*
Ehlers–Danlos syndrome, *171*
Electroencephalogram (EEG), seizure disorder, 22
Electrolyte disorders, 116–120
Electromyography (EMG)
amyotrophic lateral sclerosis, 18
Emergency problems, 223–246
Emphysema, 280–281
Encephalitis, 13–14
Endocervicitis, 361
Endocrine disorders
diabetes insipidus, 102
syndrome inappropriate antidiuretic hormone, 102–103
Endocrine glands, disorder
hypoglycemia, 100–101
Endocrinology, 91–120
Endometriosis, 356–357
End-organ hypertensive effects, 249–250

Endoscopic retrograde cholangiopancreatography (ERCP), 307
Enuresis, 327
Epididymitis, 344
Epidural hematoma, *27*
Epiglottitis, *189*
Epistaxis, 85
Epley maneuver
vertiginous disorders, 81
Epstein-Barr virus. *See* Infectious mononucleosis
Erb's palsy, *394*
Error types, 407–408
Erysipelas, 143–144, *144*
Erythema chronicum migrans, Lyme disease in, 218, *219*
Erythema infectiosum, *200*
"slapped cheek" appearance of, *201*
Erythema nodosum
with inflammatory bowel disease, *313*
Erythroblastosis fetalis, 398
Escherichia coli infection, *189*
Esophageal varices, 298–299
Esophagus
cancer of, 298
foreign body in, *227*
Esotropia, 73
Ethics
advanced directive, 409
competence, 409–410
euthanasia, 409
health care power of attorney, 409
informed consent, 410
involuntary hold, 409
minors, health care of, 410
physician-assisted suicide (PAS), 409
restraints, 409
withdrawal of care, 408
EtOH (alcohol) withdrawal, 57–58
Euthanasia, 409
Euthyroid syndrome, 94
Exophthalmos, 95
Exotropia, 73
Eye injuries
blunt trauma to, 225–226
chemical burns of, 224–225
foreign body in, 224
Eyelid, disorder, *71*

Facial fractures, *178, 234*
Factitious disorder, *50*
Familial adenomatous
    polyposis (FAP), colorectal
    cancer, 319
FAST ultrasound, internal
    injuries, *235*
Female infertility, 368–369
Female reproductive system,
    diseases of, 347–369
Fetal strips, basics of, 373–374
Fibrillation
    atrial, 260–261
    ventricular, 262, *262*
Fibroadenoma and fibrocystic
    changes, benign masses of
    the breast, 349
Fibula fracture, *179*
Fitz-Hugh–Curtis mechanism, 354
Fluid disorders, 116–120
Follicular thyroid cancer, 92
Folliculitis, 145–146
Food poisoning, 227–228
    intestinal infection, *186*
Foot disease, 208
Forced expiratory volume in
    1 second (FEV1)
    asthma, 282
Foreign bodies
    ear in, *227*
    esophagus, *227*
    eye in, *224*
    larynx in, *227*
    nose in, *227*
    pharynx in, *227*
    trachea in, *227*
Fractional excretion of sodium
    (FENa)
    hyponatremia, 116
    renal failure, 333
Fractures, *178–179*
    boxer's, *178*
    clavicle, *179*
    Colle's, *178*
    comminuted, *179*
    compound, *179*
    facial, *178, 234*
    fibula, *179*
    greenstick, *178*
    hip, *179*
    oblique, *179*
    pelvis, 234–235
    rib, *179*
    Salter-Harris, *178*
    skull, 177–178

spiral, *179*
tibia, *179*
vertebral body, *179*
Fragile X syndrome
    mental retardation, 20
Frostbite, 235–236

Gabapentin (Neurontin), 24, 49
Gallstones, 305–307
Ganglion cyst, 169
Gardnerella, of vulva/vagina, *363*
Gastritis, 301
Gastroenteritis, intestinal
    infection, *186*
Gastroenterology, 297–322
Gastrointestinal bleeding,
    316–317
    lower, 316
    peptic ulcer disease, 316
    upper, 316
Gastroschisis, *392*
Genital warts, *204*
Gestational diabetes
    mellitus, 383–385
    complications of, 383
    White classification
        system of, 384–385, *384*
Giardia lamblia, intestinal
    infection, 186
Glasgow Coma Scale, 36
Glaucoma, 66–67
    closed-angle, *67*
    open-angle, 66
Gleason score, prostate cancer, 340
Glomerulonephritis, 330, *330–331*
Glucose-6-phosphatase deficiency,
    malaria in, 218
Glucose tolerance test (GTT),
    383, *384*
Goiter, toxic multinodular,
    hyperthyroidism, 96
*Gonorrhea, 204. See also Neisseria
    gonorrhea*
Goodpasture's syndrome, *330*
Gout, 113–114
Graded exercise training, 265
Graves disease, hyperthyroidism,
    95, 96
Greenstick fracture, *178*
Greif. *See* Bereavement
Grey Turner sign, pancreatitis, 302
Group B *Streptococcus*,
    intrapartum, 378
Guillain–Barré syndrome,
    25–26, 214

HACEK organisms,
    endocarditis, 271
Haemophilus influenzae
    infection, *189*
Hallucinogens, *229*
Hand, infectious tenosynovitis
    of, 168–169
Hand disease, 208, *209*
Hashimoto's thyroiditis, 93
Headache, *33*
    worst in life, subarachnoid
        hemorrhage, 26
Health care of minors, 410
Health care power of attorney, 409
Health maintenance
    vaccination, 410, *411*
Hearing loss, 82–83
Heart block, 258–259
    first-degree, 258, *259*
    second-degree, *259*
    third-degree, *259*
Heart failure, congestive,
    256–257
Heat stroke, 239
Heberden's nodes, 182, *183*
Helicobacter pylori infection
    gastritis, 301
    peptic ulcer disease, 300
HELLP syndrome, 385, *386*
Hematology, 123–138
Hematoma, surgery
    complication, *242*
Hemolytic disease
    to Rh isoimmunization,
        398–399
Hemolytic uremic
    syndrome, 137–138
Hemophilia, 135–136
Hemorrhage
    abnormal uterine, 357–358, *358*
    complicating surgery, 240–241
    "dot and blot", diabetes in, 63
    dysfunctional uterine, *358*
    gastrointestinal, 316–317
    postpartum, 376–377, *376, 377*
    subarachnoid, 26–27
    subgaleal, *394*
Hemorrhoids, 321–322
Hepatitis, *206*
Hepatitis B markers, *206, 207*
Hereditary angioneuroctic edema,
    immune deficiency, *120*
Hernia, 317–318, *317, 318*
    diaphragmatic, *392*
    direct inguinal, *317*

Hernia (*Cont.*)
  incarcerated, *317*
  indirect inguinal, *317*
  inguinal, *343*
  reducible, *317*
  strangulated, *317*
Herpes simplex virus, 196–198
  encephalitis, 13–14
  meningitis, 13
Highly active antiretroviral therapy
      (HAART), *191*
Hip dysplasia, *173*
Hip fracture, *179*
Hirschprung's disease, *392*
Histoplasmosis, *205*
Histrionic disorder, *60*
HIV infection, 190–192
Hodgkin's lymphoma, 123–124
Hordeolum, *71*
Horner's syndrome, 285, *286*
Human herpesvirus 8 (HHV8),
      Kaposi's sarcoma, 194
Human immunodeficiency virus
      (HIV), 190–192
  prophylaxis in, 191, *192*
Human papillomavirus
      (HPV), 147–148
Hyaline membrane
      disease, 394–395
Hydrocele, *343*
Hydrops fetalis, 398
Hydroxy iminodiacetic
      acid (HIDA) scan,
      gallstones, *306*
Hymen, imperforate, 364
Hyperaldosteronism, 105–106
Hypercholesterolemia, 270
Hypercoagulable states,
      134–135
Hyperkalemia, 118
Hyperlipidemia, 92, *113*, 329
Hypernatremia, 117
Hyperopia, *68*
Hyperparathyroidism, 101
Hypertension, 248–249
  classifications of, *248*
  end organ effects, 249–250
  pulmonary, 292–293
  secondary, 250–251
Hyperthyroidism, 95–96
Hypertriglyceridemia, 302
Hypertrophic cardiomyopathy,
      255–256
Hypertrophic obstructive
      cardiomyopathy (HOCM).

See Hypertrophic
      cardiomyopathy
Hypertrophic scar formation,
      153, 242
Hypervolemia, 119–120
Hypochondriasis, *50*
Hypoglycemia, 100–101
Hypokalemia, 117–118
Hypomania, bipolar in, 49
Hyponatremia, 116–117
  SIADH in, 102–103
Hypothermia, 236–237
Hypothyroidism, 92–94
Hypotonic (flaccid) bladder, 324
Hypovolemia, 118–119
Hysterectomy. *See* Total abdominal
      hysterectomy/bilateral
      salpingectomy (TAH/BSO)
Hysterosalpingogram, 368

Idiopathic hypertrophic
      subaortic stenosis.
      See Cardiomyopathy,
      hypertrophic
Idiopathic thrombocytopenic
      purpura, 136–138
IgA deficiency, immune
      deficiency, *120*
IgA nephropathy, *330*
Immunity deficiency, *120*
Imperforate hymen, 364
Impetigo, 146
Impingement, 165, *166*
Imrie (Glasgow) rating scale,
      pancreatitis, 302
Incarcerated hernia, *317*
Incidence, 405
Incomplete abortion, *382*
Incontinence. *See* Stress
      incontinence in female
Incubation periods and
      infectivity, *221–222*
Indirect inguinal hernia, *317*
Inevitable abortion, *382*
Infection, postoperative, 241
Infectious diseases, 185–215
Infectious Diseases Society
      of America
      pulmonary tuberculosis, 287
Infectious endocarditis, 270–272
  Duke's criteria for, 271, *272*
Infectious mononucleosis, 209–211
Infective arthritis, 179–180
Infertility
  female, 368–369

male, 345–346
Inflammatory bowel disease,
      312, *312*, 313
  Crohn's disease vs ulcerative
      colitis, 312
  erythema nodosum with, *313*
  pyoderma gangrenosum
      with, *313*
Influenza, 278–280
Informed consent, 410
Inguinal hernia, *343*
Inhalants, *229*
Insomnia, 35
Insulin, diabetes mellitus, *97*, 98
Intelligence Quotient (IQ)
  mental retardation, 19, *20*
Internal injury, 234–235
Intestinal infection, *186*
Intestinal obstruction, 310
Intraocular pressure,
      glaucoma in, 66
Intrapartum antibiotic prophylaxis
      (IAP), 378
Intrapartum group B
      Streptococcus, 378
Intrauterine growth retardation
      (IUGR), 393
Involuntary hold, 409
Iodine deficiency,
      hypothyroidism, 93
  radioactive, 94
Iron deficiency anemia
      (IDA), 129
Irritable bowel syndrome,
      314–315
Ischemic stroke, 29–30
I/T ratio, neonatal sepsis, 398

Jarisch–Herxheimer reaction,
      syphilis in, 203
Jaundice, in newborn, 399–340
  kernicterus, *400*
Joint committee of the American
      Thoracic Society (ATS)
      pulmonary tuberculosis, 287

Kanavel's signs, infectious
      tenosynovitis of the
      hand, 168
Kaposi's Sarcoma, 194
Kawasaki's disease, *200*
Keloid and hypertrophic scar,
      153, 242
Keratocanthoma, *153, 154*
Kernicterus, *400*

Kernig's and Brudzinski's signs
    (meningitis), 12
Kidney
    diseases of, 323–336
    malignant neoplasm of, 327–328
Klinefelter's syndrome, 387
Klumpke's palsy, 394
Knee, internal derangement
    of, 164, 165
Koplik's spots, on oral buccal
    mucosa, 199
Krukenberg tumor, 300, 350
KUB (kidney/ureters/bladder)
    plain film, 335

Labor, 373
    and delivery. See also Childbirth
        complications of, 379, 385–386
        with minor or no
            complications, 372–375
    stages of, 373
Labrynthitis, 80
Laceration, perineal
    types of, 374–375
Lachrymal system, disorder, 71
Laryngeal carcinoma, 88–89
Larynx, foreign body in, 227
Lateral collateral ligament
    (LCL), 165
Lead poisoning, anemia, 129
Le Fort facial fracture, 178, 234
Legg–Calvé–Perthes disease, 173
Leiomyoma, of uterus, 355–356
Leukemia
    acute lymphocytic leukemia
        (ALL), 127–128
    acute myelogenous leukemia
        (AML), 127–128
    chronic lymphocytic leukemia
        (CLL), 127–128
    chronic myelogenous leukemia
        (CML), 127–128
Leukotriene antagonists
    allergic rhinitis, 84
Levodopa-carbidopa, 17
Levothyroxine, thyroid
    disorders, 94
Lewy bodies
    Parkinson's disease, 17
Lhermitte's sign, multiple
    sclerosis, 17
Lichen sclerosis, 364
Lip cancer, 89
Lipid metabolism,
    disorders, 112–113

Lipoma, 153
Liver
    malignant neoplasm of,
        307–308
Lockjaw (trismus). See Tetanus
Lou Gehrig's diesease (ALS), 18
Lower gastrointestinal
    bleeding, 316
Lower postvaginal wall, vaginal
    prolapse of, 363
Lund and Browder chart,
    burns in, 243
Lungs
    malignant neoplasm of, 285–286
Lyme disease, 218
Lymphadenopathy, 211
Lysergic acid diethylamide
    (LSD), 59, 413

Macular degeneration, 64–65
Magnesium, metabolism of, 115
Magnesium sulfate, therapy,
    preeclampsia/eclampsia
    in, 386
Major depressive episodes/disorders,
    47–48
Malaria, 216–218
Male infertility, 345–346
Male reproductive system,
    diseases of, 339–346
Malignant intracranial
    neoplasm, 30–31
Malignant melanoma, 150–152
Malignant metastases, 177
Malignant neoplasm. See also
    Cancer
    of brain, 30–31
    of bladder, 323–324
    of breast, 348–349
    of bronchus and lung,
        285–286, 286
        paraneoplastic syndromes
            and, 286
    of cervix, 358–359
    of kidney, 327–328
    of liver, 307–308
    of ovary, 350–351
    of pancreas, 304–305
    of prostate cancer, 340–341
    of stomach, 300
    of uterus, 355
    of vagina, 362
    of vulva, 362
Malingering, 50
Malnutrition

kwashiorkor, 108, 108
marasmus, 108, 109
mineral deficiencies, 110
protein-energy, 108–109
vitamin deficiencies, 109–110
Mania, bipolar in, 48
Manning criteria, irritable bowel
    syndrome, 314
Marfan syndrome, 171
Marijuana, 59, 413
Mast cell stabilizers
    allergic rhinitis, 84
Mastectomy
    modified radical, 349
    radical, 349
    segmental, 349
    simple, 349
Mastitis, 350
Mastoiditis, 77–78
Mean arterial pressure
    (MAP), subarachnoid
    hemorrhage, 27
Measles, 198–199
Meconium aspiration, 395–396
Medial collateral ligament
    (MCL), 165
Medicinal and biologic substances
    effects of, 231–232
Medullary thyroid cancer, 92
Meigs' syndrome, 350
Meningitis, 12–13
Meniscal tear, 165
Menometrorrhagia, 358
Menopause, 367–368
Menorrhagia, 358
Mental retardation, 19–20
Meta-analysis, 408
Metabolic/immunity disorders, 111
    gout, 113–114
    lipid metabolism, 112–113
    mineral metabolism, 114–115
    phenylketonuria, 111
Metastasis, malignant
    musculoskeletal, 177
Methicillin-resistant Staphylococcus
    aureus (MRSA)
    cellulitis, 143, 144
    skin abscess, 143
Metrorrhagia, 358
Middle ear effusion (MEE)
    hearing loss, 82
    otitis media, 79
Migraine, 31–32
Miller Fisher test, 16
Mineral deficiencies, 110

Mineral metabolism,
    disorders, 114–115
  calcium, *115*
  magnesium, *115*
  phosphorus, *115*
Minimal change disease, *330*
Mini-Mental Status Exam
  Alzheimer's disease, 15
  dementia, 55
Minor withdrawal, *57*
Miosis, 285
Missed abortion, *382*
Mobitz type heart block
  type I, *259*
  type II, *259*
Molluscum contagiosum, 211
Mononucleosis. *See* Infectious
    mononucleosis
Mood stabilizers, 49
Movements, cardinal,
    delivery in, 374
Mouth disease, 208, *209*
Multiple endocrine neoplasia type
    II (MEN II), 92
  pheochromocytoma, 107
Multiple fetuses, 388
Multiple myeloma, 125–126
Multiple sclerosis, 17–18
Mumps, 207
  orchitis of, *208*
  parotitis of, *208*
Murphy's sign
  gallstones, 305
  primary sclerosing
    cholangitis, 307
Muscular fatigability, 24
Musculoskeletal system,
    159–183
Myasthenia gravis, 24–25
Mycoses, *205*
Myocardial infarction,
    acute, 251–253
Myocarditis, 258
Myopia, *68*
Myositis, *170*
Myxedema coma, hypothyroidism,
    92, 94

Narcissistic disorder, *60*
Nasal malformations, *85*
National Institutes of Health
    (NIH), polycystic ovarian
    syndrome, 352
National Osteoporosis Foundation
    (NOF), 172

Negative predictive value
    (NPV), 405
Neisseria gonorrhea
  cervicitis/endocervicitis, 361
  epididymitis, 344
  orchitis, 344
  pelvic inflammatory disease, 354
  prostatitis, 342
  urethritis, 325
Neisseria meningitidis, 12
Neonate. *See* Newborn
Neoplasm of the breast
  benign, 349–350
  malignant, 348–349
Neoplasm of the small intestine,
    benign, 308
Nephrolithiasis. *See* Urinary
    calculus
Nephrotic syndrome, 328–329
Neurofibromatosis, 157–158
  bilateral acoustic, 157
  von Recklinghausen
    disease, 157
Neurogenic bladder, 324–325
  hypotonic (flaccid), 324
  spastic (contractile), 324, 325
Neuroleptic malignant
    syndrome, 41
Neuroleptics
  atypical, 41
  typical, 41–42
Neurology, 7–37
Newborn, 391–401
  feeding problem in, 400–401
  transient tachypnea of, 397
New York Heart Association
    classification of CHF, 257
N-methyl-D-aspartate (NMDA)
    receptor antagonists
  Alzheimer's disease, 15
Non-Hodgkin's
    lymphoma, 124–125
Nonmedicinal substance ingestion
    treatment of, *230*
Non-solid malignancies, 123
Normal pressure hydrocephalus, 16
Nose, foreign body in, *227*
Number needed to treat
    (NNT), 407
Nystagmus, 73–74

Obsessive-compulsive disorder,
    44–45, *60*
Obstruction, intestinal, 310
Obturator sign, appendicitis, 309

Oculocephalic/oculovestibular
    reflex, brain death in, 37
Odds ratio (OR), 406
Oligomenorrhea, *358*
Omphalocele, *392*
Onychomycosis, 142–143
Ophthalmic manifestations of
    diabetes, 63–64
Ophthalmology, 63–75
Opioids, *229*
Oppositional defiant disorder, *52*
Oral cavity cancer, 89
Orbital cellulitis, 72–73
Orchitis, 344
Osteoarthritis, 182–183
Osteomyelitis, 219–221
Osteoporosis, 172–173
  Cushing's disease, 103
  hyperthyroidism, 95
Otitis media, 79, *189*
Outcomes, table of, 405
Ovarian cyst, 351–352
Ovary
  malignant neoplasm of, 350–351

Pacemaker, 255, 256
Pancreas
  malignant neoplasm of,
    304–305
Pancreatitis
  acute, 302–304
    Ranson's criteria for,
      302, *303*
Panic attacks, 42–43
Papillary thyroid cancer, 92
Pap smear, abnormal, 359–360
Paralysis, 22, 25, 55, 92
Parametritis, acute, 354–355
Paraneoplastic syndromes
  with lung malignancy, *286*
Paranoid disorder, *59*
Paraplegia, 20–21
Parathyroid gland, disorders
  hyperparathyroidism, 101
Parkinson's disease, 16–17
Parkland formula, burns in, 244
Patau syndrome, *387*
Patent ductus arteriosis
    (PDA), *273*, 274
Pelvic cellulitis, 354–355
Pelvic inflammatory disease. *See*
    Pelvic cellulitis
Pelvis fracture, 234–235
Peptic ulcer disease, 300–301
Perianal abscess, 320–321

Pericarditis, 254–255
Perinatal period, conditions
 originating in, 391–394
 birth trauma, *394*
 congenital anomalies, *392*
 intrauterine growth
  retardation, 393
 postterm infant, 393
Perinuclear antineutrophil
 cytoplasmic antibody
 (p-ANCA), ulcerative
 colitis, 307, *312*
"Periodic lateralized epileptiform
 discharges" (PLEDs),
 encephalitis, 14
Peripheral vascular disease, 265
Perirectal abscess, 320–321
Peritonitis, 315–316
Peritonsillar abscess, 83
Personality disorders, *59–60*
Pertussis, 294–295
Pharyngeal cancer, 89
Pharynx, foreign body in, *227*
Phencyclidine hydrochloride
 (PCP), *59*
Phenylketonuria, 111
 mental retardation, 19
Pheochromocytoma, 107
Phobias, 44
Phosphorus, metabolism of, *115*
Physician assisted suicide, 409
Pink puffers, 280
Pneumoconiosis, 283–285
Pneumocystis carinii
  pneumonia, 192–193
Pneumomediastinum, 396
Pneumonia, *189*, 278, *279*
Pneumothorax, 396
 spontaneous, 294
Podagra, gout, 114
Poisoning, 228–229
Poliomyelitis, 9
 postpoliomyelitis progressive
  muscular atrophy
  (PPMA), 9
 postpolio syndrome (PPS), 9
Polycystic ovarian syndrome
 (PCOS), 352–353
Polycythemia, 133
Polymalgia rheumatica, *170*
Polymenorrhea, *358*
Polymyositis, *170*
Polyp
 gastrointestinal, 319
 nasal, 84, *85*

Positive predictive value
 (PPV), 405
Postconcussive syndrome, 56
Posterior cruciate ligament
 (PCL) tear, *165*
Postictal state, seizure disorder,
 21, 22
Postherpetic neuralgia, 195
Postoperative infection, 241
Postpartum fever, 379
Postpartum hemorrhage, 376–377
 characteristics of, *377*
 classification of, *376*
Postpoliomyelitis progressive
  muscular atrophy
  (PPMA), 9
Postpolio syndrome (PPS), 9
Poststreptococcal
  glomerulonephritis, *341*
Postterm infant, 393
Postterm pregnancy, *379*
Posttraumatic stress
  disorder, 45–46
Pott's disease, tuberculosis, 287
Preeclampsia, 385–386. *See also*
  Eclampsia
 classification of, *386*
Pregnancy, 371–389
 cesarean, 380, *381*
 loss, 381–382, *382*
 second trimester of, 382
 supervision of
  maintenance schedule,
  371, *372*
Premature rupture of membranes
 (PROM), *379*
Premenstrual Dysphoric
 disorder, 365–366
Premenstrual tension, 365–366
Presbyopia, *68*
Preseptal cellulitis, ocular, 72
Preterm rupture of
  membranes, *379*
Pretibial myxedema, *95*
Prevalence, 405, *406*
Primary sclerosing cholangitis, 307
Prion caused disease. *See*
  Creutzfedt-Jakob disease
Progestin challenge test,
  amenorrhea, 366, *367*
Prolonged rupture of
  membranes, *379*
Prostate cancer, 412
 malignant neoplasm of,
  340–341

Prostate specific antigen, (PSA),
  prostate cancer, 340, 412
Prostatitis, 342
Proteinuria, 385
 nephrotic syndrome, *329*
 preeclampsia, *386*
Pseudomonas infection, *189*
 conjunctivitis, 70
 cystic fibrosis, 290
 hot tub folliculitis, 145
Psoas sign, appendicitis, 309
Psoriasis, 155–157
Psychiatry, 39–60
Psychotic disorders, *43*
Pterygium, 74
Ptosis, 285
Pulmonary embolism, 291–292
Pulmonary hypertension,
  292–293
Pulmonary tuberculosis, 287–288
Pulseless electrical activity
 (PEA), 263
p-Value, 407
Pyelonephritis, 326
Pyoderma gangrenosum
 with inflammatory bowel
  disease, *313*
Pyogenic granuloma, *153, 154*

Quadriplegia, 20–21
Quadruple screen, pregnancy,
  supervision of, *372*
Quinsy. *See* Peritonsillar abscess

Rabies, 10–11
 prophylaxis after animal
  bite, 10
Radiofrequency ablation, of
  accessory pathways, 264
Randomized control trial, 408
Ranson's criteria, pancreatitis,
  302, *303*
Rape/crisis adjustment, 232–233
Raynaud's disease/phenomenon,
  266–267
Red flag symptoms
 disc herniation, 175
 irritable bowel disease, 314
Reducible hernia, *317*
Reed–Sternberg cells, 124
Relative risk (RR), 406
Relative risk reduction
  (RRR), 406
 vs ARR, 407
Renal colic, 334–335

Renal failure
  acute, 332–334
    classification of, *333*
  chronic, 331–332
Renin–angiotensin cycle, *106*
Respiratory distress syndrome
      (RDS), 394–395
Respiratory problems, after
      birth, 394–398
  meconium aspiration, 395–396
  neonatal sepsis, 398
  pneumomediastinum, 396
  pneumothorax, 396
  respiratory distress syndrome
      (RDS), 394–395
  transient tachypnea, of
      newborn, 397
Respiratory system, diseases
      of, 275–295
Restraints, 409
Retinal detachment, 65
Retinal disorders, 65
Reye syndrome, 207
Rhabdomyolysis, 169–170
Rheumatoid arthritis,
      162–164
Rhinovirus, 213
Rh isoimmunization
  hemolytic disease
      due to, 398–399
  Rhogam use, 399
Rib fracture, *179*
Rinne test
  hearing loss, 82, 83
  labrynthitis, 80
RIPE therapy
  pulmonary tuberculosis, 288
Rocker bottom feet, *387*
Rocky mountain spotted
      fever, 215–216
Roseola, *200*
Rotator cuff tear, 165, *166*
Rovsing's sign, appendicitis, 309
Rubella, *200, 201*

Saline, nasal spray, 87
  allergic rhinitis, *84*
Salter–Harris fractures, *178*
Sarcoidosis, 288–289
  staging of, *288*
Scabies, 139–140
Scadding's classification,
      sarcoidosis in, 288
Scar, hypertrophic and keloid,
      153, 242

Schizoaffective disorder, *43*
Schizoid disorder, *59*
Schizophrenia, 40–42, *43*
Schizophreniform disorder, *43*
Schizotypal disorder, *59*
Seborrheic keratosis, *153, 154*
Second trimester, pregnancy
      loss, 382
Seizures, *57*
  absence, 22
  conversion, 22
  disorder, 21–22
  generalized tonic/clonic, 21
  partial, 21
  status epilepticus, 22
Selective estrogen receptor
      blocker (SERB), breast
      cancer, 339, 349
Selective estrogen receptor
      modulator (SERM). *See*
      Selective estrogen receptor
      blocker (SERB)
Selective serotonin reuptake
      inhibitors (SSRI's), 46, 48,
      51, *60*, 366
Semen analysis, male
      infertility, 345
Sensitivity, 405
Sepsis, *132*
  neonatal, 398
Septicemia, 132
Septic shock, *132*
Severe combined
      immunodeficiency (SCID),
      immune deficiency, *120*
Sexually transmitted diseases
      (STDs), *204*
Sheehan's syndrome, 376
Shingles. *See* Varicella zoster
Shoulder
  afflictions of, 165–166
  dystocia, 380, *380*
Sickle cell anemia, 130–132
Single liveborn
  before admission to hospital, 388
Sinusitis, 86–87
Sitz bath, 321
Skin abscess, 145
Skull fracture, 177–178
Sleep disorder, Insomnia, 35
Slipped capital femoral epiphysis
      (SCFE), *173*
Small cell carcinoma, *286*
Small intestine
  benign neoplasm of, 308

Smoking cessation, 413–414
Somatization disorder, *50*
Somatoform disorders, *50*
Spastic (contractile) bladder,
      324, 325
Specificity, 405
Spinal stenosis, 176
Spironolactone, 106, 142, 250, 366
Spondylosis, 174
Spontaneous bacterial peritonitis.
      See Peritonitis
Spontaneous pneumothorax, 294
Sprain, ankle, 181–182
Squamous cell carcinoma,
      148–149, *286*
  actinic keratosis in, 148
  esophagus, 298
  vaginal cancer, 362
Staphylococcal infections, *188*
Statins, cholesterol disorders, 270
Status epilepticus, seizure
      disorders, 22
Steroids
  croup, 276
  intranasal, allergic rhinitis, *84*
  Lichen sclerosis, topical, 364
  multiple sclerosis, 18
  nephrotic syndrome, 329
  paraplegia/quadriplegia, 20
  rheumatoid arthritis, 164
  sarcoidosis, 289
  systemic lupus
      erythematosus, 162
  Wegener's granulomatosis, 295
Stimulants, *229*
  in ADD and ADHD, 53
Stomach
  malignant neoplasm of, 300
Strabismus, 73
Strangulated hernia, *317*
Streptococcal infections, *188*
Streptococcal sore throat, 187
  clinical tool, 187
Stress incontinence, in
      female, 335–336
Stridor, croup, 275, 276
Stroke, ischemic, 29–30
Stye (hordeolum), *71*
Subacute sclerosing panencephalitis
      (SSPE), measles in, 199
Subarachnoid hemorrhage, 26–27
Subdural hematoma, *27*
Subgaleal hemorrhage, *394*
Substantia nigra, Parkinson's
      disease, 17

Superficial
     thrombophlebitis, 267–268
Superior vena cava syndrome, *286*
Surgery, complications of, *240, 242*
Suture abscess, surgery
     complication, *242*
Sweat chloride test, 290
Syncope, 33–34
Syndrome inappropriate
     antidiuretic hormone
     (SIADH), 102–103
  brain abscess, 14
  encephalitis, 14
Syphilis, 202–203
Systemic inflammatory response
     syndrome (SIRS), *132*
Systemic lupus
     erythematosus, 160–162

Tabes dorsalis, syphilis in, 202
Tachycardia, ventricular, 261–262
Tardive dyskinesia, 58, 60
Temporomandibular joint
     syndrome, 88, 180–181
Tendonitis, 167–168
Tenosynovitis, infectious of the
     hand, 168–169
Tension, headache, *33*
Terminal complement deficiency,
     immune deficiency, *120*
Testicular cancer, 341
Testicular masses, 343
Testicular torsion, 344
Tetanus, 8
  wound prophylaxis, *8,* 226
Tetralogy of Fallot, *273*
Thallasemia, 129
Thiamine, 58
Threatened abortion, *382*
Thrombolytic medications
  acute myocardial infarction, 252
  ischemic stroke, 30
Thrombophlebitis,
     superficial, 267–268
Thrombotic thrombocytopenic
     purpura, 137–138
Thyrocalcitonin, 92
Thyroid gland
  diseases
     malignant lesions, 92
  disorders
     hyperthyroidism, 95–96
     hypothyroidism, 92–94
Thyroiditis, 93
  subacute, 96

Tibia fracture, *179*
Tinea, 203
Tinnitus, 81–82
TORCHES infections, of
     pregnancy, *219*
  cerebral palsy, 22
Torsion, testicular, 344
Total abdominal
     hysterectomy/bilateral
     salpingoectomy (TAH/BSO)
  leiomyoma of the uterus, 356
  ovarian cancer, 351
  uterine cancer, 355
Toxic effects, of substances, *229*
Toxoplasmosis, 213–214
  brain abscess, in, 14
Trachea, foreign body in, *227*
Tracheoesophageal fistula, *392*
Transfusion reaction, *133–134*
  allergic, *134*
  delayed, *133*
  immediate, *133*
  transfusion related acute lung
     injury (TRALI), *134*
Transient ischemic attack, 28–29
Transient tachypnea, of newborn
     (TTN), 397
Transjugular intrahepatic
     portacaval shunt (TIPS)
  esophageal varices, 299
Transurethral resection of the
     prostate (TURP)
  benign prostatic
     hypertrophy, 343
  prostate cancer, 341
Trauma, 223–246
Traveler's diarrhea,
     gastroenteritis, 189
Tremor, 34
  Parkinson's disease, 17
Triads
  abdominal aortic aneurysm, 264
  autistic disorder, 54
  Charcot's, 305, 322
  hemolytic uremic syndrome, 137
  Horner's syndrome, 285, *286*
  multiple myeloma, 125
  normal pressure hydrocephalus,
     16, 37
  Virchow's, 268, *291*
Trichomonas, of vulva/vagina, *363*
  cervicitis, 361
Trichomoniasis, *204*
Tricyclic antidepressants (TCA's),
     32, 46, 48, 180, 315, 366

Trigeminal neuralgia, 23–24
Triple screen, pregnancy,
     supervision of, 372
Tumor
  Krukenberg, 300, 350
Turner's syndrome, *387*
Twinning. *See* Multiple fetuses
Tympanostomy, otitis
     media in, 79

Ulcerative colitis
  vs Crohn's disease, *312*
  primary sclerosing
     cholangitis, 307
Uncomplicated cystitis,
     325–326
United States preventive services
     task force (USPSTF), 66, 172,
     319, 340, 346, 410, 412
Upper gastrointestinal
     bleeding, 316
Upper postvaginal wall, vaginal
     prolapse of, 363
Urethritis, 325
Uric acid excretion test, gout, 114
Urinary calculus, 334–335, *335*
Urinary tract, diseases of,
     323–336
Urolithiasis. *See* Urinary calculus
Uterine bleeding,
     abnormal, 357–358
Uterine prolapse, 357
Uterus
  leiomyoma of, 355–356
  malignant neoplasm of, 355

Vaccination, 410, *411*
Vagina
  malignant neoplasm of, 362
Vaginal walls, prolapse of,
     363, *363*
Vaginitis, 362, *363*
Valvular disease, 270, *271*
Varices, esophageal, 298–299
Varicella, 195–196
Varicella zoster, 196
Varicocele, *343*
Varicose veins, 269
Vasovagal (neurocardiogenic)
     syncope, 34
Venous thrombosis, 268–269
Ventricular fibrillation, 262, *262*
Ventricular septal defect, 273
Ventricular tachycardia,
     261–262, *262*

Ventriculo-peritoneal shunt
(VP), 37
normal pressure
hydrocephalus, 16
Vertebral body fracture, *179*
Vertiginous disorders, 81
Video-assisted thoracoscopic
surgery (VATS)
lung cancer, 286
spontaneous pneumothorax, 294
Viral pneumonia
vs bacterial, *279*
Viral warts, 147–148
Virchow's triad, *291*
Visual disturbances, *68*
Visual field defects, *69*
Vitamin deficiencies, *109–110*
von Recklinghausen disease,
neurofibromatosis, 157
VP shunting. *See*
Ventriculo-peritoneal shunt

Vulva
malignant neoplasm of, 362
Vulvovaginitis, 362, *363*

Warfarin (Coumadin)
pulmonary embolism, 292
venous thrombosis, 269
Warts
genital, *204*
viral, 147–148
Water deprivation test, diabetes
insipidus, 102
Water's view xray
sinusitis, 86
Weber test
hearing loss, 82, *83*
labrynthitis, 80
Wegener's granulomatosis,
295, *341*
West Nile virus, 214–215
White classification system

of gestational diabetes
mellitus, 384–385, *384*
Whooping cough. *See* Pertussis
Wiskott–Aldrich syndrome,
immune deficiency, *120*
Withdrawal of care, 408
Wolff–Parkinson–White (WPW)
syndrome, 263–264
World Health Organization
(WHO)
osteoporosis, *172*, 184
Wounds and bites, 226

X-linked (Bruton's)
agammaglobulinemia,
immune deficiency, *120*
Xray, neck, croup in,
276, 296

Zollinger–Ellison (ZE) syndrome
peptic ulcer disease, 300

INDEX